Springhouse Review for

MEDICAL-SURGICAL NURSING CERTIFICATION

FOURTH EDITION

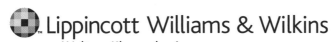

Lippincott Williams & Wilkins
a Wolters Kluwer business
Philadelphia · Baltimore · New York · London
Buenos Aires · Hong Kong · Sydney · Tokyo

STAFF

Executive Publisher
Judith A. Schilling McCann, RN, MSN

Editorial Director
H. Nancy Holmes

Clinical Director
Joan M. Robinson, RN, MSN

Art Director
Mary Ludwicki

Editorial Project Manager
Jennifer Kowalak

Clinical Project Manager
Carol A. Saunderson, RN, BA, BS

Editors
Naina D. Chohan, Julie Munden

Clinical Editors
Pamela Kovach, RN, BSN;
Jennifer Meyering, RN, MSN, CCRN

Copy Editor
Linda Hager

Designer
Linda Jovinelly Franklin

Digital Composition Services
Diane Paluba (manager), Joyce Rossi Biletz,
Donna S. Morris

Manufacturing
Beth J. Welsh

Editorial Assistants
Megan L. Aldinger, Karen J. Kirk, Linda K. Ruhf

Design Assistant
Georg W. Purvis IV

Indexer
Ellen Brennan

The clinical treatments described and recommended in this publication are based on research and consultation with nursing, medical, and legal authorities. To the best of our knowledge, these procedures reflect currently accepted practice. Nevertheless, they can't be considered absolute and universal recommendations. For individual applications, all recommendations must be considered in light of the patient's clinical condition and, before administration of new or infrequently used drugs, in light of the latest package-insert information. The authors and publisher disclaim any responsibility for any adverse effects resulting from the suggested procedures, from any undetected errors, or from the reader's misunderstanding of the text.

MSNC4010906 – 070411

Library of Congress Cataloging-in-Publication Data

Springhouse review for medical-surgical nursing certification. — 4th ed.
   p. ; cm.
   Includes bibliographical references and index.
   1. Nursing—Examinations, questions, etc. 2. Surgical nursing—Examinations, questions, etc. I. Lippincott Williams & Wilkins. Springhouse Division. II. Title: Review for medical-surgical nursing certification.
   [DNLM: 1. Nursing--Examination Questions. 2. Nursing—Outlines. 3. Perioperative Nursing—Examination Questions. 4. Perioperative Nursing—Outlines.   WY 18.2 S76955 2007]
   RT55.A47 2007
   610.73076--dc22
ISBN13: 978-1-58255-507-2
ISBN10: 1-58255-507-9 (alk. paper)   2006019520

Contents

Contributors and consultants

Katrina D. Allen, RN, MSN, CCRN
ADN Nursing Faculty
Faulkner State Community College
Bay Minette, Ala.

Doris Bartlett, BSN, MS
Assistant Professor
Bethel College
Mishawaka, Ind.

Nancy Berger, RN, BC, MSN
Instructor
Charles E. Gregory School of Nursing
Raritan Bay Medical Center
Perth Amboy, N.J.

Lawrence Carey, PharmD
Assistant Professor, Physician Assistant Studies
Philadelphia (Pa.) University

Lillian Craig, MSN, RN, FNP-C
Family Nurse Practitioner
Borger, Tex.
Nursing Instructor
Oklahoma Panhandle State University
Goodwell, Okla.

Vivian C. Gamblian, RN, MS
Professor of Nursing
Collin County Community College District
McKinney, Tex.

Sharon L.G. Lee, APRN, MS
Faculty
BryanLGH College of Health Sciences
Lincoln, Neb.

Phyllis Magaletto, MSN, APRN, BC
Instructor
Cochran School of Nursing
Yonkers, N.Y.

Ann S. McQueen, MSN, CRNP
Family Nurse Practitioner
Health Link Medical Center
Southampton, Pa.

Mariann M. Montgomery, RN, MSN
Associate Professor of Nursing
Kent State University, Tuscarawas
New Philadelphia, Ohio

Pamela Moody, PhD, MSN, APRN-BC
Nurse Practitioner Consultant
Alabama Department of Public Health–Family Health Services
Tuscaloosa

Melody F. Pope, MSEd, MSN, RN, CNHA
Assistant Professor
College of the Redwoods–Del Norte Campus
Crescent City, Ca.

Monica Narvaez Ramirez, MSN, RN
Nursing Instructor
University of the Incarnate Word School of Nursing & Health Professions
San Antonio, Tex.

Kendra S. Seiler, RN, MSN
Nursing Instructor
Rio Hondo College
Whittier, Ca.

Diane Yaglowski, RN, OCN
Staff Nurse
St. Luke's Hospital & Health Network
Bethlehem, Pa.

Foreword

In my 15 years of volunteer work with nursing certification boards and panels, I have truly come to appreciate the value of certification as a mark of validation of specialized knowledge, skills, and experiences. Indeed, it's a mark of distinction as well as a way to assure the public of our expertise in specialty areas of nursing.

Medical-surgical nursing is the core of nursing care in most health care settings; it's the main focus of care in primary, acute, and long-term care settings. For those of us in the specialty, certification validates excellence among those nurses caring for patients with physiologic alterations in health status and their resulting social and behavioral problems.

The nursing profession has valued certification for over 60 years. When certification first began in 1946, it was offered to nurse anesthetists. In the late 1970s, other nursing specialties also began offering certification. Studies have confirmed that certified nurses practice in a manner more likely to improve patient outcomes. In addition, certification has been linked to improved patient safety and increased accountability, creditability, and competence. Further, certification is thought to broaden job opportunities, increase earning potential and job satisfaction, and enhance one's professional prestige. Over and over again certified nurses report an increased sense of personal accomplishment and satisfaction with their roles.

I want to personally congratulate you on assuming the risk involved in deciding to take a certification examination. I'm sure you'll experience some anxiety as you prepare for this journey. But know that others have gone before you and shared the same feelings and reactions. Be proud of your knowledge and experience. Take the next step towards certification that will earn you formal recognition for your expertise.

We have organized a valuable resource that can serve as the foundation for your examination review and preparation. The 4th edition of the *Springhouse Review for Medical-Surgical Nursing Certification* is an excellent tool to use in preparing for either the American Nurses Credentialing Center's Medical-Surgical Nurse certification examination or the Academy of Medical-Surgical Nurses certification examination. The book is organized around content areas that are similar to the test outlines. Chapter 1 offers you information on the certification examinations including eligibility requirements, test content outlines, and test-taking strategies. Having this knowledge should help to decrease your anxiety. Chapter 2 covers foundations of nursing including the nursing process, roles of the nurse, collaborative practice, case management, nursing research, performance improvement, risk management, consultation, patient education, and delegation. Chapter 3 focuses on legal and ethical aspects of nursing, such as nurse practice acts, common legal concerns, and health care regulation and policies. Key principles of medical-surgical nursing are covered in Chapter 4 including growth and development and assessment and therapeutic communication. Chapter 5 focuses on principles of wound care. Disruptions in homeostasis such as stress, shock, inflammation and infection, fluid/electrolyte/acid-base imbalances, and pain are all reviewed in Chapter 6. Chapters 7 through 18 are dedicated to a review of each body system including disorders of the cardiovascular, hematologic, respiratory, neurologic, musculoskeletal, GI, skin, endocrine, renal and urinary tract, reproductive, and immune systems, as well as eye, ear, and nose disorders. Chapter 19 includes information related to preoperative, intraoperative, and postoperative care, as well as common postoperative complications. Additional useful resources are included in the appendices, as well as a posttest that's designed similar in form and content to the actual examination so you can evaluate your readiness to take the certification examination.

I wish you success as you begin your journey toward certification—a mark of distinction and formal recognition of your nursing excellence.

Lynore DeSilets, EdD, RN, BC
Assistant Dean
Director, Continuing Education in
Nursing and Health Care
College of Nursing
Villanova (Pa.) University

CHAPTER 1

Medical-surgical nursing certification

Medical-surgical nurses are the backbone of health and wellness care in the United States. Indeed, new nursing graduates are strongly encouraged to work in a hospital as a medical-surgical nurse for 1 to 2 years to hone their skills before branching out into other areas of nursing. In 1972, the American Nurses Association (ANA) recognized this valuable specialty by certifying medical-surgical nurses through the American Nurses Credentialing Center (ANCC)—almost 151,000 nurses have been certified to date in more than 30 specialty and advanced practice areas of nursing. Further, as of 1990, a new medical-surgical nursing organization, the Academy of Medical-Surgical Nurses (AMSN), was founded to serve the specific educational needs of this group of nurses. The AMSN has also developed a certification examination to recognize the knowledge base of the practicing medical-surgical nurse.

The ANCC certification examination

The ANA offers two examinations for medical-surgical nursing certification: a basic medical-surgical nurse examination and a clinical specialist examination in medical-surgical nursing. The ANCC administers the examinations each June and October in cities throughout the United States and its territories. The tests are given in the morning and last about 4 hours.

Eligibility and application

The ANCC establishes criteria for eligibility to take the examination. Requirements for the basic examination differ from those of the clinical specialist examination. The criteria discussed in this book were in effect as of the 2006 examination. Because requirements can change, candidates should obtain the latest criteria before applying for certification. (See *ANCC certification eligibility requirements*, page 2.) The medical-surgical nursing examination is available to nurses with an associate's degree or diploma, thus establishing two levels of credentialing. Nurses certified at the baccalaureate level are designated as Board Certified, or "RN,BC"; nurses certified at the associate or diploma level are designated as Certified, or "RN,C." The credential approved for clinical nurse specialists is "APRN,BC."

After you have decided to prepare for the examination, obtain the certification catalog by writing to the American Nurses Credentialing Center, 8515 Georgia Ave., Suite 400, Silver Springs, MD 20910-3492, or by calling toll-free 1-800-284-2378. This catalog provides all the information you'll need to apply.

ANCC certification eligibility requirements

The American Nurses Credentialing Center's (ANCC) eligibility criteria for certification in medical-surgical nursing, as of 2006, are listed below. Note that the requirements for the basic nursing examination differ from those of the specialist examination.

Criteria for a medical-surgical nurse (04 associate/diploma, 38 baccalaureate)

By the time of application, you must:
1. hold a current, active unrestricted professional registered nurse (RN) license in the United States or its territories
2. have practiced the equivalent of 2 years full-time as an RN in the United States or its territories
3. have practiced as a licensed RN in medical-surgical nursing for a minimum of 2,000 hours within the past 3 years*
4. have received 30 contact hours within the last 3 years.

Criteria for a clinical specialist in medical-surgical nursing (05 clinical specialist)

By the time of application, you must:
1. hold a current, active RN license in the United States or its territories
2. hold a master's degree or higher in nursing
3. have been prepared in medical-surgical nursing through a master's degree program or a formal postgraduate master's program in nursing
4. have graduated from an accredited institution granting graduate-level academic credit for all of the course work that includes both didactic and clinical components, and a minimum of 500 hours of supervised clinical practice in medical-surgical nursing and role. †

---

*Nursing faculty may use up to 500 hours of faculty teaching or clinical supervision in medical-surgical nursing toward the practice requirement. Students may use up to 500 hours of time spent in an academic program of nursing study toward their clinical practice requirement.

†Students who graduate without 500 clinical hours in their educational program will not be allowed to make up the clinical hours postgraduation after the December 31, 2006 deadline.

Source: American Nurses Credentialing Center, Silver Spring, MD. Available at *www.ana.org/ancc.*

Examination information, catalogs, and applications may also be obtained through the ANCC Web site at *www.ana.org/ancc.*

Pay careful attention to all steps in the application process. Failure to complete any step correctly may make you ineligible to take the examination on the date you had planned. All applicants must pay a nonrefundable application fee and an examination fee, set each year by the credentialing center.

Certification test plan

After establishing your eligibility, the credentialing center will mail you a handbook that contains the current examination blueprint, or test plan. The test plan outlines the test content and the ratio (weighting) of each content area. Information about the test plan, especially its content, can provide considerable guidance in helping you organize your study plan.

In the ANCC catalog for 2006, medical-surgical examination topics included biophysical and psychosocial concepts, pathophysiology of body systems, patient care, and issues and trends. Examination topics for the clinical specialist in medical-surgical nursing included clinical practice, consultation, management, education, research, and issues and trends.

The Board on Certification for Medical-Surgical Nursing Practice, one of the many ANCC certification boards, develops the certification examination. The test objectively evaluates knowledge, comprehension, and application of medical-surgical nursing theory and practice to patient care. The committee defines the content areas covered in each test and the emphasis placed on each area.

Certified medical-surgical nurses from around the country contribute questions for each examination. The test development committee reviews each test item for accuracy, readability, and relevance to the test plan. Sample questions approved by the committee are compiled into an examination that will be used on the next test date. The clinical nurse specialist examination may be computerized in the near future.

Each test contains about 150 multiple-choice questions, usually preceded by brief clinical situations. Candidates have 4 hours to complete the test. A break usually is provided.

Test results are mailed to all candidates about 6 to 8 weeks after the examination. No results are released early or over the telephone to protect the privacy of candidates.

The AMSN certification examination

The AMSN is a professional organization for nurses who practice medical-surgical/adult health care. The organization developed the Scope and Standards of Medical-Surgical Nursing Practice; it builds on the ANA's Standards of Clinical Practice and helps to establish the responsibilities of medical-surgical nurses in all types of health care settings.

The AMSN founded the Medical-Surgical Nursing Certification Board (MSNCB) to promote and implement a certification examination for medical surgical nurses. The tests are administered every May and October in cities throughout the United States as well as the annual AMSN conference. The test lasts 4 hours.

Eligibility and application

The MSNCB establishes criteria for eligibility to take the examination. However, because requirements can change, candidates should obtain the latest criteria before applying for certification. (See *AMSN certification eligibility criteria*, page 4.) The medical-surgical certification examination does not require a BSN degree. Nurses who are certified through this examination are designated as "RN,CMSRN."

MSNCB works with a testing center, the Center for Nursing Education (C-Net). The certification catalog and examination application may be obtained by writing to C-Net, 601 Pavonia Avenue, Suite 201, Jersey City, NJ 07306. Or download an application from the Web site *www.medsurgnurse.org*.

Again, be sure to read all directions, and pay careful attention to all steps in the application process. Failure to complete the application properly may lead to ineligibility to take the examination.

AMSN certification eligibility criteria

The Academy of Medical-Surgical Nurses (AMSN) eligibility criteria, as of 2006, are listed below.

By the time of application you must:
- hold a current and unrestricted license as a registered nurse (RN) in the United States, or any of its territories

OR

- hold a current, full, unrestricted license to practice as a first-level general nurse in the country in which one's general nursing education was complete; and meet the eligibility criteria for licensure as an RN in accordance with requirements of the Commission of Graduates of Foreign Nursing Schools (CGFNS)
- have 2 full years (of the last 5 years) of experience practicing as a RN in an adult medical-surgical clinical setting
- have accrued a minimum of 3,000 hours of clinical practice as a staff nurse, clinical nurse specialist, clinical educator, faculty member, manager, or supervisor.

Source: Academy of Medical-Surgical Nurses, Pitman, N.J. Available at *www.medsurgnurse.org*.

Certification test plan

If the application is completed properly, an examination permit is mailed approximately 2 weeks before the test. The permit will include the test center address and the time you should report to the center. You must have the examination permit to be admitted to take the exam.

The test consists of 200 multiple-choice questions that focus on the nursing care of acutely ill, hospitalized, and adult patients. The questions cover patient problems from all the physiologic systems and also various domains of nursing practice.

The candidate is notified of examination results by mail approximately 8 weeks following the examination.

Preparing for the certification examination

To ensure success on the examination, you must know how to analyze questions and use specific strategies to help you select the best response. Readiness for taking the test involves three areas of preparation: intellectual, physical, and emotional.

Intellectual preparation involves a complete review of all the topics that will be covered on the examination. This book provides you with an organized source for that review. Supplement its use with other sources, such as current medical and nursing literature, particularly if the subject isn't one you deal with every day in your practice. If you take a review course, pay special attention to unfamiliar material being discussed, and ask the instructor for clarification when necessary. You also may want to discuss topics covered in the review course with other participants or organize a study group to review difficult material after the course is over.

Take the posttest included in this book, and then review the correct answers. This test exposes you to questions from all content areas covered on the certification examination. Reviewing the reasons for incorrect answers can suggest areas for further study, thereby helping you to avoid repeating these mistakes on the actual test.

Physical preparation for the examination may seem obvious, but many candidates ignore its importance. Staying up all night before the test to cram last-minute information clearly is a mistake. Sound physical preparation also involves applying to take the test well in advance and securing all the necessary documents to ensure your eligibility. Keep your test permit in a safe place, and remember to take it with you to the examination. If you live near the examination site, visit it in advance to determine travel time and familiarize yourself with parking facilities. Nothing can affect your performance more adversely than arriving late in a state of high anxiety. Make overnight reservations early if you must travel a long distance. Staying close to the test location will promote a good night's sleep and prompt arrival. If you are sensitive to room temperature, take a sweater; it's easy to put on or remove quickly. Take mints or hard candy to relieve a dry mouth. Finally, eat a light but nourishing breakfast. It will give you the energy you need to perform at an optimum level.

Emotional preparation significantly influences test performance. Be confident. Think positively. Look at the examination as a way of demonstrating your mastery of the subject matter. After all, you have been practicing medical-surgical nursing for many years. You have a wealth of knowledge about most of the test content. You have taken standardized tests before, the most memorable being the NCLEX-RN (state boards). Everyone is anxious before an important examination. The feeling is normal, even beneficial. Anxiety keeps you alert, motivates you to study, and helps you concentrate. However, too little or too much anxiety can affect performance. Think about past experiences when you have been anxious during a test. If you recall being too anxious, now is the time to learn some simple relaxation exercises, such as rhythmic breathing and progressive muscle relaxation. Guided imagery, such as imagining yourself successfully answering all the questions on the test, can be helpful. Remind yourself of relaxation techniques that worked in the past. They can work again. During the test, avoid becoming distracted by others who may be exhibiting anxious behavior. Concentrate on the test in front of you, and keep your feelings under control. Positive feelings will help you relax and keep your confidence high. Don't be bothered by people who seem to have finished the test early. Tell yourself that they have just given up and probably didn't complete the examination.

Test-taking strategies

You can improve your chances of passing standardized multiple-choice examinations by using techniques that have proved successful for others. These techniques include knowing how timed examinations are administered, understanding all the parts of a test question, and taking specific steps to ensure that you have selected the correct answer.

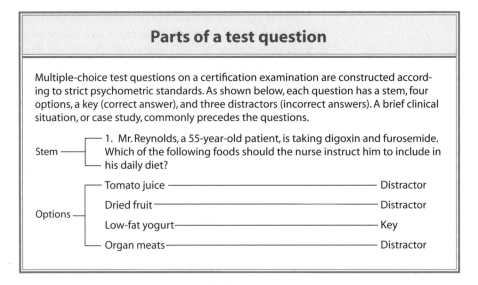

Parts of a test question

Multiple-choice test questions on a certification examination are constructed according to strict psychometric standards. As shown below, each question has a stem, four options, a key (correct answer), and three distractors (incorrect answers). A brief clinical situation, or case study, commonly precedes the questions.

Stem ——
1. Mr. Reynolds, a 55-year-old patient, is taking digoxin and furosemide. Which of the following foods should the nurse instruct him to include in his daily diet?

Options ——
Tomato juice —————————————— Distractor
Dried fruit —————————————— Distractor
Low-fat yogurt —————————————— Key
Organ meats —————————————— Distractor

Time management is crucial when taking a standardized test because you receive no credit for unanswered questions. Consequently, you should try to pace yourself to finish the test on time. Remember, you'll have about 1 minute to answer each question. Don't spend too much time on any one question. Instead, place a light pencil mark next to it and come back later, if time is available. Other questions may stimulate your recall of the correct answer for the question you left unanswered. Also keep in mind that you aren't penalized for guessing. If you have no idea of the correct answer, select any option; you have a 1 in 4 chance of being correct.

All questions on a certification examination are carefully crafted and pretested to ensure readability and uniformity. Understanding the components of a question can help you analyze what it's asking, which increases the likelihood that you'll respond correctly. The diagram above shows the parts of a multiple-choice question. Note how clearly the question is written, with no unnecessary words in the stem. Each option is relatively uniform in length. (See *Parts of a test question.*)

Read every question carefully. If a clinical situation precedes the question, study the information given. Watch for key words (such as most, first, best, and except). They are important guides to which option you should select. For example, if a question reads, "Which of the following nursing actions should the nurse perform first?" you may find that all the options are appropriate for the patient's condition but only one clearly takes precedence over the others.

As you read the stem, try to anticipate the correct answer. Look at the options to see if your answer is listed. If so, it's probably correct.

If you don't see your expected answer in the options, read all the options again before you select one. If you select an option before reading all of them, you'll deny yourself the opportunity to evaluate all the choices. Try to find an option that most closely resembles the one you thought would be correct. If you don't find one, look for the best option available. Remember, you are looking for the best answer among those given. It may not be what you think is the best response, but it's all you have to work with.

For some questions, you may see two options that seem correct, and you can't decide between them. Look at them again. There must be a difference. Read the stem again. You may discover something you didn't see before that will help you make a selection. If not and you still can't choose, make an educated guess, and place a light mark by the question, so you can return to it later.

Despite thorough preparation, you may not know the answer to some questions. Relax. Remember that you are an expert practitioner and possess a wealth of information. Think of patient cases you have had, and recall information about them that you can apply to the question. Tell yourself the principle involved, and recall what you know about applying that principle to practice situations. At the very least, this will help you eliminate some of the options that are probably wrong. Now you have narrowed down the selection to perhaps two options. This should make your choice easier.

If time remains when you answer the final item, return to the questions that you marked for later review or didn't answer. Erase the mark and answer the question, or review your answer for possible change. Don't be afraid to change a selection if you later think of a better choice. Finally, remember to erase any marks in your test book that don't belong there. Your examination will be scored by computer, and extraneous marks could affect the scoring.

Taking the certification examination shows confidence in your knowledge of medical-surgical nursing. An organized study program, such as the one provided on the following pages, will help ensure that you are fully prepared to take the test.

Foundations of nursing

❖ **Nursing process**
- History of the nursing process
  - ◆ In the 1970s, the American Nurses Association (ANA) mandated that the nursing process be part of nursing practice and instituted a five-step process (assessment, diagnosis, planning, implementation, and evaluation)
  - ◆ In 1982, the North American Nursing Diagnosis Association now know as NANDA International (NANDA-I) was established to develop, review, and update nursing diagnoses; this organization meets every 2 years
- Purpose of the nursing process
  - ◆ The nursing process provides a basis for problem solving, clinical decisions, and individualized patient care
  - ◆ It uses the scientific method of observation, measurement, data collection, and data analysis to evaluate the needs of patients and their families
  - ◆ The nursing process provides an organized and universal method of communication for nurses in education, practice, and research
  - ◆ Through the nursing process, nurses have adopted a body of knowledge that's unique to nursing; this knowledge encompasses illness, illness prevention, and health maintenance
- Standards of practice
  - ◆ The Standards of Clinical Nursing Practice are directly related to the nursing process
    - ▶ Standard I ("The nurse collects patient health data") relates to step 1 of the nursing process (assessment)
    - ▶ Standard II ("The nurse analyzes the assessment data in determining diagnosis") relates to step 2 of the nursing process (diagnosis)
    - ▶ Standard III ("The nurse identifies expected outcomes individualized to the patient") and Standard IV ("The nurse develops a care plan that prescribes interventions to attain expected outcomes") relate to step 3 of the nursing process (planning)
    - ▶ Standard V ("The nurse implements the interventions in the care plan") relates to step 4 of the nursing process (implementation)
    - ▶ Standard VI ("The nurse evaluates the patient's progress toward outcomes") relates to step 5 of the nursing process (evaluation)
  - ◆ These clinical standards use the steps of the nursing process to help achieve the standards of practice that have been set forward by state nurse practice acts and the ANA standards of professional performance

as well as the Academy of Medical-Surgical Nurses Scope and Standards of Nursing Practice

◆ These varying standards help assure quality nursing care and provide the gauge by which to measure quality

■ Steps of the nursing process

◆ Assessment

▶ Assessment is the collection and organization of data

▶ Data collection involves the formation of a database from the patient interview, patient history, subjective data (what the patient says or believes), objective data (vital signs, laboratory results), and physical assessment (inspection, palpation, percussion, auscultation)

▶ Data organization involves clustering related findings, reviewing the amount and completeness of data, and evaluating it through comparison with normal or baseline data

▶ Data documentation involves recording all data on the patient's chart and comparing it with research and medical findings

◆ Diagnosis

▶ Diagnosis is the identification of actual or potential health problems as indicated by the assessment data; it's also defined as the responses to actual or potential health problems

▶ The diagnostic statement consists of three parts: identifying the problem or need, identifying the cause of the problem or need ("related to"), and identifying related signs and symptoms ("as evidenced by")

▶ A sample diagnostic statement is "ineffective breathing pattern related to fatigue, as evidenced by shortness of breath, shallow respirations, and tachycardia"

▶ Nursing diagnoses are organized in a taxonomy based on human response patterns (see NANDA nursing diagnoses, page 336); they also may be grouped by functional health patterns (health perception–health management; nutritional-metabolic; elimination; activity-exercise; sleep-rest; cognitive-perceptual; self-perception–self-concept; role-relationship; sexuality-reproductive; coping–stress tolerance; and value-belief)

◆ Planning

▶ Planning involves determining expected outcomes, setting priorities, establishing goals, selecting appropriate interventions, and documenting care

▶ Priorities can be based on Maslow's hierarchy of needs (in which physical needs, such as oxygen and safety, take priority over psychosocial needs, such as self-esteem and self-actualization) or other factors

▶ Goals are established by identifying the desired outcomes; short-term and long-term goals can be defined and are measurable and time-specific

▶ Specific nursing interventions are selected to develop an individualized care plan; interventions should specify times, frequencies, and amounts

---

Practice roles

No matter what the practice setting, the nurse can assume various roles.

Caregiver

As a caregiver, the nurse assesses the patient, analyzes his needs, develops nursing diagnoses, and plans, delivers, and evaluates nursing interventions.

Advocate

As an advocate, the nurse helps the patient and his family members interpret information from other health care providers and make decisions about health-related needs.

Educator

As an educator, the nurse educates the patient and his family members by providing knowledge of health-promoting activities, disease-related conditions, and specific treatments. Education can take place in planned individual or group sessions or informally when caring for the patient.

Coordinator

As a coordinator, the nurse coordinates the patient's care plan with various health care providers. Many organizations recognize this nursing role, which requires good communication and management skills, by appointing nurses as case managers for patients.

Discharge planner

As a discharge planner, the nurse assesses the patient's needs at discharge, including the patient's support systems and living situation. The nurse also links the patient with available community resources.

Change agent

As a change agent, the nurse works with the patient and staff members to address organizational and community concerns. This role demands a knowledge of change theory, which provides a framework for understanding the dynamics of change, human responses to change, and strategies for effecting change.

▶ The care plan is documented so that all health care team members know the patient's individualized plan
◆ Implementation
  ▶ Implementation involves providing actual care to the patient
  ▶ Data collection and assessment continue during this step
◆ Evaluation
  ▶ To provide effective care, the goals, outcomes, and appropriateness of interventions must be evaluated on an ongoing basis in relation to the care plan
  ▶ During evaluation, the care plan is revised as needed in terms of nursing diagnoses, goals, outcomes, and interventions

❖ **Roles of the nurse**
  ■ General information
   ◆ Nursing's goal is to promote, restore, and maintain the health of people, who are regarded as holistic beings
   ◆ Although the expectations for providing nursing care have expanded and increased, this goal has remained constant
  ■ Roles
   ◆ In adapting to changing health care needs, nurses assume various roles in health care settings (see *Practice roles*)
   ◆ Each role has specific responsibilities, but some facets of these roles are common to all nursing positions

❖ **Collaborative practice**
- General information
  - ◆ Successful collaboration requires respect for the unique contribution of each member of the health care team
  - ◆ An interdisciplinary approach to care serves the patient's needs best
- Nurse-physician collaboration
  - ◆ Collaboration is facilitated when nurses and practitioners work together regularly
  - ◆ Methods of encouraging nurse-physician collaboration include scheduling times to develop and sustain working partnerships, communicating openly and directly, and agreeing to discuss conflicts when they arise
- Collaboration with other members of the health care team
  - ◆ Collaboration with other health care providers, such as social workers, nutritionists, and physical, occupational, and respiratory therapists, requires an understanding of their roles
  - ◆ General knowledge of these roles can be achieved by reading relevant articles and by communicating directly with members of these groups
  - ◆ Interdisciplinary case conferences allow team members to learn about other health professionals' contributions to patient care; such conferences reflect a facility's commitment to collaborative practice

❖ **Case management**
- General information
  - ◆ Case management is a system of patient care delivery that focuses on achieving outcomes within specific time frames and using resources appropriately
  - ◆ It includes the entire episode of illness, crossing all settings in which the patient receives care
  - ◆ Its expense limits its use to complex and costly cases
  - ◆ Research shows that nursing case management improves quality of care and reduces health care costs
- Case management versus managed care
  - ◆ Case management differs from managed care, although both systems are designed to reduce costs and achieve quality outcomes
  - ◆ Case management provides continuity of the care provider by linking people across clinical settings
  - ◆ Managed care provides continuity of the care plan by linking tasks, shifts, and departments within the organization
- Goals of case management
  - ◆ The goals of case management are the same regardless of setting
  - ◆ An organization may designate individual case managers or group practice case managers; the latter can represent practitioner or clinical nurse specialist practices
- Role of case managers
  - ◆ Case managers are accountable for patient and cost outcomes and may provide administrative, educational, and research services
  - ◆ They collaborate with the attending physician, patient, family members, and other service providers

◆ They evaluate the patient's physical and mental health, functional capability, support systems, and financial resources
  ❙ Interdisciplinary teams or individual providers perform the assessments, with the case manager coordinating the process
  ❙ Standardized instruments for collecting data are key to coordinating care
◆ With the patient and family, case managers formulate a care plan that includes mutually agreed-on goals with measurable objectives so that outcomes can be evaluated (critical pathways)
◆ They help provide the patient with appropriate resources to fulfill the care plan; case managers troubleshoot for the patient if problems arise
◆ They use performance improvement to evaluate the quality and cost-effectiveness of patient care
■ Characteristics of case managers
◆ The ANA recommends that nurse case managers hold a baccalaureate degree in nursing and have 3 years of clinical experience; however, many organizations prefer nurses with master's degrees who are clinical specialists in the areas related to the patient's condition
◆ Successful case managers possess expert clinical knowledge and skills, can set realistic goals and outcomes, and clearly understand the financial aspects of health care systems and strategies for quality improvement
◆ They skillfully communicate, negotiate, and collaborate with other health care providers and know what resources are available in health care institutions and the community

❖ **Nursing research**
■ General information
◆ For nursing research to achieve full impact, its findings must be applied in practice; nurses in administration, research, and practice must collaborate to create an environment in which nurses raise questions about policies, look for solutions to problems, and develop protocols for testing innovations in nursing care
◆ The level of participation in research varies with the nurse's educational background
◆ An associate degree or diploma in nursing qualifies the nurse to assist in identifying clinical problems in nursing practice, to collect data in a structured format, and to work with a professional nurse in applying research findings
◆ A baccalaureate degree in nursing allows the nurse to identify clinical problems that need further research, to critique research findings for use in practice, to collect data, and to implement research findings
◆ A master's degree in nursing permits the nurse to act as clinical expert in collaborating with an experienced researcher and to provide leadership for integrating findings in clinical nursing practice
◆ A doctoral degree allows the nurse to formulate nursing knowledge through research and theory development and to conduct funded independent research projects

- Types of research
  - ◆ *Quantitative research* is a deductive process that aims to describe, explain, and test hypotheses and examine cause-and-effect relationships that apply to a wider universe; this type of research emphasizes facts and data to validate or extend existing knowledge
  - ◆ Specific terms are associated with quantitative research
    - ▶ *Control* involves the use of design techniques to decrease the possibility of error, thereby increasing the potential for findings that accurately reflect reality
    - ▶ *Hypothesis* is a formal statement of the expected relationships between two or more variables
    - ▶ *Sampling* is the selecting of subjects that are representative of the population being studied
    - ▶ *Randomization* is a sampling procedure used to provide each member of the study population with an equal chance of being selected for an intervention
    - ▶ *Independent variable* describes the treatment or experimental variable that's manipulated or varied by the researcher to create an effect on the dependent variable
    - ▶ *Dependent variable* is the response, behavior, or outcome that the researcher hopes to predict or explain; changes in the dependent variable are presumed to be caused by the independent variable
  - ◆ *Qualitative research* is an inductive process that aims to understand, describe, and identify the meaning of phenomena for a particular context; this type of research emphasizes the development of new insights, theory, and knowledge
  - ◆ Specific terms are associated with qualitative research
    - ▶ *Bracketing* requires the researcher to lay aside what's known about the experience being studied and be open to new insights
    - ▶ *Intuiting and reflecting* refer to focused awareness on the phenomena under study
    - ▶ *Theoretical sampling* is the selecting of subjects on the basis of concepts that have theoretical relevance to an evolving theory
    - ▶ *Saturation* describes the point at which data collection is ended because continuing would result in "more of the same"
- Research process
  - ◆ The quantitative research process consists of 10 steps: formulating the problem, reviewing related literature, developing a theoretical framework, identifying research variables, formulating research questions or hypotheses, selecting the research design, defining the population and sampling procedures, developing a plan for data collection and analysis, implementing the research plan, and communicating findings
  - ◆ The qualitative research process follows different steps
    - ▶ The initial literature review is less exhaustive to avoid oversensitizing the researcher to the subject matter; after key concepts emerge, a more extensive literature review is conducted, and its insights are woven into the analysis

▶ A theoretical framework is seldom used because the goal of qualitative research is to develop concepts, constructs, models, or theories based on the data; a theoretical framework can result from data analysis

▶ Variables aren't preselected for study; they become evident as data collection proceeds

▶ Research questions are broad at first and then become more focused as data are collected; hypotheses aren't formulated

▶ Guidelines for data collection exist, but the direction of the research can change as dictated by the data

❖ **Performance improvement and benefits**
■ Performance improvement (PI)
  ◆ PI ensures a specified degree of excellence in patient care through continuous measurement and evaluation; it's used to implement change, not to identify problems or solutions
  ◆ It's a continuous three-stage cycle: measurement of observed nursing practice, comparison of observed practice with expectations (standards of practice), and implementation of change to reconcile discrepancies between observations and expectations
  ◆ Three approaches are used to evaluate the quality of care
    ▶ *Structure evaluation* examines the components of services, such as the setting and environment, which affect quality of care
    ▶ *Process evaluation* examines the activities and behaviors of the health care provider such as the nurse
    ▶ *Outcome evaluation* measures demonstrative changes in the patients' behaviors and attitudes
  ◆ Two types of review are used to evaluate the quality of care
    ▶ *Retrospective review* is a critical examination of past or completed health care delivery to a specified patient population; chart audits, postcare conferences, interviews, and questionnaires are used for this type of review
    ▶ *Concurrent review* is a critical examination of a patient's movement toward desired alterations in health status (outcomes) and patient care management (process) while patient care and treatment are in progress; chart audits, interviews, observation, and inspection of the patient are the usual sources of data
  ◆ Before a PI program is implemented, written descriptions are needed of the scope of services provided to patients, the structure of the PI committee and its relation to other committees, the person responsible for PI activities, the procedures to be followed, the methods by which assessments are made, and the type of documentation necessary
■ Benefits
  ◆ PI programs benefit nurses and patients
  ◆ They help describe the scope of nursing practice and the effectiveness of nursing interventions in improving and maintaining patient health
  ◆ They give patients an opportunity to critique the care received, which helps ensure accountability for the care provided

❖ Risk management and related reports
- Risk management
  - ◆ Risk management seeks to prevent accidents and injuries and control liability
  - ◆ It has three main goals
    - ❭ Decrease the number of claims by promptly identifying and following up on adverse events
    - ❭ Reduce the frequency of preventable injuries and accidents leading to lawsuits by maintaining or improving the quality of care
    - ❭ Control costs related to claims by pinpointing trouble spots early and working with the patient and his family
  - ◆ Risk managers identify, analyze, and evaluate risks within their facility and formulate plans to decrease the frequency and severity of accidents and injuries
- Occurrence reports
  - ◆ An occurrence, or incident, report is filled out when an event occurs that's inconsistent with a health care facility's ordinary routine, regardless of whether an injury occurs
  - ◆ Examples of events that require an incident report to be filed include medication errors, injuries from medical equipment (such as a burn), falls (even if the patient wasn't injured), and accidents and injuries involving family members, visitors, or staff members
  - ◆ An occurrence report has two functions
    - ❭ It informs the administration of the incident, so the risk manager can work to prevent similar incidents
    - ❭ It alerts the administration and the facility's insurance company to a potential claim and the need for further investigation
  - ◆ An occurrence report should be objective and include the names of the persons involved and any witnesses, the patient's account of what happened, factual information about the event, the consequences to the patient, who discovered the patient, your immediate action, who was notified and at what time, and the patient's response to the event
  - ◆ An occurrence report shouldn't include your assumptions, opinions, suggestions, or accusations

❖ Consultation
- General information
  - ◆ In a consultation, the nurse draws on internal and external resources to resolve a patient problem; *formal consultation* uses a written agreement that follows specific steps, whereas *informal consultation* relies on a verbal agreement between colleagues or other staff members
  - ◆ As health care organizations decentralize, staff nurses will become more involved in consultations
- Models of consultation
  - ◆ *Patient-centered case consultation* provides expert advice on handling a particular patient or group of patients
  - ◆ *Consulted-centered case consultation* focuses on work difficulties with patients, which are used as a learning opportunity

◆ *Program-centered administrative consultation* provides expert advice on developing new programs or improving existing ones

◆ *Consulted-centered administrative consultation* considers work problems in the areas of program development and organization

■ Formal consultation process

◆ The process begins with the initial contact, in which clear communication and an understanding of the consultation's goal are particularly important

◆ The second step is to formulate a contract, which establishes the framework for the process and helps minimize misunderstandings

◆ The negotiating process is followed by problem identification and diagnostic analysis, which results in a plan of action

◆ The plan of action is implemented, and feedback is obtained

◆ Finally, the consultant provides findings and recommendations

■ Informal consultation

◆ Informal consultation occurs among colleagues and requires the same principles and skills as those of formal consultation

◆ Increased specialization in nursing has resulted in more nurse clinicians tapping the expertise of other nurses to improve patient care

◆ The decision whether to implement the recommendations of the consultant rests with the individual or group who sought the consultation

❖ Patient teaching

■ General information

◆ The educational process uses a problem-solving approach similar to that of the nursing process

◆ Assessment and evaluation are continuous, so that planning and teaching strategies can be adapted to fit the situation

■ Educational process

◆ The educational process involves the development of a teaching plan based on a patient's and family's needs

◆ The patient's educational needs and type of teaching plan depend on the patient's current knowledge and perceived need, education and reading ability, environment (including culture and support systems), readiness to learn, and learning style

◆ The teaching plan outlines the learning objectives, content, and teaching methods to be used

◆ During implementation, the nurse must document activities and monitor progress so that changes can be made quickly if needed

◆ The effects of teaching can be evaluated by testing skills with return demonstrations, creating hypothetical situations and testing the patient's response, and letting the patient explain his understanding of a topic

◆ If further education is needed, the nurse can refer a patient to other resources in the community

- Documentation
  - ◆ The nurse documents all teaching activities
  - ◆ The nurse also documents when the patient isn't ready to learn because of difficulty coping with an illness, uncontrolled pain, or other factors
  - ◆ The nurse documents the data on which patient assessment is based and includes the action taken
- Practical aspects of teaching
  - ◆ Teaching by nurses may be informal and may occur while the nurse performs other activities
  - ◆ Accurate assessment of a patient's needs is the key to effective and efficient use of nursing time
  - ◆ Negotiating with patients on educational needs acknowledges their responsibility in the process and is more effective in the long term
  - ◆ To meet patient and family learning needs, the nurse can use creative methods, such as waiting-room teaching sessions and printed materials and other media
  - ◆ Before patients are discharged, the nurse must ensure that they're aware of the critical information pertaining to their condition and document this in the medical record

❖ Delegation

- General information
  - ◆ Delegation occurs when a nurse assigns tasks and the authority to complete those tasks to other personnel, such as unlicensed assistive personnel (UAP)
  - ◆ The ANA defines a *UAP* as an individual trained to function in an assistive role to the registered professional nurse in the provision of patient care activities, as delegated by and under the supervision of that nurse
  - ◆ Further definition and clarification regarding delegation of nursing tasks may be defined by Nurse Practice Acts in individual states
- Delegation process
  - ◆ The nurse should know facility policy regarding delegation and only delegate tasks (but not the nursing process) that the UAP is competent to perform
  - ◆ UAPs make observations, collect clinical data, and report findings to the nurse
  - ◆ Responsibility for the task is delegated but not the accountability, so the nurse should receive regular updates from the UAP, ask specific questions, and make frequent rounds of patients
  - ◆ The nurse must evaluate the task and the outcome and ensure that they're accurately documented in the medical record

Review questions

1. The registered nurse has an unlicensed assistant working with her for the shift. When delegating tasks, the nurse understands that the unlicensed assistant:

○ **A.** interprets clinical data.

○ **B.** collects clinical data.

○ **C.** is trained in the nursing process.

○ **D.** can function independently.

Correct answer: B Unlicensed personnel make observations, collect clinical data, and report findings to the nurse. Option A is incorrect because the registered nurse, who has learned critical thinking skills, interprets the data. Option C is incorrect because though unlicensed assistants are trained to perform skills, they don't learn the nursing process. Option D is incorrect because unlicensed assistants don't function independently; they're assigned tasks by a registered nurse who retains overall responsibility for the patient.

2. When performing an assessment, the nurse identifies the following signs and symptoms: impaired coordination, decreased muscle strength, limited range of motion, and reluctance to move. These signs and symptoms indicate which nursing diagnosis?

○ **A.** Health-seeking behaviors

○ **B.** Impaired physical mobility

○ **C.** Disturbed sensory perception

○ **D.** Deficient knowledge

Correct answer: B Impaired physical mobility is a limitation of physical movement and is defined by the patient's signs and symptoms. Options A, C, and D are nursing diagnoses with different defining signs and symptoms.

3. When prioritizing a patient's care plan based on Maslow's hierarchy of needs, the nurse's first priority would be:

○ **A.** allowing the family to see a newly admitted patient.

○ **B.** ambulating the patient in the hallway.

○ **C.** administering pain medication.

○ **D.** using two nurses to transfer the patient.

Correct answer: C   In Maslow's hierarchy of needs, pain relief is on the first layer. Activity (option B) is on the second layer. Safety (option D) is on the third layer. Love and belonging (option A) are on the fourth layer.

4. When a nurse asks another nurse for advice on handling a particular patient problem, she's seeking what type of consultation?

○ **A.** Patient-centered case consultation

○ **B.** Consulted-centered case consultation

○ **C.** Program-centered administrative consultation

○ **D.** Consulted-centered administrative consultation

Correct answer: A Patient-centered case consultation (option A) provides expert advice on handling a particular patient or group of patients. Consulted-centered case consultation (option B) focuses on work difficulties with patients, which are used as a learning opportunity. Program-centered administrative consultation (option C) provides expert advice on developing new programs or improving existing ones. Consulted-centered administrative consultation (option D) considers work problems in the areas of program development and organization.

Legal and ethical aspects of nursing

❖ **Nurse practice acts**
  ■ State statutes
    ◆ Each state has statutes, or nurse practice acts that define the levels of nursing (for example, advanced practice nurse [nurse practitioner, clinical nurse specialist, certified nurse midwife, certified nurse anesthetist], registered nurse, licensed practical nurse, and nursing assistant); they're the most important laws governing nurses and nursing practice
      ▶ Most statutes set licensure requirements for each level of nursing
      ▶ They may prescribe minimum educational qualifications for licensure
    ◆ Regulatory boards created by the nurse practice acts govern nursing practice in the state
    ◆ Nurse practice acts may provide for a board of nursing accreditation and approval of educational programs in the state
  ■ Disciplinary actions
    ◆ The state board of nursing may take action against a nurse who violates the nurse practice act or the licensing board's regulations (see *Common legal concerns for nurses*)
      ▶ A nurse can be disciplined for habitual substance abuse affecting the ability to practice, fraud or deceit in obtaining a nursing license, incompetence, criminal felony conviction, and unprofessional conduct
      ▶ Other actions or conditions that would inhibit the nurse's safe and effective nursing practice also are grounds for discipline
    ◆ A licensed nurse has a limited property right to her license
      ▶ The state must follow specific procedures to determine if a nurse's license should be revoked to protect public safety
      ▶ The licensee must be notified of the complaint, must have an opportunity to respond to the complaint and present evidence, and must be allowed to have a hearing before an impartial panel and to appeal the panel's decision
  ■ Possible sanctions
    ◆ The nurse's license may be revoked
    ◆ The license may be suspended for a predetermined time
    ◆ The license may be suspended for an undetermined time, and the nurse may reapply after completing a course of study or treatment
    ◆ Conditions may be placed on the license to limit the nurse's practice

Common legal concerns for nurses

Three areas commonly cause legal problems for nurses: confidentiality, consent to treatment, and the right to refuse treatment.

Confidentiality

Confidential information is any information that the patient communicates to the nurse or practitioner for diagnosis or treatment with the expectation that it won't be disclosed. Nurses have an ethical and legal duty to avoid disclosing such confidential information to unauthorized people who aren't involved in the patient's care and treatment.

A nurse who discloses confidential information without the patient's permission may be subject to a lawsuit or disciplinary action for unprofessional conduct. The nurse can be liable for invasion of privacy, defamation, intentional or negligent infliction of emotional distress, or breach of an implied contract of secrecy. Some states provide a statutory penalty against health care providers who violate the patient's right to confidentiality.

However, confidential information can be disclosed under certain circumstances. For example, the nurse must disclose such information when authorized by a patient (but only to the extent authorized), when a patient is a danger to himself or others, or when required by law for a reportable communicable disease or suspected abuse. In some cases, the court may order disclosure of confidential patient information.

Consent to treatment

The law presumes that adults are legally capable of consenting to treatment. To provide a valid consent, a patient must be mentally capable of understanding the nature and consequences of treatment. Expressed consent is obtained orally or in writing; implied consent is obtained by the patient's voluntarily submitting to treatment. Medical treatment performed without a patient's expressed or implied consent may result in legal claims of battery or negligence.

Therefore, informed consent should be obtained before a patient undergoes an invasive procedure, receives anesthesia or blood, or undergoes procedures that carry a significant risk of harm. Informed consent requires the health care provider (physician, nurse practitioner, physician assistant, nurse midwife) to provide appropriate information. The adequacy of this information is evaluated by two questions: Did the health care provider provide information that a reasonably competent health care provider in the same situation would provide? Did the patient receive sufficient information such that a reasonable person in the same circumstances could make an informed decision? If a patient receives appropriate information and refuses care or treatment against medical advice, the physician or health care provider is responsible for documenting that the informed consent conversation took place, the general facts discussed, and the patient's decision.

Exceptions to informed consent

Informed consent isn't required if a delay to obtain consent for emergency treatment would cause imminent harm that outweighs the risk of treatment, if the patient would be substantially harmed by disclosing the risks of treatment, if the patient waives the right to consent and asks not to be informed, or if compulsory treatment is mandated by law or a court order.

Right to refuse treatment

Adults are presumed to be legally capable of refusing treatment. In fact, mentally competent patients with terminal conditions can refuse life-sustaining treatment without creating legal liability for their health care providers.

The Patient Self-Determination Act of 1990 encourages persons to express their wishes about life-sustaining treatment should they become legally incapacitated. The act requires health care facilities that participate in Medicare and Medicaid to develop programs to inform patients about advance directives, such as living wills and durable powers of attorney and do-not-resuscitate (DNR) orders. Under this act, the health care facility must provide patients with written materials explaining their rights under their state laws to make decisions concerning medical care, including the right to accept or refuse treatment and the right to execute an advance directive. A living will expresses a patient's wishes about withholding or withdrawing life-sustaining treatment. A durable power of attorney designates a person to make health care decisions, including termination of life support, for a patient who can no longer do so. A DNR order authorizes health care personnel not to initiate resuscitative measures. The Patient Self-Determination Act specifically prohibits covered health care facilities from conditioning the provision of care or discriminating against an individual based on whether the individual has executed an advance directive.

When a patient is no longer mentally capable of making health care decisions, a court order, statute, or law may authorize a surrogate decision maker to accept or refuse medical treatment for the patient based on the patient's prior documentation or expressed wishes.

♦ The nurse may voluntarily surrender the license or enter into a consensual agreement with the nursing board, agreeing to limitations on the license or supervision of practice for a time

♦ The nurse may receive a disciplinary warning or reprimand

❖ Legal concepts of responsibility

- Individuals
  ♦ In the absence of mental or legal incapacity, a person is responsible for his own actions; a nurse, as a professional, is legally accountable for her nursing assessment and care
  ♦ Although the nurse may be individually accountable, other people or entities also may be legally responsible for a nurse's negligence
- Employers and supervisors
  ♦ An employer is automatically liable for its employees' actions within the scope of their employment; the employer is thereby encouraged to hire competent employees
  ♦ A nurse in a management or supervisory position may be liable for the actions of a negligent nurse under her supervision; liability can result if the supervisor didn't adequately assess the nurse's competence or the assignment's requirements, didn't adequately supervise the nurse's performance, or knew the nurse's limitations and didn't provide adequate training or staffing
- Independent contractors
  ♦ An independent contractor is one who contracts with another to do a specific job; in nursing, the private duty nurse who is employed by an agency but hired on a per diem basis by a health care facility is the most common example of an independent contractor
  ♦ The independent contractor's actions aren't directly controlled by the employer; the contractor has independent discretion in performing the job
  ♦ The employer may not be liable for the negligent actions of an independent contractor unless the employer knew or should have known of the independent contractor's incompetence
- Corporations
  ♦ A health care facility is obligated to carefully monitor the credentials and competence of employees and independent contractors
  ♦ A health care facility that doesn't ensure its workers' competence may be liable for injuries caused by the workers' negligence

❖ Possible civil actions

- Torts
  ♦ A tort is a civil action for damages for injury to a person, property, or reputation
  ♦ Torts are classified as unintentional or intentional
- Unintentional torts
  ♦ *Professional negligence* and *professional malpractice* are the most common legal claims against nurses

◗ Negligence is the failure to exercise the degree of care that a person of ordinary prudence would exercise under the same circumstances; for example, if a nurse notices water on the floor of a room and doesn't wipe it up, and the water causes a patient to fall and injure himself, this constitutes negligence

◗ The plaintiff in a negligence suit must prove that the nurse's actions caused harm

◗ Professional malpractice or professional negligence requires a plaintiff to introduce proof of duty, breach of duty, proximate cause, and damages or harm; proof of the nurse's standard of care is critical to establishing the first three elements

◗ Unlike negligence cases, professional negligence cases require expert testimony as to the duty of care, its breach, and its causal relationship to the injury

◆ A nurse also can be sued for *negligent infliction of emotional distress*

◗ In many states, a plaintiff can be awarded damages for severe emotional distress resulting from a nurse's negligent actions

◗ Some states require that the plaintiff have physical manifestations of the emotional distress, such as palpitations, gastric discomfort, or insomnia

■ Intentional torts

◆ *Assault* is an act that places a patient in fear of harmful or offensive touching

◆ *Battery* is touching a patient without justification or permission

◆ *Defamation* results when a nurse communicates false information verbally (slander) or in writing (libel) about a patient that damages the patient's reputation or causes the patient to be shunned or avoided by the community

◆ *Invasion of privacy* occurs when a nurse gives unauthorized access to the patient or information about the patient; taking photographs of a patient without permission is an invasion of privacy

◆ *Fraud* and *misrepresentation* are false or misleading statements by the nurse that the patient relies on to his detriment

◆ *False imprisonment* is unjustifiable restriction of patient movement

◆ *Intentional infliction of emotional distress* results when a nurse's actions produce distress so severe that no reasonable person could be expected to endure it

■ Contract actions

◆ Contract actions are determined by whether the parties performed obligations agreed to in a contract

◆ A breach of contract results when one party fails to perform as required by the contract

◆ Nurses are most commonly involved in employment contracts and malpractice insurance contracts

❖ Possible defenses to a health care negligence suit

■ Comparative and contributory negligence

◆ With comparative negligence (the more common defense), the jury compares the degree of negligence of the parties or of various defendants and apportions damages (that is, compensation or indemnification) accordingly

◆ With contributory negligence, because the plaintiff's conduct contributes to the cause of his injury and falls below the standard by which individuals are expected to conform, he can't recover damages, even though the defendant violated a duty of care to the plaintiff and would be liable

■ Statutes of limitation

◆ A statute of limitation sets a time limit within which the legal action must be brought; a nurse can't be sued for negligence if the claim is made after the time limit expires

◆ Statutes of limitation for health care negligence are established by the state legislature

◆ These statutes may not apply in some cases, such as those involving fraudulent concealment of negligence or later discovery of negligence

■ Good Samaritan laws

◆ All states have Good Samaritan laws to protect people who render assistance at the scene of an emergency

◆ Some statutes protect all citizens; others cover only specified health care providers

◆ Those protected under Good Samaritan laws are liable only for grossly negligent acts

■ Statutory defenses

◆ Many states have statutes that prescribe special procedures for health care negligence cases

◆ A suit may be dismissed if the statutory requirements aren't met

❖ Professional liability insurance for nurses

■ Types of policies

◆ A *claims-made policy* provides coverage for claims made during the policy period

◆ An *occurrence policy* provides coverage for negligence that occurs during the policy period

■ Obligations of the insurer and the insured

◆ Insurers must provide and pay for legal counsel to defend the nurse in the lawsuit and must pay damages (within coverage limits) for which the nurse is judged liable

◆ The nurse must notify the insurer that a claim has been made and must assist as needed in preparing the defense (see *Reducing nursing liability*)

❖ Ethical aspects of nursing

■ General information

◆ Ethics is a branch of philosophy that examines values, actions, and choices to determine right and wrong

Reducing nursing liability

The nurse can take measures to reduce liability in several areas.

Liability area	Prevention measures
Competent practice	• Know your practice area, and stay current in the field. • Recognize your strengths and limitations. • Be familiar with the American Nurses Association's Standards of Practice and the standards of practice of appropriate specialty groups. • Build a good relationship with your patients. • Review and follow your facility's nursing policies and procedures.
Charting	• Record information accurately, promptly, and legibly. • Use only approved abbreviations. • Record the assessment of the patient completely. • Record all nursing actions and the patient's responses to them. • Correct errors by drawing a single line through them and initialing the line; don't obliterate the error. • Never falsify, alter, or destroy a patient's record.
Access to medical records	• Release copies of medical records to the patient on proper request and to others authorized by the patient. • Release human immunodeficiency virus or acquired immunodeficiency syndrome test results as required by state law. • Don't release alcohol or other substance abuse counseling records unless explicitly authorized; a general authorization is insufficient. • Don't release protected documents to the patient, such as incident reports and peer-review materials.
Common sources of injuries Falls	• Assess every patient's risk of falling; closely monitor patients at high risk.
Medications	• Keep current about commonly used drugs in your practice. • Read package insert information before administering unfamiliar drugs. • Be vigilant when preparing and administering drugs. • Question all unusual orders. Recheck orders questioned by the patient.
Restraints	• Exhaust all alternative methods of care before considering restraints. • Regularly monitor restrained patients. • Follow institutional policy regarding restraints.
Inadequate patient education	• Assess the patient's knowledge before and after teaching. • Use written and verbal teaching methods. • Use return demonstration of physical skills.
Abandonment	• Don't leave a patient without arranging for continuing care. • Be clear when transferring patient care. • Document the completion of treatment.
Malfunctioning equipment	• Check equipment regularly. • Have malfunctioning equipment fixed or replaced immediately. • Notify appropriate authorities of the problem and the action taken.

▶ Nursing ethics is part of normative ethics, a type of ethics that's based on the criteria by which people make moral judgments

▶ As the basis for professional codes of ethics, ethical theories attempt to provide a system of principles and rules for resolving ethical dilemmas

▶ The American Nurses Association's "Code of Ethics for Nurses" provides guidance for carrying out nursing responsibilities consistent with the ethical obligations of the profession

◆ Morality involves rules of conduct about right and wrong

▶ It's based on norms of conduct determined by society

▶ Society's moral codes guide what people ought to do; professional codes, such as the code of ethics for nurses, communicate the goals and ideals of a profession

◆ Although *ethics* and *morals* are theoretically distinct terms, they're used interchangeably to describe right and wrong actions

■ Professional code of ethics for nurses

◆ Nurses have a contract with society to behave in accordance with rules dictated by society and the nursing profession

◆ Whereas nurse practice acts set the legal standards for safe nursing practice, the code for nurses delineates nursing's moral ideals, provides guidelines for ethically principled behavior, and holds nurses morally accountable for their actions (see *Code of Ethics for Nurses*)

■ Ethical theories

◆ *Deontology* holds that an act's moral rightness is determined by the inherent duty one has to act in accordance with rules and principles

▶ It presumes that the rightness of an act is determined by the intent to conform with a moral rule, not by the consequences of the act

▶ Immanuel Kant is a principal deontologic theorist

◆ *Utilitarianism* holds that an act's moral rightness is determined by its ability to produce good consequences and to avoid harmful ones

▶ It presumes that the rightness of an act is determined by its consequences, not by the person's intent

▶ John Stuart Mill and Jeremy Bentham are utilitarian theorists

■ Ethical principles

◆ *Autonomy* is a state of being self-regulating, self-defining, and self-reliant

▶ Immanuel Kant believed that all people are worthy of unconditional positive regard (Kantian principle of "respect for persons"); he also introduced the concept of freedom of will

▶ John Stuart Mill believed that a person should be respected for his freedom of thought and action

▶ The principle of autonomy, that actions and choices shouldn't be restricted by others, has many clinical applications

• A patient's right to informed consent derives from the principle of autonomy

• The principle of "respect for persons" dictates that a patient has a right to treatment and a right to refuse treatment

---

Code of Ethics for Nurses

The American Nurses Association's "Code of Ethics for Nurses" provides ethical standards of conduct and guidelines for all aspects of nursing practice.

1. The nurse, in all professional relationships, practices with compassion and respect for the inherent dignity, worth, and uniqueness of every individual, unrestricted by considerations of social or economic status, personal attributes, or the nature of health problems.

2. The nurse's primary commitment is to the patient, whether an individual, family, group, or community.

3. The nurse promotes, advocates for, and strives to project the health, safety, and rights of the patient.

4. The nurse is responsible and accountable for individual nursing practice and determines the appropriate delegation of tasks consistent with the nurse's obligation to provide optimum patient care.

5. The nurse owes the same duties to self as to others, including the responsibility to preserve integrity and safety, to maintain competence, and to continue personal and professional growth.

6. The nurse participates in establishing, maintaining, and improving health care environments and conditions of employment conducive to the provision of quality health care and consistent with the values of the profession through individual and collective action.

7. The nurse participates in the advancement of the profession through contributions to practice, education, administration, and knowledge development.

8. The nurse collaborates with other health professionals and the public in promoting community, national, and international efforts to meet health needs.

9. The profession of nursing, as represented by associations and their members, is responsible for articulating nursing values, for maintaining the integrity of the profession and its practice, and for shaping social policy.

Reprinted with permission from *Code of Ethics for Nurses with Interpretive Statements.* © 2001, American Nurses Association, Washington, D.C.

- Advance directives, such as living wills and durable powers of attorney for health care, maintain a patient's autonomy
- *Beneficence* is a moral principle that holds that individuals should promote good
  - Based on the duty to help, beneficence requires nurses to act in their patients' best interests
  - This principle may create a duty when the law doesn't
  - This principle often conflicts with the principle of autonomy—for example, a nurse may violate the autonomy principle by preventing a patient from acting on suicidal impulses (a beneficent act)
- *Nonmaleficence* mandates that a nurse doesn't harm others or put them at risk for harm; this principle causes many debates about euthanasia, withholding and withdrawing treatment, and the use of artificial hydration and nutrition
- *Justice* is a moral concept that maintains equals should be treated equally and those who aren't equal should be treated according to their differences; it's used when there are scarcities or competition for resources or benefits
- *Veracity* obligates the nurse to be truthful with patients

◆ *Privacy* requires the nurse to restrict access to the patient appropriately; *confidentiality* requires the nurse to deny access to information about the patient

◆ *Fidelity* refers to a nurse's faithfulness in keeping a promise; in practice, the nurse makes an implied promise to care for a patient

■ Ethical dilemmas

◆ An ethical dilemma arises when a nurse must choose between competing claims or select from equally undesirable alternatives

◆ When faced with an ethical dilemma, the nurse should apply a rational decision-making process by gathering all the facts, identifying the problem or dilemma, listing possible actions, choosing the most appropriate action, and evaluating the results of the action

❖ Organ donation

■ Uniform Anatomical Gift Act

◆ This legislation was approved in 1968 by the National Conference of Commissioners on Uniform State Laws

◆ It allows people to control the disposition of their organs after death

■ United Network for Organ Sharing (UNOS)

◆ UNOS maintains the nation's organ transplant waiting list under contract with the Health Resources and Services Administration of the U.S. Department of Health and Human Services (DHHS)

◆ UNOS's organ-sharing policy, Required Request, increases the probability of a successful transplant

▶ Legalized in 1987, this initiative requires that the family of every potential organ and tissue donor be asked about donating their family member's organs

▶ Its purpose is to ensure that no potential donor is missed and that the family of every potential donor understands the option to donate

■ Centers for Medicare and Medicaid Services (CMS) (formerly the Health Care Financing Administration)

◆ CMS requires health care facilities to report all deaths to the regional organ procurement organization (OPO)

◆ The OPO then enters donor information into the UNOS computer

■ Organ collection

◆ For most organs—such as the heart, liver, kidney, and pancreas—the patient must be pronounced brain dead and kept physically alive until the organs are harvested

◆ Such tissue as the eyes, skin, bone, and heart valves may be taken after death

■ Nursing interventions

◆ Follow your facility's policy for identifying and reporting a potential organ donor

◆ Contact your local regional OPO when a potential donor is identified

▶ Typically, a specially trained person from your facility along with someone from your regional OPO will speak with the family about organ donation

◗ The OPO coordinates the donation process after a family consents to donation

❖ Health care regulation and policies

■ Agency for Healthcare Research and Quality (AHRQ) (formerly the Agency for Health Care Policy and Research)

◆ AHRQ works collaboratively with the public and private sectors to improve quality and safety of patient care

◆ As part of the DHHS, AHRQ supports research designed to improve the quality of health care, advance the use of information systems, reduce health care cost, improve patient safety, decrease medical errors, and broaden access to essential services

◆ AHRQ supports the development of evidence reports through its 12 evidence-based practice centers and the dissemination of evidence-based guidelines through the AHRQ's National Guideline Clearinghouse

■ Reimbursement

◆ Reimbursement for health care services involves numerous plans (private and governmental), methods of coverage, and options depending on an individual's income, employment status, and age

◆ Each type of plan differs in coverage, payment terms, medical treatment procedures, and choice of health care providers

◆ Common types of private plans include indemnity plans, preferred provider organizations (PPOs), health maintenance organizations (HMOs), and point-of-service (POS) plans

◗ An indemnity, or fee-for-service, plan allows the individual to use any health care facility or practitioner

● The individual submits a claim, and the insurance company reimburses him or the health care provider

● Indemnity plans are flexible but carry higher premiums than other types of health coverage

● Typically, the individual must meet a deductible before reimbursement begins

◗ A PPO provides a network of hospitals, practitioners, and clinics that discount their fees to insurance companies in exchange for being part of a network

● If an individual chooses to use a provider outside the network, he'll most likely pay a higher deductible

● This type of plan is typically less expensive but doesn't offer the flexibility of an indemnity plan

◗ An HMO is a network of providers that deliver all the medical services an individual requires

● Except in emergencies, any use of health care providers outside the HMO must be authorized by the HMO, or services may not be reimbursed

● HMOs don't require the individual to pay a deductible, but most do require a small co-payment

- POS is an HMO option whereby the primary health care provider may refer an individual to a health care provider outside the HMO network with minimal or no additional cost

◆ Government reimbursement programs include Medicare and Medicaid

▶ The CMS is the federal agency that provides health insurance through Medicare and Medicaid

▶ Medicare, authorized by Congress in 1965, is a federal health insurance plan for people age 65 or older, some disabled people younger than age 65, and people with end-stage renal disease

- Part A of Medicare pays for hospital care, skilled nursing facility care, hospice care, and some skilled nursing home care for most people when they turn age 65; it is funded by Medicare taxes
- Part B pays for practitioners, services, outpatient hospital care, and some other medical services not covered in part A, such as physical and occupational therapy, and some home health care and supplies; part B requires most enrollees to apply monthly
- Part C—In 1997, Congress created Medicare Advantage (Part C) formerly known as Medicare + Choice. Individuals with Medicare Parts A and B can choose to receive all of their health care through one of these provider organizations such as HMOs, PPOs, POS, or private fee for service plans
- Part D—Beginning January 1, 2006, individuals with Medicare, regardless of income, health status, or prescription drug usage, will have access to prescription drug coverage

▶ Medicaid became a law in 1965 under Title XIX of the Social Security Act to provide medical care to eligible needy individuals

- Medicaid is jointly funded by the federal and state governments to assist states in the provision of adequate medical care to needy individuals
- The Medicaid program varies considerably state to state and within each state over time

■ Occupational Safety and Health Administration (OSHA)

◆ In 1970, Congress approved the Occupational Safety and Health Act that placed safety and health enforcement under the federal agency called OSHA

◆ OSHA ensures compliance of standards through an inspection program, with penalties for violations

◆ OSHA established the National Institute for Occupational Safety and Health to conduct research and training in occupational safety and health in workplaces covered by OSHA

■ Joint Commission on Accreditation of Healthcare Organizations (JCAHO)

◆ JCAHO is an independent, nonprofit organization

◆ It sets standards in areas such as patient rights, patient safety, health care provider credentialing, management of human resources, management of information, leadership and management, performance improve-

ment, utilization management, emergency care, and environmental protection
 ◆ It also evaluates health care organizations—such as hospitals (including general, psychiatric, pediatric, and rehabilitation), health care networks, home care agencies, long-term care facilities, assisted living residences, behavioral health care organizations, ambulatory care providers, and clinical laboratories—in those areas and then grants or denies accreditation
 ◆ Health care organizations that don't receive JCAHO accreditation don't receive reimbursement from insurance companies and Medicare
■ Health Insurance Portability and Accountability Act (HIPAA)
 ◆ In 1996, Congress approved HIPAA, which is intended to limit the ability of an employer to deny an employee with preexisting medical conditions health insurance coverage
  ▶ The U.S. Department of Health and Human Services has developed privacy rules that include, but are not limited to, electronic medical records; these privacy rules apply to all health care providers who transmit information electronically; these rules prohibit the release of personal health information without permission

Review questions

1. A nurse needs assistance transferring a confused, elderly patient to bed. The nurse leaves the patient to find someone to assist her with the transfer. While the nurse is gone, the patient falls and hurts herself. The nurse is at fault because she hasn't:

○ **A.** properly educated the patient about safety measures.

○ **B.** restrained the patient.

○ **C.** documented that she left the patient.

○ **D.** arranged for continual care of the patient.

Correct answer: D By leaving the patient, the nurse is at fault for abandonment. The better courses of action are to turn on the call bell or elicit help on the way to the patient's room. Options A and C are incorrect because neither excuses the nurse from her responsibility for ensuring the patient's safety. Option B is incorrect because restraints are only to be used as a last resort, when all other alternatives for ensuring patient safety have been tried and have failed; moreover, restraints won't ensure the patient's safety.

2. The nurse is caring for a patient admitted to the emergency department after a motor vehicle accident. Under the law, the nurse must obtain informed consent before treatment unless the patient:

○ **A.** is mentally ill.

○ **B.** refuses to give informed consent.

○ **C.** is in an emergency situation.

○ **D.** asks the nurse to give substituted consent.

Correct answer: C The law doesn't require informed consent in an emergency situation when the patient can't give consent and no next of kin is available. Option A is incorrect because even though a patient who is declared mentally incompetent can't give informed consent, mental illness doesn't by itself indicate that the patient is incompetent to give such consent. Option B is incorrect because a mentally competent patient may refuse or revoke consent at any time. Option D is incorrect because although the nurse may act as a patient advocate, the nurse can never give substituted consent.

3. Which of the following acts committed by a nurse is an intentional tort?

○ **A.** Battery

○ **B.** Breach of confidentiality

○ **C.** Negligence

○ **D.** Abandonment

Correct answer: A Battery, touching a patient without justification or permission, is an intentional tort. Option B is incorrect because although a nurse who breaches a patient's confidentiality can be subject to a lawsuit or disciplinary action, the act isn't an intentional tort. Option C is incorrect because negligence, the failure to exercise the degree of care that a person of ordinary prudence would exercise under the same circumstances, is an unintentional tort. Option D is incorrect because although abandonment is a liability for nurses, the act isn't an intentional tort.

4. OSHA is responsible for:

○ **A.** compensating workers injured in the workplace.

○ **B.** providing rehabilitation for workers injured in the workplace.

○ **C.** inspecting high-hazard workplaces for compliance with protective standards.

○ **D.** disciplining workers injured in the workplace.

Correct answer: C OSHA is responsible for preventing work-related injuries, illnesses, and deaths. Options A and B are incorrect because it's the responsibility of workers' compensation to compensate workers for injuries occurring in the workplace and to provide rehabilitative services. Option D is incorrect because it's the employer's responsibility to improve the safety and health of employees. Employers who violate OSHA standards are subject to fines and penalties.

5. A patient became seriously ill after a nurse gave him the wrong medication. After his recovery, he files a lawsuit. Who is most likely to be held liable?

○ **A.** No one because it was an accident

○ **B.** The hospital

○ **C.** The nurse

○ **D.** The nurse and the hospital

Correct answer: D Nurses are always responsible for their actions. The hospital is liable for negligent conduct of its employees within the scope of employment. Consequently, the nurse and the hospital are liable. Therefore, options B and C are incorrect. Option A is incorrect because although the mistake wasn't intentional, standard procedure wasn't followed.

Principles of medical-surgical nursing

❖ **Adult growth and development**
- General information
  - ◆ Growth refers to the increase in physical size and changes in physical appearance and body function that occur with aging
  - ◆ Development refers to changes in a person's psychological, intellectual, and social functioning
- Principles of growth and development
  - ◆ Growth and development occur from conception until death
  - ◆ These processes are influenced by heredity and environment
  - ◆ These processes are continuous and orderly, yet each person experiences them in a unique way
- Theories of growth and development
  - ◆ Psychosocial, behavioral, social-learning, cognitive, and humanist theories describe human growth and development
  - ◆ In Erik Erikson's psychosocial theory, each person goes through predictable, age-related stages
    - ▶ Each stage involves a key conflict or core problem that may be completely, partially, or unsuccessfully resolved
    - ▶ Healthy personality development is associated with positive resolution of key conflicts (see *Stages of adult development*)
- Death and dying
  - ◆ Many factors influence an adult's views of death: ethnic, social, and cultural background; religious beliefs; personal values; previous experiences with death; and developmental stage
  - ◆ Young and middle-age adults usually spend little time considering the possibility of their own death; they view it as an intrusion or an injustice and are most concerned with who will take care of their family if they should die
  - ◆ Older adults begin to consider the possibility of death and tend to view it as a phase of life; although some older adults welcome death as freedom from pain, others fear dying alone or suffering needlessly
  - ◆ Each person responds to death in his own way; there are no right or wrong responses
  - ◆ The circumstances of a death can influence a person's response
    - ▶ Sudden, unexpected deaths may be harder to accept than those that have been anticipated for some time
    - ▶ A premature death, such as that of a child, is harder to accept than that of an elderly person

Stages of adult development

As adults age, they enter different stages of physical, cognitive, and psychosocial development and face various challenges and health problems and concerns.

Development	Challenges	Health problems and concerns
Young adulthood (ages 18 to 35) Physical • By his mid-20s, a person reaches adult height, and body systems are fully developed. • Young adults are at peak physical strength, maximum physiologic reserve, and prime reproductive capability. Cognitive • With stimulation, young adults continue to develop their intellectual abilities. Psychosocial • The key conflict is "intimacy versus isolation." • Young adults struggle to form commitments without losing their identity. • With positive resolution, the young adult develops satisfying, intimate relationships. • With negative resolution, the young adult becomes self-absorbed and focuses only on his own needs.	• Selecting and preparing for a vocation • Becoming financially independent • Establishing a new living arrangement • Managing a home • Selecting a marriage partner • Choosing an alternative lifestyle such as homosexuality • Developing a satisfactory sex life • Becoming a parent and raising children • Finding a congenial social group • Assuming civic responsibilities	*Health problems* • Childbirth or infertility • Substance abuse • Stress and stress-related illnesses such as peptic ulcer disease • Sexually transmitted diseases • Accidents and injuries *Health concerns (when illness occurs)* • Loss of independence and disruption of lifestyle • Disruption of employment and loss of employment benefits such as health insurance • Decreased self-esteem
Middle adulthood (ages 36 to 65) Physical • Middle-aged adults experience a slow decline in body functions. The rate of decline varies greatly and is affected by heredity, diet, exercise, rest, and stress. • Typical physical changes include hair thinning and graying, skin wrinkling, diminished eyesight and hearing, menopause, decreased metabolism, weight gain, decreased strength and endurance, loss of bone mass and density, muscle and joint stiffness, and decreased libido. Cognitive • Intellectual performance remains relatively stable. Psychosocial • The key conflict in middle age is "generativity versus stagnation." • Middle-aged adults need to be productive and accept responsibility for their family, work, and community. • With positive resolution, the middle-aged adult is productive and satisfied with life. • With negative resolution, the middle-aged adult becomes egocentric, stagnant, and dissatisfied.	• Maintaining satisfactory employment • Preparing for retirement • Adjusting to the physical changes of middle age • Developing satisfying relationships with grown children, friends, and other adults • Helping children become responsible, happy adults • Resolving the empty-nest crisis as children leave home • Becoming a grandparent • Relating to aging parents • Developing leisure activities • Maintaining social and civic responsibilities	*Health problems* • Chronic diseases (such as arthritis, hypertension, coronary artery disease, osteoporosis, diabetes, and lung disease) and depression, anxiety, or other emotional problems • Cancer, particularly of the lung, breast, colon, rectum, and prostate • Substance abuse • Accidents and injuries *Health concerns* • Loss of job and employment benefits such as health insurance • Awareness of mortality and fear of early death • Ability to meet commitments to children, aging parents, and community • Concerns about retirement and retirement benefits

(continued)

Stages of adult development *(continued)*

Development	Challenges	Health problems and concerns
Older adulthood (age 66 and older) Physical • The maximum life span is age 110; the average is age 80. • The body systems of older adults function adequately unless stressed, which taxes their decreased physiologic reserves. • Older adults experience decreased strength, endurance, cardiac output, vital capacity, GI motility, and skin elasticity and secretions; weakened muscles and joints; bone and muscle loss; diminished eyesight and hearing; and altered renal function. Cognitive • Intellectual abilities generally remain stable. • Normal changes include increased response time and minor short-term memory loss; other cognitive changes warrant investigation. Psychosocial • The key conflict in older adulthood is "integrity versus despair." • Older adults focus on a life review and acceptance of the worth of their life. • With positive resolution, the older adult is satisfied with his accomplishments. • With negative resolution, the older adult has feelings of hopelessness, regret, and despair.	• Adjusting to retirement and an altered financial situation • Maintaining satisfactory housing arrangements • Adjusting to the death of a spouse, family members, and friends • Adjusting to decreased physical strength • Adjusting to declining health • Adjusting to mental changes and short-term memory loss • Maintaining social relationships • Finding leisure activities	*Health problems* • Chronic diseases (especially arthritis, cardiovascular disease, cerebrovascular disease, cancer, diabetes, osteoporosis, Alzheimer's disease, glaucoma, benign prostatic hyperplasia, pneumonia, and other respiratory disease), fractures, and cataracts • Greater susceptibility to adverse drug reactions • Longer recovery from illness • Vague or atypical symptoms of illness *Health concerns* • Loss of functional abilities • Disruption of current lifestyle and living arrangements

♦ Elisabeth Kübler-Ross described a typical pattern of response to death (see *Dealing with death and dying*)

❖ Assessment
- ■ General information
  - ♦ A nursing assessment includes a comprehensive health history, thorough physical examination, and (when applicable) review of diagnostic test results
  - ♦ A thorough, accurate nursing assessment is critical in determining appropriate nursing diagnoses
- ■ Health history
  - ♦ Excellent communication techniques and interviewing skills are the key to obtaining a good health history
  - ♦ The nurse begins the history by obtaining *biographic data:* name, address, age, date of birth, sex, race, marital status, education, occupation, and financial status

Dealing with death and dying

Elisabeth Kübler-Ross discovered that most people pass through five stages in response to death and dying. Although some individuals experience the stages in a different order and others revisit some stages, knowledge of these stages can help the nurse evaluate — and deal with — a patient's responses to death and dying.

Stages of death and dying

1. *Denial and isolation:* the initial response characterized by shock and disbelief
2. *Anger:* expressions of rage and resentment
3. *Bargaining:* attempts to strike a bargain, typically with God, in exchange for prolonged life
4. *Depression:* feelings of loss, grief, and intense sadness
5. *Acceptance:* a quiet stage characterized by a gradual, peaceful withdrawal from life

Nursing implications

For a dying patient's psychosocial and spiritual needs
- Help the patient make final plans.
- Help the patient control personal routines and affairs as long as possible.
- Provide opportunities for reminiscence and validation of self-worth.
- Support the patient's expression of difficult feelings.
- Use touch as a communication tool, if acceptable to the patient.
- Provide for formal spiritual support, such as clergy visits or last rites.

For a dying patient's physical needs
- Regularly perform routine personal care measures, such as turning, positioning, bathing, and grooming.
- Be alert for constipation, a common problem.
- Anticipate bowel and bladder incontinence as death nears.
- Be sensitive to individual preferences for lighting and noise control.
- Use pain medications and comfort measures as needed to maintain patient comfort.
- Offer favorite liquids and soft foods; appetite wanes as death nears.
- Remember that hearing is the last sense to be lost.

For family members' psychosocial and spiritual needs
- Allow flexible visitations.
- Encourage family members to participate in patient care.
- Recommend rest breaks for family members.
- Visit the patient regularly, and perform routine personal care activities while family members are present.
- Encourage the family to personalize the patient's room.
- Provide for bereavement follow-up.
- Recognize the need for formal counseling in difficult situations.
- Encourage the use of support groups when available.

◆ The nurse then determines the patient's *chief complaint* or reason for seeking health care

◆ Next, the nurse obtains a *history of current illness,* including a description of the symptom's location, duration, frequency, intensity, precipitating factors, and relieving factors

◆ The nurse continues by ascertaining a *personal history*

  ❱ The personal history includes childhood illnesses and childhood and recent immunizations

  ❱ It also includes questions about disorders, such as allergies, heart disease, and diabetes; accidents; and emotional problems or mental illness

  ❱ It investigates prior hospitalizations, surgery, and transfusions

  ❱ It assesses work history, including occupational exposure to toxins or other harmful substances

  ❱ If the patient is female, it addresses age at menarche, age at menopause, and pregnancy history

▶ The personal history evaluates lifestyle and health habits, including sexual orientation and activity; alcohol and tobacco use; diet; over-the-counter, herbal, and recreational drug use; and sleeping patterns

▶ It explores prescription medication use

◆ Then the nurse obtains a *family history*

▶ It ascertains the ages of the patient's parents and the number, sex, and age of siblings

▶ It also inquires about a family history of various diseases and emotional problems or mental illness

◆ The nurse concludes the history with a *review of physical status*

▶ *General:* Assess overall health status, malaise, fatigue, chills and fever, night sweats, recent weight gain or loss, and increased sensitivity to heat or cold

▶ *Skin, hair, and nails:* Ask about skin disease or rash, urticaria, acne, psoriasis, alopecia, hirsutism, pigmentation changes, jaundice, and increased skin dryness or moisture

▶ *Head:* Inquire about trauma, headache, vertigo, syncope, and change in level of consciousness (LOC)

▶ *Eyes:* Investigate visual acuity, use of glasses or contact lenses, photophobia, diplopia, night blindness, nystagmus, eye infections, eye pain, and halos around lights

▶ *Ears:* Assess tinnitus, ear infections, ear pain, ear discharge, loss of hearing, use of hearing aids, and occupational or lifestyle exposure to damaging sounds

▶ *Nose:* Ask about problems with smell, frequent colds, sinus infections or pain, and epistaxis

▶ *Mouth:* Have the patient discuss condition of teeth, use of dentures or partial plates, bleeding or swollen gums, frequent sore throats, hoarseness, and difficulty swallowing

▶ *Neck:* Evaluate for pain, tenderness, and swelling

▶ *Cardiovascular:* Inquire about edema, dyspnea, orthopnea, number of pillows needed when supine, cough, chest pain, intermittent claudication, hypertension, palpitations, anemia, varicosities, and results of the last electrocardiogram and blood cholesterol levels

▶ *Respiratory:* Learn about any dry or productive cough, color of sputum, hemoptysis, dyspnea, wheezing, and last chest X-ray

▶ *GI:* Discuss dietary intake, polyphagia, polydipsia, anorexia, nausea, vomiting, heartburn, bowel habits, diarrhea, constipation, change in stool color, blood or mucus in stool, flatulence, hemorrhoids, location and intensity of abdominal pain, jaundice, and ascites

▶ *Genitourinary:* Check into nocturia, frequency, burning, decreased urinary stream, hesitancy, pain, dribbling, polyuria, and incontinence

▶ *Musculoskeletal:* Assess for joint pain or stiffness, decreased mobility, edema, and heat or tenderness

▶ *Neurologic:* Ask about seizures, headaches, fainting spells, decreased LOC, paresis or paralysis, paresthesia, aphasia, tremor, head injuries, and loss of memory

◗ *Mental status:* Inquire about mood swings, anxiety, depression, insomnia, and suicidal ideation

◗ *Reproductive*

● *Male:* Ask about testicular self-examination, penile discharge, sexually transmitted diseases, sexual activity, safer sex practices (such as the use of latex condoms with spermicide and having one known partner), impotence, and infertility

● *Female:* Inquire about age of menarche; date, duration, and flow of last menses; vaginal discharge; sexually transmitted diseases; sexual activity; use of birth control; safer sex practices; age of menopause; last Papanicolaou test; breast tenderness or discharge; breast self-examination; and last mammogram

■ Physical examination

◆ To perform an effective physical examination, the nurse must be proficient in the following techniques

◗ *Inspection* uses the senses of sight and smell to observe the patient, such as when the nurse observes a patient's gait or smells a fruity odor on the patient's breath

◗ *Palpation* uses the sense of touch to gather data, such as when the nurse takes a radial pulse or feels the breasts for lumps

◗ *Percussion* involves striking one object against another to generate a vibration that produces an audible sound wave, such as when the nurse taps over clear lung fields (resonance), a body organ (dullness), or an air-filled stomach (tympany)

◗ *Auscultation* uses the sense of hearing to listen for sounds, usually with a stethoscope, produced by body organs, such as when the nurse takes an apical pulse or listens over the carotid artery for a bruit

◆ The nurse usually conducts the physical examination from head to toe and from least to most sensitive areas

◗ The nurse begins with a *general assessment*

● Check height, weight, and vital signs

● Observe general appearance and grooming, breath and body odor, overall mental state, posture, and ability to move

◗ Next, the nurse examines the *head*

● Note condition of scalp and hair and distribution of hair

● Note head size and contour and facial symmetry

◗ Then the nurse checks the *eyes*

● Check visual acuity, visual fields, and extraocular movements

● Note condition of conjunctivae, sclerae, and eyebrows

● Check pupil size and reaction to light and corneal reflex

● Examine the retinas using an ophthalmoscope

◗ The nurse continues by assessing the *ears*

● Observe ear size, shape, and position

● Examine the tympanic membrane with an otoscope, noting color, landmarks, external canal condition, and any wax or foreign bodies

● Conduct hearing screening tests

– For the *Weber's test,* hold a vibrating tuning fork at the middle of the patient's forehead, and check for equal distribution of sound; the sound should be equal on both sides; lateralization indicates abnormality

   — For the *Rinne test,* hold a vibrating tuning fork over the mastoid process; when the vibration stops, place the tuning fork near the external ear; the patient should still be able to hear the vibration

▶ Then the nurse assesses the *nose*
- Observe nares for patency, appearance, and septal deviation
- Test for sinus tenderness and the ability to discriminate smells

▶ The nurse examines the *mouth and throat* next
- Note condition of the teeth and use of dentures or partial plates
- Observe mucous membranes, tongue, tonsils, and pharynx
- Determine the patient's ability to discriminate different tastes
- Test for the gag reflex and ability to move the uvula
- Palpate the lymph nodes

▶ The nurse evaluates the *neck*
- Observe for mobility
- Palpate thyroid for size and shape
- Palpate trachea for midline placement
- Auscultate for carotid bruits

▶ The nurse assesses the *heart*
- Inspect for visible pulsations and jugular vein distention
- Palpate for point of maximal impulse at the fifth intercostal space, at the midclavicular line
- Palpate for thrills or ventricular heave
- Auscultate heart sounds and assess apical pulse for rate, rhythm, and quality

▶ The nurse also assesses the *lungs*
- Inspect chest for size, shape, and symmetrical excursion
- Note use of accessory muscles
- Palpate for symmetrical excursion and tactile fremitus
- Auscultate for breath sounds

▶ Next, the nurse checks the *breasts*
- Observe for symmetry, dimpling, or retraction
- Palpate for masses and palpable lymph nodes

▶ Then the nurse evaluates the *abdomen*
- Inspect for size, contour, and scars
- Auscultate all quadrants for bowel sounds
- Percuss for tympany and area of dullness at liver margin
- Palpate for tenderness or masses; the liver, spleen, and kidneys normally aren't palpable

▶ The nurse assesses the *musculoskeletal system*
- Note symmetry, alignment, and joint range of motion
- Palpate for tenderness, muscle tone, and crepitus in joints

▶ The nurse also assesses the *nervous system*
- Note LOC, orientation, speech, and gait
- Check deep tendon and plantar reflexes
- Check sensory perceptions of pain, touch, position, vibration, and temperature

- Test cranial nerve function
- Test motor system for muscle tone and strength
❱ The nurse then examines the *genitalia*
- For a male patient, inspect general appearance, circumcision (if any), pubic hair distribution, urethral opening, scars, swelling, and discharge; also palpate for tenderness, descended testicles, masses, swelling, and palpable inguinal lymph nodes
- For a female patient, inspect external genitalia and pubic hair distribution, check vaginal mucosa and cervix with a speculum, and perform bimanual examination of uterus and ovaries
❱ Finally, the nurse assesses the *rectum*
- Inspect for hemorrhoids and fissures
- Note stool color
- Palpate rectum for shape, tenderness, and internal hemorrhoids; for male patient, palpate posterior prostate for symmetry and tenderness

❖ Therapeutic communication
- ■ General information
  - ◆ Therapeutic communication is as important for a medical-surgical nurse as for a psychiatric and mental health nurse
  - ◆ A therapeutic relationship facilitates application of the nursing process and is based on the patient's needs
    - ❱ It focuses on the patient; personal issues that interfere with a nurse's ability to relate to a patient must be resolved through peer supervision or counseling
    - ❱ It's influenced by the nurse's style of interaction (see *Interaction styles affecting therapeutic communication,* page 42)
- ■ Uses of therapeutic communication
  - ◆ Therapeutic communication enhances the patient's coping skills by helping the patient become an integral part of the treatment plan, actively participate in recovery, and try new health-promoting behaviors
  - ◆ It decreases patient defensiveness by building a trusting nurse-patient relationship; it also helps the nurse identify health problems, such as substance abuse, and promotes cooperation with nursing interventions
  - ◆ It can clarify issues, which reduces misunderstandings and facilitates the design of an individualized care plan
  - ◆ It can promote healing (see *Therapeutic communication techniques for medical-surgical nursing,* page 43)
- ■ Types of messages
  - ◆ *Constructive messages* confirm the patient's importance, keep the lines of communication open, and allow for further data collection; examples include "What would you like from me?" "What do you think about…?" and "I can see you're in pain; let's talk about your options for managing it"
  - ◆ *Destructive messages* negate the patient's importance, close the lines of communication, and put all parties on the defensive; examples include

Interaction styles affecting therapeutic communication

Interaction styles range from defensive to sympathetic to holistic. To enhance therapeutic communication, the nurse should strive to achieve a holistic style.

Defensive style

Nurses who interact defensively have an intense need to be perfect and feel a need to justify everything. They're closed, they withhold information, and they don't risk exposing personal vulnerabilities. They tend to blame their patients and feel frustrated when the patients don't "measure up."

This interaction style can produce anxiety, defensiveness, fatigue, guilt, frustration, and burnout.

Sympathetic style

Nurses who interact sympathetically have poor boundaries and can't clearly separate their own emotional responses from the patient's needs and wants. Sympathizers tend to project their own feelings onto others. They take on others' burdens as their own and feel a need to make everything turn out right. They experience a sense of personal failure if the patient's problem isn't resolved.

This interaction style can cause an emotional outflow of energy, emotional exhaustion, and a sense of futility.

Holistic style

Nurses who interact holistically have healthy ego boundaries: They understand what belongs to their patients and what belongs to them. Holistic nurses provide an atmosphere for patient growth and allow it to happen in whatever manner is meaningful to their patients.

This interaction style can lead to self-awareness, centeredness, differentiation of nurse and patient needs, controlled energy outflow, vitality, tranquility, and satisfaction.

"The doctor ordered this," "There are other patients on this floor besides you," and "We're doing the best we can"

- Patient perceptions
  - ◆ Patients are affected not only by what they know about their situation but also by how they perceive it
  - ◆ Therapeutic communication allows the nurse to assess the patient's knowledge of his condition; examples include "What's your understanding of your condition?" "What have you been told about your condition?" and "What questions do you have about your condition?"
  - ◆ Therapeutic communication allows the nurse to assess how the patient perceives his condition; examples include "What are your thoughts about what's happening to you?" "How does this illness affect your life?" and "Based on your condition, what do you anticipate happening?"
  - ◆ Therapeutic communication lets the nurse assess how the patient feels about his health; examples include "How do you feel about your condition?" and "On a scale of 1 to 5, how comfortable are you with knowing that you have…?"
- Steps to therapeutic communication
  - ◆ Respect privacy
  - ◆ Convey unconditional positive regard; patients need to feel valued no matter how they look or act

Therapeutic communication techniques for medical-surgical nursing

The medical-surgical nurse can use various techniques to achieve therapeutic communication.

Technique	Description	Example
Broad opening	General statement or question designed to encourage the patient to talk about whatever is most important at the moment	Patient (in bed): "Hello." Nurse: "How are you doing?" or "How is it going?"
Clarification	Seeking validation for what was said	Nurse: "What do you mean when you say…?" or "You're awfully quiet today. What's going on?"
Concreteness	Seeking further information by asking how, what, where, when, and who, which helps the nurse gather more information and helps the patient become more objective about a situation	Patient: "They said…" Nurse: "Who said…?" Patient: "I feel so bad." Nurse: "Tell me how you feel bad."
Confrontation	Calling the patients' attention to discrepancies in their communication patterns or discrepancies between what they say and do	Patient: "I don't have any concerns about…" Nurse: "You say you aren't concerned, but I notice your muscles are tense" or "You say you don't have any concerns, yet you've asked me the same question four times."
Empathy	Putting yourself temporarily in another's position	Patient: "I should never have agreed to this surgery." Nurse: "Sounds like you're having second thoughts."
Focusing	Helping the patient direct attention to something specific	Patient: "This is so complicated, I don't know where to begin. How will I ever learn how to take care of…" Nurse: "For now, I want you to concentrate on…"
Reflection	Paraphrasing what the patient has said	Patient: "I'm useless. I can't even scratch my own nose." Nurse: "You're convinced you'll never be able to do anything for yourself."
Silence	Refraining from speech to gather information, collect personal thoughts, or give the patient an opportunity to speak when ready	Patient: "It's so awful to lose your husband" (weeps vigorously). Nurse: remains quietly with the patient but doesn't try to take away the patient's pain.

◆ Choose words carefully; the use of *why* can sound accusatory, and other words can hinder self-disclosure
◆ Use an appropriate sequence of questions
  ▶ First, ask for descriptions; for example, "Tell me about the pain"
  ▶ Second, ask what the patient thinks about the situation; for example, "What do you think this pain is all about?"
  ▶ Third, ask the patient how he feels about the situation; for example, "How do you feel about having this pain?"
◆ Use the nursing process in a culturally relevant way
  ▶ Assess the patient's health beliefs and practices to avoid misunderstandings and noncompliance

▶ Formulate a culturally relevant etiology statement in the nursing diagnosis to allow development of individualized care plans

▶ Devise plans or goals that are compatible with the patient's values; incompatible plans will frustrate the patient and the nurse

▶ Use culturally relevant interventions; whenever possible, interweave the patient's usual health practices with scientific health practices

▶ Evaluate outcomes within the context of the patient's background

◆ Establish a therapeutic environment

  ▶ Address the reality of the patient's experience

    • If a patient asks, "Am I going to die?" an appropriate nursing response is "Tell me why you're asking that question"

    • Avoid responses that close off exploration, such as "You'll have to ask your doctor" or "Yes, you know your illness is terminal"

  ▶ Provide patients with the information that they need about their condition and the health care system

    • Tell patients what to expect from the system and the nurse, and explain what's expected of them

    • Tell them who has access to information about their condition

    • Inform them of the unit rules

    • Explain procedures and medications

    • Provide the names of personnel associated with their care

  ▶ Empower patients

    • Include them in care conferences

    • Ask them what they think of the care plan, what they want the nurse to know about them, and what they expect from the nurse

  ▶ Anticipate patients' needs

    • Begin discharge planning when a patient enters care, and include significant others in the planning

    • Provide written materials; most patients are moderately anxious and comprehend only fragments of information at a time

    • Allow for privacy and space needs

    • Conserve patients' energy for healing; don't expect or require them to do more than is realistic

    • Don't wait for patients to tell you of their needs such as a need for pain medication; ask about their needs regularly

    • Arrange for diversionary activities as patients recover

  ▶ Be accountable to patients

    • Keep patients informed of care plans

    • Ask them about care, and determine if they would like to change anything

Review questions

1. The nurse is assessing pain in a patient with appendicitis. Which initial statement or question will be most effective in eliciting information?

○ **A.** "Tell me how you feel."

○ **B.** "Point to where you're feeling pain."

○ **C.** "Does your pain medication relieve your pain?"

○ **D.** "Coughing makes your pain worse, doesn't it?"

Correct answer: A Asking the patient to describe how he's feeling is an open-ended question, allowing for the widest range of responses. Asking the patient to point to his pain (option B) may be an important follow-up question but is too limiting to be the nurse's first question. Asking if pain medication relieves his pain (option C) is a closed question requiring only a yes or no response and should be avoided. Option D is leading as well as closed. It suggests to the patient that coughing should make his pain worse.

2. When performing an abdominal assessment, the nurse should follow which examination sequence? Place the following in proper order.

○ **A.** Auscultation

○ **B.** Inspection

○ **C.** Palpation

○ **D.** Percussion

Correct answer: B, A, D, C The correct sequence for abdominal assessment is inspection, auscultation, percussion, and palpation because this sequence prevents altering bowel sounds with palpation before auscultation. The correct sequence for all other assessments is inspection, palpation, percussion, and auscultation.

3. To maintain a therapeutic environment with a patient and his family, the nurse can use communication techniques such as clarification. An example of clarification is:

○ **A.** "How is it going?"

○ **B.** "You say you aren't concerned, but you've asked me many questions on this same subject."

○ **C.** "What do you mean when you say…?"

○ **D.** "For now, I would like to concentrate on…"

Correct answer: C Option C is an example of clarification or seeking validation. Option A isn't a communication technique. Option B is an example of confrontation, which calls attention to discrepancies in what the patient is saying. Option D is an example of focusing or helping the patient direct his thoughts.

4. In the stages of death and dying as defined by Elizabeth Kübler-Ross, loss, grief, and intense sadness are symptoms of:

○ **A.** depression.

○ **B.** denial.

○ **C.** anger.

○ **D.** acceptance.

Correct answer: A Loss, grief, and intense sadness indicate depression. Denial (option B) is indicated by the refusal to admit the truth or reality. Anger (option C) is manifested by rage and resentment. Acceptance (option D) is evidenced by a gradual, peaceful withdrawal from life.

Principles of wound care

❖ Introduction
■ Skin, the body's largest organ and the outer covering of the body, serves as a protective barrier against microorganisms
■ The skin is subject to injury from various external and internal factors
   ◆ *External factors* include extremes of heat and cold, mechanical forces such as pressure and shearing, allergens, chemicals, radiation, and excretions and secretions (for instance, from an ostomy or draining wound)
   ◆ *Internal factors* include emaciation, drugs, altered circulation and impaired oxygen transport, altered metabolic state, and infections

❖ Definitions
■ *Angiogenesis* is the formation of new granulation vessels
■ *Cellulitis* is the inflammation of cellular or connective tissue
■ *Colonization* refers to the presence of bacteria that cause no local or systemic indications of infection
■ *Dehiscence* is the separation of the layers of a surgical wound
■ *Eschar* is thick, leathery, necrotic, devitalized tissue
■ *Friction* is the mechanical force exerted when skin rubs against a coarse surface such as bed linens
■ *Full thickness* describes a wound that involves skin loss with extensive destruction, tissue necrosis, or damage to muscle, bone, or supporting structures
■ *Infection* is the invasion and multiplication of microorganisms in body tissue in a sufficient quantity (greater than 1 million organisms per gram of tissue) to overwhelm tissue defenses; an infection can produce purulent exudate, odor, erythema, warmth, tenderness, edema, pain, fever, and an elevated white blood cell (WBC) count
■ *Maceration* is the softening of tissue by wetting or soaking; it can produce skin degeneration and disintegration if left uncontrolled
■ *Partial thickness* describes a wound that involves damage to epidermal and, possibly, dermal skin layers
■ *Sloughing* is the separation of necrotic tissue from viable tissue
■ *Shearing* is trauma caused by tissue layers sliding against one another; it results in disruption or strangulation of blood vessels and can result in skin tear injuries
■ A *wound* is any disruption to the anatomic or physiologic function of tissue

❖ Types of wounds

- An *acute* wound heals uneventfully within an expected time frame unless underlying systemic conditions interrupt the process; examples include surgical incisions and trauma wounds
- A wound is *chronic* when underlying pathophysiology causes the wound or interferes with the course of healing; several types exist (see *Characteristics of acute and chronic wounds*)

❖ Wound-healing process

- A dynamic process that restores anatomic and functional integrity, wound healing works on a continuum from injury to healing
  - ◆ In *healing by primary intention,* the wound is surgically closed (such as with sutures, staples, glue, or Steri-Strips), and healing occurs by fibrous adhesion; granulation tissue isn't apparent, and there's little or no scar tissue
  - ◆ In *healing by secondary intention,* the wound's edges are too far apart to be surgically closed, and there's marked tissue loss; the wound is instead closed naturally by the formation and adhesion of granulation tissue and epithelialization
  - ◆ In *healing by tertiary intention,* there's a delay in wound closure, resulting in granulation of the wound edges; later surgical closure results in more scar formation
- Wound healing consists of several phases
  - ◆ The *injury* is a break in the skin's integrity
  - ◆ *Hemostasis* is a brief period of vasoconstriction at the site of injury as the body attempts to prevent excessive bleeding
  - ◆ The *inflammatory phase* starts right after the injury and lasts from 2 to 6 days; this defensive reaction to tissue injury involves increased blood flow and capillary permeability and aids in phagocytosis or autolytic debridement; it's marked by increased heat, redness, swelling, and pain in the affected area
  - ◆ During the *proliferative phase,* granulation tissue forms and epithelialization begins
    - ▶ Granulation tissue is a pink-to-red, moist tissue that contains new blood vessels, collagen, fibroblasts, and inflammatory cells; the tissue fills the open deep wound and acts as a kind of scaffolding for the eventual migration of epithelial cells
    - ▶ During epithelialization, epithelial cells migrate across the wound's surface, forming a layer of new tissue; these cells look silvery and form a perimeter around the granulation tissue
  - ◆ As *epithelial closure* occurs, the wound contracts and begins to close
  - ◆ During the final *maturation phase,* collagen reorganizes and strengthens, a process that continues for months and sometimes years; chronic wounds may regain 50% of their original tensile strength after 2 to 3 weeks, but they'll ultimately regain only 70% to 75% of their original strength

Characteristics of acute and chronic wounds

The following chart summarizes the type and cause, location, related signs and symptoms, and appearance of acute and chronic wounds. Specific nursing measures vary with the type of wound.

Type and cause	Location	Related signs and symptoms	Appearance
Surgical wound • Sterile incision, which is then closed with glue, staples, sutures, or Steri-Strips • Heals by first intention	• Anywhere on body • Usually follows integumentary cleavage line, which enhances healing	• Vary with type of surgery	• Even, sharp wound margins • Clean, with no drainage or scab formation
Arterial ulcer (ischemic ulcer) • Insufficient arterial perfusion to an extremity • Risk increasing with history of peripheral vascular disease, diabetes mellitus, or advanced age	• Between toes (web space) or on tips of toes • Over phalangeal heads • Around lateral malleolus • On areas subjected to trauma or rubbing from shoes	• Thin, shiny, dry skin • Thickened toenails • Pallor in affected limb on elevation and dependent rubor • Cyanosis • Decreased temperature in affected limb • Absent or diminished pulses in affected limb • Severe pain	• Punched-out appearance of wound edges • Gangrene or necrosis • Deep, pale wound bed • Blanched, purpuric • Signs of cellulitis • Minimal exudate
Diabetic ulcer • Peripheral neuropathy • Risk increasing with history of diabetes mellitus or arterial insufficiency	• On plantar aspect of foot • Over metatarsal heads • Under heels	• Diminished or absent sensation in foot • Foot deformities • Increased temperature in foot without sweating • Atrophy of subcutaneous fat • Altered gait • Signs of peripheral vascular disease	• Even, well-defined wound margins • Depth of wound bed variable, possibly with undermining • Signs of cellulitis or underlying osteomyelitis • Variable amounts of exudate • Possible necrosis • Possible granulation tissue
Venous ulcer • Disturbance in return blood flow from legs • Risk increasing with history of valve incompetence, perforating veins, deep vein thrombophlebitis or thrombosis, previous ulcers, obesity, or advanced age	• On medial lower leg and ankle • Above medial malleolus	• Firm edema • Dilated superficial veins • Dry, thin skin • Evidence of previously healed ulcer • Lack of pain sensation at wound site • Possible dermatitis	• Irregular wound margins • Superficial wound bed • Ruddy, granular tissue • Moderate to heavy exudate

(continued)

Characteristics of acute and chronic wounds *(continued)*			
Type and cause	**Location**	**Related signs and symptoms**	**Appearance**
Pressure ulcer • Excessive pressure (either high pressure over a short time or low pressure over a longer time) that causes localized tissue damage • Risk increasing with history of advanced age, inadequate tissue perfusion, incontinence, or prolonged immobility	• On bony prominences, especially sacrum and heels • On areas where friction and shear can damage tissue	• Possible local pain • Foul-smelling odor	• Stage I: reddened skin that won't return to normal color (discoloration in dark-skinned patients), warmth, edema, induration, and hardness • Stage II: superficial ulcer that involves epidermis and possibly dermis; may look like abrasion, blister, or shallow crater • Stage III: deep crater, possibly with undermining of adjacent tissue, that may extend through subcutaneous tissue down to underlying fascia • Stage IV: deep crater, possibly with undermining of adjacent tissue, that extends through full thickness of skin and causes extensive destruction, tissue necrosis, and possible damage to muscle, bone, and supporting structures (tendons and joint capsules); sinus tracts may form

❖ **Factors that affect wound healing**
- Local factors
  - ◆ Moisture—for instance, from incontinence—leads to skin maceration and edema, making the epidermis more susceptible to abrasion; the chemicals and bacteria in urine and stool also cause tissue breakdown
  - ◆ Necrotic debris and other foreign material in a wound interfere with optimal healing and must be removed; by increasing the bacterial count, dead tissue increases the risk of infection
  - ◆ Infection at a level of more than 1 million organisms per gram of tissue inhibits granulation and epithelialization
- Systemic factors
  - ◆ Aging has a profound impact on all body systems; it affects wound healing by decreasing the inflammatory response, delaying angiogenesis, decreasing collagen synthesis and degradation, slowing epithelialization (resulting in a thinner epidermal layer), decreasing cohesion between the epidermal and dermal layers, decreasing the function of sebaceous glands (resulting in dryness), and altering the function of melanocytes (resulting in skin discoloration)

The role of nutrition in wound healing

The following chart outlines the role protein, calories, and vitamins and minerals play in wound healing.

Nutrient	RDA/Healthy adults	Effects of deficiency	Effects on healing
Protein	0.8/kg	Impairs all aspects of healing and host defenses	Improves tissue integrity; increase to 1.5 to 2 g/kg needed for healing
Calories	• Resting: 1,500 • Sedentary: 2,000 • Very active: 3,500	Muscle wasting	May need to increase fivefold for positive nitrogen balance to promote healing
Vitamin C	60 mg	Collagen instability; decreased tensile strength	Necessary for collagen synthesis; not stored in body so deficiency occurs quickly
Vitamin A	1,000 mcg	Decreased epithelialization, collagen synthesis, resistance to infection by way of decreased macrophage production	Supplementation reverses effects of glucocorticoids
Vitamin B_6	2 mcg	Decreased protein synthesis	Decreased collagen synthesis, thereby increasing tensile strength
Vitamin B_{12}	2 mcg	Decreased protein synthesis	Decreased collagen synthesis, thereby increasing tensile strength
Folate	200 mcg	Decreased protein synthesis	Enables transport of oxygen; decreased absorption in elderly patients so supplementation may be necessary
Zinc	15 mg	Decreased immunity, collagen synthesis	Enables protein synthesis and tissue repair; healing improving after supplementation in true deficiency

◆ Malnutrition delays or prevents healing by depriving the body of the nutrients it needs to combat the physiologic stress of infection and to meet the increased metabolic demands of tissue repair; patients with chronic or difficult-to-heal wounds have special dietary needs (see *The role of nutrition in wound healing*)

◆ Dehydration can hasten debilitation and death; a patient with a large wound can lose far more than 1 L of water per day, the water loss of a healthy adult

◆ Vascular insufficiency can lead to poor healing and the development of leg ulcers

❥ Arterial insufficiency results in an inadequate blood supply, which can lead to tissue hypoxia, infection, and death

❥ Cardiovascular insufficiency leads to systemic hypoxemia, which impedes wound healing

◗ Venous insufficiency—impaired flow toward the heart and elevated pressure in the venous system—leads to the leakage of fibrinogen around capillaries into the dermis; this results in formation of a fibrin layer that blocks tissue oxygenation, nutrient exchange, and waste removal

■ Metabolic factors

◆ A patient with diabetes mellitus requires strict maintenance of normal blood glucose levels for proper wound healing, particularly for the acute phase of tissue repair, during periods of stress, after surgery, and for combating sepsis; poorly controlled diabetes results in notoriously slow and complicated wound healing for several reasons

◗ Impaired circulation caused by thickening of the capillary basement membrane results in reduced local blood flow

◗ Reduced sensation from diabetic neuropathy significantly reduces sensation in the lower extremities, making patients less aware of injuries and serious infections

◗ Hyperglycemia impairs the inflammatory response and collagen synthesis and produces leukocyte dysfunction, which increases the risk of infection

◆ Renal failure or insufficiency increases the risk of infection and wound dehiscence and delays granulation

◆ A newly recognized disorder, reperfusion injury is thought to result from the uncontrolled release of free radicals (superoxide anion, hydroxyl radicals, and hydrogen peroxide) when ischemic tissue is reperfused or reoxygenated; oxygen-free radicals can cause damage to cell membranes, lipids, proteins, blood vessels, and deoxyribonucleic acid and can trigger the inflammatory process

■ Neurologic factors

◆ The absence of pain sensation can lead to significant tissue damage from pressure or trauma; a patient who doesn't feel pain can't respond to alleviate the pain

◆ Immobility and impaired sensory perception contribute to pressure ulcer development and delayed healing

■ Psychological factors

◆ Stress, depression, and sleep disorders can alter the immune response

◆ A stressed, depressed, or sleep-deprived patient is less likely to participate in self-care, including wound care

◆ The sleep deprivation that can result from many psychological disorders interferes with the restorative properties of rest and sleep

◆ Some patients with severe psychiatric disorders may deliberately injure themselves or interfere with wound care measures

■ Immunologic deficiencies

◆ Immunologic deficiencies impair many aspects of the inflammatory phase of healing

◆ Such deficiencies also predispose patients to infection

■ Clotting disorders

◆ Clotting disorders interfere with the coagulation cascade critical in wound healing

◆ Platelet aggregation normally initiates hemostasis and the release of chemotactic and growth-promoting substances, but clotting factor deficiencies (for instance, from hemophilia, malnutrition, or hepatic disease), thrombocytopenia, and anticoagulation therapy can prolong bleeding into a wound and delay healing

■ Other factors

◆ Glucocorticoid therapy (for instance, with prednisone or hydrocortisone) can interfere with healing by suppressing the inflammatory response, preventing macrophages from migrating into the wound, reducing fibroblast and endothelial cell activity, and delaying contraction and epithelialization

◆ Medications, including anti-inflammatory drugs, cancer-fighting agents, anticoagulants, and antiprostaglandins, interfere with the normal healing process

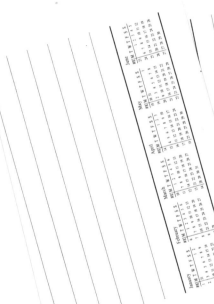

;ing assessment

■ ⌐neral assessment

Determine the patient's age

Ask about urinary and fecal incontinence

Note any chronic illnesses that can interfere with wound healing, in-'uding diabetes mellitus, chronic obstructive pulmonary disease, and ar-⌐iosclerotic heart disease

Assess the patient's nutritional status, including general appearance ⌐nd skin turgor, and hydration status; look for signs of weight loss

Make sure the patient's laboratory values fall within the normal ⌐ige: serum albumin level, 3.5 to 5 g/dl; serum transferrin level, 200 to ⌐ mg/dl; total lymphocyte count, 1,800 to 3,000 µl; and thyroxine-⌐ing prealbumin level, 20 to 30 mg/dl

⌐sess the patient's oxygenation and circulation status, noting indica-⌐ f respiratory and circulatory impairment and peripheral vascular ⌐ ; ask if he smokes

⌐ss the patient's immune status; ask about corticosteroid use, and ⌐ patient has been diagnosed with cancer and is undergoing ⌐ ⌐rapy; determine whether he tests positive for the human im-⌐eficiency virus

⌐ about use of medications, including steroids, nonsteroidal anti-inflammatories, immunosuppressants, antineoplastics, anticoagulants, and antiprostaglandins

◆ Determine the patient's stress level, asking about family support and community resources

■ Wound assessment

◆ Determine the wound's cause

◆ Note the wound's location

◆ Measure the wound's length, width, and depth in centimeters

◆ Determine the wound's stage

◆ Observe the wound margins, looking for undermining, tunneling, and sinus tracts

- ◆ Look for exudate in the wound, observing the amount and type (serous, serosanguineous, sanguineous, or purulent); note any odor
- ◆ Assess the tissue in the wound bed
  - ❯ Granulation tissue will look beefy red
  - ❯ Epithelial tissue will look pearly pink
  - ❯ Sloughing necrotic or devitalized tissue will look soft and yellow-gray; eschar necrotic tissue will look thick and black
- ◆ Note signs of infection, including induration, fever, erythema, edema, an elevated WBC count, and purulent drainage

❖ **Management**
- ■ Prevention of pressure ulcers
  - ◆ Identify patients at risk, including bedridden and chair-bound patients and patients who have difficulty repositioning themselves
  - ◆ Using a valid risk assessment tool, assess at-risk patients for pressure ulcers on admission and at regular intervals; document your assessment on the Braden or Norton scale
  - ◆ Identify risk factors that contribute to skin breakdown, including immobility, incontinence, nutritional deficiencies, and an altered level of consciousness
- ■ Prevention of vascular ulcers
  - ◆ Identify patients at risk, including those with chronic diseases such as diabetes mellitus, and cardiovascular, renal, and neurologic disease
  - ◆ Identify risk factors that can contribute to vascular ulcers, including aging, malnutrition, and therapy with such drugs as glucocorticoids, anti-inflammatories, antineoplastics, anticoagulants, and antiprostaglandins
- ■ Prevention of skin tear injuries
  - ◆ Identify patients at risk, especially elderly patients and those with a history of skin tears
  - ◆ Use a valid skin integrity risk assessment tool and a classification system such as Payne-Martin
- ■ Early intervention
  - ◆ Treat the underlying disorder—for example, monitor blood glucose levels, administer insulin or an oral antidiabetic, and teach proper nutrition to the patient with diabetes
  - ◆ Minimize skin exposure to moisture from incontinence, perspiration, or wound drainage
  - ◆ Clean skin as soon as it becomes wet, and bathe the patient regularly
    - ❯ Avoid soap that dries the skin
    - ❯ Use warm, not hot, water
    - ❯ Use cream on dry, scaly skin
    - ❯ Don't rub reddened areas over bony prominences
  - ◆ Use topical moisture barriers to protect skin from urine and feces
  - ◆ Make sure the patient receives adequate protein, calories, vitamins, and minerals
  - ◆ Encourage daily activity and, if possible, exercise

◆ If the patient is bedridden, take steps to minimize pressure on vulnerable skin areas
  ▶ Reposition the patient—from back to side, to opposite side, to back—at least every 2 hours
  ▶ When the patient is on his side, make sure he isn't lying directly on the trochanter
  ▶ Use pillows or foam wedges to keep bony prominences from direct contact with the bed
  ▶ Avoid massaging the skin over bony prominences
  ▶ Take steps to reduce shearing and friction
    • Use the sheet to lift or reposition the patient in bed; don't drag the patient up in bed
    • Have an overhead trapeze bar installed for a patient who has enough strength in his upper extremities to reposition himself
    • Use a slide board for transferring the patient from a bed to a stretcher
    • Place sheepskin directly under the patient (unless he's incontinent)
    • Elevate the head of the bed to no more than 30 degrees, unless contraindicated
  ▶ Lift the patient's heels off the bed, or use a device that totally relieves pressure on the heels
  ▶ Consider using a pressure-reducing or pressure-relieving mattress for a patient who is at high risk for developing pressure ulcers
◆ If the patient is chair bound, take steps to minimize pressure on vulnerable skin areas
  ▶ Make sure the patient shifts his weight frequently
  ▶ Seat the patient on a 4″ pressure-reducing, high-density foam pad—not a doughnut-type device
  ▶ Consider postural alignment, distribution of weight, balance and stability, and pressure relief when positioning a patient in a chair or wheelchair
  ▶ Use elbow and heel pads to protect skin and minimize friction
■ Treatment
  ◆ Protect the wound from further trauma
    ▶ Use pressure-reducing devices
    ▶ Reduce friction and shear
      • Elevate the head of the bed no more than 30 degrees
      • Use a sheet to reposition the patient in bed
      • Remove dressings gently
    ▶ Use nonadhering dressings or those with minimal adherent
    ▶ Use wraps, such as a stockinette or soft gauze, to protect areas at high risk of skin tearing
  ◆ Prevent infection and promote a clean wound base
    ▶ Cover the wound to protect it from infection
    ▶ Remove or debride any necrotic tissue

● *Mechanical debridement* is the manual removal of devitalized tissue using physical forces, such as whirlpooling, wet-to-dry gauze dressings, and wound irrigation

● *Sharp debridement* is the removal of foreign material or devitalized tissue with a sharp instrument, such as a scalpel or scissors

● *Autolytic debridement* uses synthetic dressings to cover the wound; this allows the enzymes naturally present in the wound fluid to digest devitalized tissue

● *Chemical* or *enzymatic debridement* involves the topical application of a proteolytic substance (such as enzymes) to break down devitalized tissue

▶ Use pressurized irrigation (a 35-ml syringe with a #19 angiocatheter) to clean the wound surface or cavity; use a noncytotoxic agent such as normal saline solution

▶ Absorb excess exudate with collagen or calcium alginates or absorbent powders, beads, or paste

▶ Pack dead space with collagen or calcium alginates or moistened saline nonwoven gauze dressings

◆ Use a moisture-retentive dressing that keeps the wound bed moist but leaves the surrounding skin dry

▶ Use one of the following dressings for a wound with light to moderate exudate

● A *transparent film* is a clear, adherent, nonabsorptive, polymer-based dressing that is permeable to oxygen and water vapor but not to water

● A *hydrogel* is a nonadherent dressing composed of water and a polymer that has some absorptive properties

● A *polyurethane foam dressing* is made up of a spongelike polymer; it can be adherent and has some absorptive properties

● A *thin hydrocolloid* is an adhesive, moldable wafer made of a carbohydrate-based material, usually with a backing that's impermeable to oxygen, water, and water vapor; the thin version has some absorptive properties

▶ For a wound with moderate to heavy exudate, use a polyurethane foam dressing, a collagen or calcium alginate dressing (a nonwoven, absorptive dressing made from seaweed), or a thick hydrocolloid dressing, which is more absorbent than the thin dressing

◆ Take steps to improve the patient's overall condition

▶ Provide nutritional support

● Arrange for a nutritional consultation

● Provide nutritional supplements as needed

● Make sure the patient is hydrated

▶ Maintain the patient's oxygenation and circulation

● If the patient experiences venous insufficiency, use compression to optimize venous return

● If the patient is diabetic, take steps to control his blood glucose level

- Institute measures to optimize the patient's arterial blood supply and avoid circulatory impairment
  - ❱ Help the patient reduce his stress level by involving him and his family in his care; contact the appropriate community resources
- ◆ Minimize the patient's pain
  - ❱ Provide sufficient analgesia before, during, and after dressing changes
  - ❱ Choose dressings that maximize the time between dressing changes and that cause minimal tissue trauma
  - ❱ Teach the patient relaxation techniques and guided imagery to help control pain and maximize the effects of pain medication

Review questions

1. A patient with an arterial ulcer over the left lateral malleolus complains of pain at the ulcer site. The nurse caring for this patient understands that the pain is caused most commonly by which of the following?

○ **A.** Infection

○ **B.** Exudate

○ **C.** Ischemia

○ **D.** Edema

Correct answer: C Severe pain at an arterial ulcer site typically results from ischemia caused by reduced arterial blood flow. Option A is incorrect because infection is a complication of arterial ulceration that may not occur in all patients with arterial ulceration. Option B is incorrect because arterial ulcers have minimal exudate. Option D is incorrect because edema isn't present with arterial ulcers.

2. A patient, age 54, is admitted with a diagnosis of venous ulceration unresponsive to treatment. Which of the following is the nurse most likely to find during an assessment of a patient with venous ulceration?

○ **A.** Gangrene

○ **B.** Heavy exudate

○ **C.** Deep wound bed

○ **D.** Pale wound bed

Correct answer: B Moderate to heavy exudate is one characteristic of a venous ulcer. Other characteristics include irregular wound margins, superficial wound bed, and ruddy, granular tissue. Options A, C, and D are incorrect because they're characteristics of arterial ulcers.

3. The nurse is providing care for a patient who has a sacral pressure ulcer with a wet-to-dry dressing. Which guideline is appropriate when caring for a patient with a wet-to-dry dressing?

○ **A.** The wound should remain moist from the dressing.

○ **B.** The wet-to-dry dressing should be tightly packed into the wound.

○ **C.** The dressing should be allowed to dry before it's removed.

○ **D.** A plastic sheet-type dressing should cover the wet dressing.

Correct answer: C   A wet-to-dry dressing should be allowed to dry and adhere to the wound before being removed. The goal is to debride the wound as the dressing is removed. Option A is incorrect because the wet-to-dry dressing isn't applied to keep a wound moist; a moist saline dressing is applied to keep a wound moist. Option B is incorrect because tightly packing a wound damages the tissues. Option D is incorrect because a wet-to-dry dressing should be covered with a dry gauze dressing, not a plastic sheet-type dressing.

4. The nurse is assessing the laboratory values of a patient with an abdominal wound healing by secondary intention. Which of the following laboratory values indicates that the patient is receiving adequate nutrition?

○ **A.** Serum albumin level of 2.5 g/dl

○ **B.** Prealbumin level of 18 mg/dl

○ **C.** Transferrin level of 244 mg/dl

○ **D.** Total lymphocyte count of 1,900 μl

Correct answer: D   A total lymphocyte count greater than 1,800 μl indicates adequate nutrition. Options A, B, and C are incorrect because these laboratory values indicate poor nutrition.

Disruptions in homeostasis

CHAPTER 6

❖ **Stress**
  ■ General information
    ◆ Stress is the body's response to stressors or stimuli that are perceived as threatening
    ◆ Stressors can be *biophysical* (such as disease, trauma, and overexertion), *chemical* (such as pollution, drugs, and alcohol), *psychosocial* (such as job loss, divorce, and bankruptcy), or *cultural* (such as traveling, being separated from family members during hospitalization, and delegating decision making to health care providers)
    ◆ The body responds to stress physiologically and psychologically
  ■ Selye's stress theory
    ◆ Hans Selye's theory describes a general adaptation syndrome that consists of three stages of a hormonally controlled stress response
      ❱ The first stage is the alarm reaction, in which the person is alerted to the presence of a stressor and the need to act
      ❱ The second stage is resistance
        • In this stage, the pituitary gland secretes corticotropin
        • Corticotropin stimulates the production of glucocorticoids and mineralocorticoids, which promote and inhibit inflammation, allowing the body to protect or surrender tissue
      ❱ If resistance continues and the body doesn't adapt, the third stage is exhaustion, which can lead to disease or death
    ◆ According to Selye, stress can result from positive or negative events
  ■ Physiologic stress responses
    ◆ Physiologic responses to stress involve the central nervous system, hypothalamus, sympathetic nervous system, anterior and posterior pituitary gland, adrenal medulla, and adrenal cortex
      ❱ Hormones and catecholamines are secreted or stimulated by these organs in response to a stressor
      ❱ Their release results in the body's fight-or-flight response to stress
    ◆ The initial reaction to stress is increased alertness in preparation for fight or flight
    ◆ Blood vessels dilate, heart rate increases, the rate and depth of respiration increase, and bronchodilation occurs; these reactions increase the oxygen supply to organs and muscles
    ◆ The arterioles in the skin, kidneys, and abdominal viscera constrict; blood is shunted from the GI tract and periphery to the brain, heart, and major muscles

◆ Gluconeogenesis increases; decreased insulin secretion and increased fatty acid metabolism increase the amount of glucose available for energy

◆ Localized sweat production increases, and muscles become tense

◆ Pain tolerance increases as endorphins (endogenous opiates) are released

◆ Repeated physiologic stress responses can damage the body, resulting in problems such as kidney failure, gastric ulcers, and exacerbation of an existing disorder

◆ The body's level of physiologic response to stress varies according to the stimuli; most physiologic stress responses aren't helpful in coping with the daily stresses of life

■ Psychological stress responses

◆ Psychological stress responses result when the body's ability to adapt to change is exceeded; a person adapts to psychological stress through coping strategies, such as problem solving, reappraising stressors, and rehearsing responses to stress

◆ The body's psychological response to stress varies according to the stressor's intensity and duration and the perceived control over the stressor

▶ Psychological stress can cause physical manifestations, such as hypertension and digestive disorders, and psychological manifestations, such as anxiety attacks and eating disorders

▶ When psychological stress exceeds a person's coping abilities, crisis (extreme psychological disequilibrium) may occur

■ Nursing assessment of stress

◆ The nurse should identify the source and duration of the stress, the patient's resources and coping strategies, and the effects of the stress on the patient and family members

◆ Sources of stress include illness and hospitalization

▶ Stressors related to illness include pain, fear of loss of a body part or function, fear of prognosis, and fear of disfigurement

▶ Stressors related to hospitalization or treatment include perceived loss of control, increased dependence, change in environment, loss of roles as worker and provider for family, change in routine, and lack of trust in the caregivers

◆ The duration of the stress depends on the stressor, which can be acute or chronic, intermittent or continuous

◆ External resources include family members and significant others; internal resources include past experiences with illness or hospitalization, education, and spirituality

◆ Coping strategies consist of past methods that have been effective for the patient, such as information seeking, relaxation techniques, prayer, counseling, physical or mental activity, meditation, discussion of options, and review of events or event rehearsal

◆ Repeated stress responses can have physical effects

▶ Immediate responses include rapid speech, restlessness, rapid heart rate, light-headedness, and palpitations

◗ Long-term responses include headaches, neck and stomach aches, muscle cramps, and changes in eating, elimination, and sleep patterns
◆ Repeated stress responses can cause psychosocial symptoms, including changes in family or working relationships, denial or anger, hopelessness, silence, or the inability to make decisions
◆ The nurse can use life-event questionnaires to measure stressors in a patient's life and hardiness scales to determine a patient's ability to cope with or adapt to stress
■ Nursing interventions
◆ Physical interventions reduce tension and support organ function
◆ Massage, heat application, warm baths, stretching exercises, and physical activity can reduce muscle tension, serve as distractions, and increase the ability to put stressors in perspective
◗ Activities to protect organ function include monitoring for complications such as ileus and GI bleeding, checking urine output, and assessing glucose levels
◆ Educational interventions include teaching the patient or family about stress and the body's response to it and rehearsing events to prepare the patient for stress-producing events
◗ Teaching plans should include what to expect from the stress-producing situation
◗ Event rehearsal helps the patient to review an expected sequence of events and deal with anxiety-producing situations in a controlled environment before the actual event occurs
◆ Emotional support can be given through counseling, encouraging discussions, sharing feelings, verbalizing difficulties, and supporting family problem solving; helping patients to separate themselves from the issue can help maintain their self-esteem
◆ Social support activities include evaluating financial status, assisting with insurance forms, providing referrals for home health care assistance, and evaluating spirituality needs (with appropriate referrals to clergy)

❖ **Shock**
■ General information
◆ Shock is an acute state of reduced perfusion of all body tissues
◆ Inadequate circulating blood volume results in decreased delivery of oxygen to tissues and decreased gas exchange in the capillaries
◆ Inadequate oxygenation leads to impaired cellular metabolism and an inability to excrete metabolic waste products
■ Pathogenesis of shock
◆ Initial stage
◗ Decrease in cardiac output leads to decrease in mean arterial pressure
◗ Sympathetic nervous system is stimulated, leading to initiation of stress response
◗ Signs and symptoms include normal to slightly increased heart rate, normal to slightly decreased blood pressure, thirst, and pale, cool, moist skin over face

◆ Compensatory stage

▶ Decrease in mean arterial pressure stimulates the sympathetic nervous system to release epinephrine and norepinephrine to try to achieve homeostasis

▶ Stimulation of alpha$_1$-adrenergic fibers causes vasoconstriction of vessels in the skin, GI organs, kidneys, muscles, and lungs, shunting blood to heart and brain

▶ Stimulation of beta-adrenergic fibers causes vasodilation of coronary and cerebral arteries, increases heart rate, and increases force of myocardial contractions, resulting in increased cardiac output

▶ Reduced renal blood flow leads to release of renin and production of angiotensin, resulting in vasoconstriction and stimulation of adrenal cortex to release aldosterone, increasing renal sodium reabsorption

▶ Increased serum osmolarity stimulates the release of antidiuretic hormone, resulting in increased water reabsorption by the kidneys and increased venous blood return to the heart and, ultimately, increased cardiac output

▶ Signs and symptoms include restlessness, normal or decreasing blood pressure, bounding or thready pulse, tachycardia, tachypnea, normal or hypoactive bowel sounds, slightly decreased urine output, and pale, cool skin (flushed and warm in septic shock)

◆ Progressive stage

▶ Compensatory mechanisms become ineffective and possibly even counterproductive

▶ Falling cardiac output and vasoconstriction cause cellular hypoxia and anaerobic metabolism; metabolic acidosis occurs as lactic acid levels rise

▶ Renal ischemia stimulates renin-angiotensin-aldosterone system, causing further vasoconstriction

▶ Fluid shifts from intravascular to interstitial space

▶ Signs and symptoms include falling blood pressure; narrowed pulse pressure; cold, clammy skin; rapid, shallow respirations; tachycardia; weak, thready, or absent pulses; arrhythmias; absent bowel sounds; anuria; subnormal body temperature (subnormal or elevated in septic shock)

◆ Irreversible stage

▶ Compensatory mechanisms are ineffective

▶ Lactic acid continues to accumulate, and capillary permeability dilation increases, resulting in loss of intravascular volume and tachycardia. This further aggravates falling blood pressure and cardiac output

▶ Coronary and cerebral perfusion declines, and organ systems fail

▶ Signs and symptoms include unresponsiveness; areflexia; severe hypotension; slow, irregular heart rate; absent pulses; slow, shallow, irregular respirations; Cheyne-Stokes respirations; and respiratory and cardiac arrest

■ Types of shock (see *Comparing types of shock*)

◆ *Cardiogenic shock* results from an inadequate pumping function that causes decreased cardiac output and stroke volume, leading to inade-

Comparing types of shock

Some assessment findings and treatments are common to all types of shock. Others are specific to the type of shock.

Assessment findings	Treatment

All types of shock
- Acid-base imbalance, such as metabolic acidosis and respiratory alkalosis
- Anuria or oliguria
- Anxiety and restlessness
- Changes in respiratory rate such as tachypnea
- Confusion, lethargy, and coma
- Cool, clammy skin
- Decreased pulse pressure and tachycardia
- Decreased urine creatinine clearance and elevated urine specific gravity
- Elevated blood urea nitrogen and serum creatinine, potassium, and lactate levels
- Elevated hematocrit (with volume depletion)
- Extreme thirst
- Hypotension
- Hypothermia (except in septic shock)

- Increase perfusion to vital organs.
- Increase peripheral perfusion.
- Decrease myocardial oxygen demand and workload.
- Relieve pulmonary congestion.
- Correct acid-base imbalances.
- Ensure adequate oxygenation.

Cardiogenic shock
- Distended neck veins
- Elevated central venous pressure (CVP)
- Peripheral edema
- Pulmonary congestion (crackles upon auscultation)

- Administer an inotropic medication, such as dobutamine or amrinone.
- Administer a vasopressor, such as dopamine, norepinephrine, or phenylephrine.
- Administer a vasodilator, such as nitroglycerine or nitroprusside.
- Administer morphine to reduce preload and afterload.
- Maintain normal pH and partial pressure of oxygen in blood.
- Intubate the patient and administer oxygen as needed.
- If the patient has no signs of pulmonary edema, infuse fluid; if the patient has signs of pulmonary edema, administer a diuretic.
- Ensure adequate relief of pain and anxiety.
- Correct electrolyte imbalances.
- Control arrhythmias.
- Use intra-aortic balloon pump therapy to reduce left ventricle's workload.

Hypovolemic shock
- Cyanosis on lips and nail beds
- Decreased CVP
- Flattened jugular veins
- Narrowed pulse pressure
- Normal breath sounds
- Obvious bleeding

- Increase intravascular volume with the appropriate solution, such as blood or a blood product, a colloid preparation, a plasma expander, or a crystalloid solution.
- Administer a vasopressor, such as norepinephrine, epinephrine, or dopamine.
- Administer an inotropic medication, such as dobutamine or amrinone.
- Maintain a patent airway, and supply oxygen as needed.

(continued)

Comparing types of shock *(continued)*

Assessment findings	Treatment
Distributive shock: septic shock Hyperdynamic phase (warm shock) • Adequate urine output • Chills and temperature above 100° F (37.8° C) • Normal or decreased blood pressure • Rapid heart rate • Signs of high cardiac output • Warm, pink extremities • Widening pulse pressure Hypodynamic phase (cold shock) • Abnormal prothrombin time, blood culture positive for infectious organisms, leukocytosis, and thrombocytopenia • Cold extremities • Narrowing pulse pressure • Oliguria • Signs of intense arterial vasoconstriction • Signs of low cardiac output	For both phases: • Initiate antibiotic therapy. • Initiate vasopressor therapy, such as dopamine or norepinephrine. • Initiate inotropic therapy such as dobutamine. • Control hypothermia and hyperthermia. • If patient develops disseminated intravascular coagulation, initiate heparin therapy. • Administer colloids or crystalloid infusions.
Distributive shock: anaphylactic shock • Abdominal pain, diarrhea, nausea, and vomiting • Feelings of impending doom • Flushing, pruritus, and urticaria • Hoarseness, inspiratory stridor, and wheezing or respiratory distress • Seizures or unresponsiveness	• Administer adrenalin and an antihistamine. • Administer a vasopressor, such as norepinephrine or dopamine. • Administer a steroid. • Administer a bronchodilator if needed.
Distributive shock: neurogenic shock • Bradycardia • Hypotension • Hypothermia	• Administer a vasopressor, such as dopamine and epinephrine. • Use a plasma expander to ensure adequate volume. • If bradycardia develops, administer atropine.

quate tissue perfusion and a precipitous drop in blood pressure and urine output; it results from such occurrences as acute myocardial infarction (MI), acute mitral insufficiency, right ventricular infarction, arrhythmias, heart failure, myocarditis, cardiac tamponade, and cardiac surgery

◆ *Hypovolemic shock* results from decreased intravascular volume in relation to the vascular bed's size; loss of blood plasma into the tissues leads to decreased circulating blood volume and venous return, reduced cardiac output, and inadequate tissue perfusion

  ❱ This type of shock is classified by the amount of blood loss: class I is an acute loss of up to 15% of blood volume; class II, 16% to 30%; class III, 31% to 40%; and class IV, more than 40%

  ❱ Absolute, or measurable, external fluid losses can be caused by hemorrhage, burns, trauma, surgery, dehydration, intestinal obstruction, diabetes mellitus, diabetes insipidus, diuretic therapy, peritonitis, pancreatitis, cirrhosis, hemothorax, and hemoperitoneum

　▶ Relative, or immeasurable, internal fluid losses in the intravascular space can be caused by venous or arterial pooling and in the extravascular space, by capillary leakage

◆ *Distributive shock* results from poor distribution of blood to the tissues, which is caused by acute vasodilation without simultaneous expansion of the intravascular volume; anaphylactic, neurogenic, and septic shock are types of distributive shock

　▶ *Anaphylactic shock* results from an antigen-antibody reaction that releases histamine into the bloodstream, which causes widespread dilation of arterioles and capillary beds and bronchial hypersensitivity; it can be caused by allergic reactions to contrast media used in diagnostic tests, drugs, foods, animal and insect bites, and blood

　▶ *Neurogenic shock* results from decreased vasomotor tone with generalized vasodilation; it can result from general or spinal anesthesia, epidural block, spinal cord injury, vasovagal syncope, barbiturate or phenothiazine ingestion, and insulin shock

　▶ *Septic shock* results from a systemic response to microorganisms in the blood, causing vasodilation with selective vasoconstriction and poor distribution of blood; it commonly stems from overt infection, localized infection that spreads to the systemic circulation, urinary tract infection, postabortion or postpartal infection, or immunosuppressant therapy

◆ *Obstructive shock* results from a physical obstruction that reduces cardiac output despite normal contractility and intravascular volume; it's caused by pulmonary embolism, dissecting aortic aneurysm, atrial myxoma, cardiac tamponade, and tension pneumothorax

■ Complications of shock

◆ Myocardial depression may be caused by decreased coronary blood flow and acidosis and can lead to arrhythmias, MI, and cardiac failure

◆ Acute respiratory distress syndrome, also known as shock lung, may result from decreased perfusion to pulmonary capillaries

◆ Renal failure may occur when prolonged renal hypoperfusion causes acute tubular necrosis

◆ Hepatic insufficiency may stem from poor perfusion to the liver and can lead to recirculation of bacteria and cellular debris

◆ Disseminated intravascular coagulation may occur because shock causes excessive consumption of clotting factors

◆ GI ulcerations may occur when reduced blood flow increases acid production

■ Nursing interventions

◆ Ensure an adequate airway

　▶ Encourage coughing and deep breathing; administer medications for pain as needed to ensure deep breathing; suction as needed; and position the patient to maintain a patent airway and maximum ventilation

❫ Turn the patient frequently, and elevate the head of the bed, unless contraindicated

❫ Administer oxygen as prescribed

❫ Perform postural drainage and chest physiotherapy to mobilize secretions

❫ Evaluate breath sounds for crackles and wheezes

◆ Maintain hemodynamic stability

❫ Assess pulse rate and rhythm

❫ Assess blood pressure for changes, using a Doppler ultrasound transducer if a sphygmomanometer doesn't provide an audible blood pressure

◆ Maintain a normal temperature

❫ Prevent hypothermia (core temperature less than 95° F [35° C]) by setting the room thermostat higher, warming the room with infrared lights, covering the patient with warmed blankets, using a warming mat as prescribed, warming lavage solutions, and using a fluid warmer when infusing I.V. solutions or blood

❫ Prevent hyperthermia (increase in body temperature and metabolic rate) by removing excess blankets, administering medications as prescribed to decrease temperature, giving a tepid sponge bath, and using a cooling mat as prescribed

◆ Maintain normal volume status to prevent fluid imbalance

❫ Assess skin turgor for signs and symptoms of dehydration

❫ Note signs of extreme thirst

❫ Monitor urine output (amount, color, and specific gravity)

❫ Monitor drainage (wound, gastric, and chest tube drainage)

❫ Check for abnormal breath sounds

❫ Assess the patient for weight gain or loss

❫ Infuse fluids as prescribed

❫ Assess blood loss, if possible

◆ Prevent complications of shock

❫ Assess nutritional status to ensure adequate caloric intake to meet metabolic demands

❫ Watch for signs of decreased tissue perfusion, such as changes in skin color and temperature, level of consciousness (LOC), peripheral pulses, and urine output

❫ Prepare for transfer to the critical care unit if the patient's status deteriorates

◆ Reduce patient and family anxiety

❫ Explain all procedures in understandable terms

❫ Medicate the patient for pain to ensure patient comfort

❫ Teach patient relaxation techniques used to reduce anxiety

❫ Give family members time to ask questions and express concerns

◆ Follow infection control policies

❖ Inflammation and infection

■ Inflammation

◆ The inflammatory process is a defense mechanism that's activated in response to localized injury or infection; also called the local adaptation syndrome, this process acts to limit the spread of infection and promote wound healing

◆ The inflammatory process occurs in three phases

▶ In the first phase, blood vessels at the injury site constrict to control bleeding; vasoconstriction is followed by the release of histamines and increased capillary permeability to encourage blood flow and attract white blood cells (WBCs) to the area

▶ In the second phase, exudate is produced, the amount of which depends on the wound's size, location, and severity; exudate is composed of cells and fluid that have escaped from blood vessels and may be serous, sanguineous, purulent, or a combination of the three

▶ In the final stage, damaged cells are repaired by regeneration or formation of scar tissue

■ Infection

◆ The infectious process results from a combination of several factors

▶ A causative agent (pathogen) must be present

▶ A reservoir must be available for the pathogen

▶ The reservoir must have a means of exit, such as the nares, feces, or wound drainage

▶ The pathogen must be transmitted directly or indirectly to the new host; direct transmission requires contact between the reservoir and the new host, whereas indirect transmission usually occurs when an inanimate object carries the pathogen

▶ The pathogen must enter the host through a portal of entry, such as the GI tract, respiratory tract, or a wound

▶ The pathogen's virulence and the host's susceptibility also affect the infection process

◆ Signs and symptoms of systemic and localized infections

▶ *Systemic infections* are generalized and produce symptoms in multiple body systems

● Prodromal symptoms, which may be vague, include malaise, weakness, fatigue, aches, and anorexia

● Progression of infection is evidenced by symptoms such as fever, tachycardia, leukocytosis with a shift in differential, and lymphadenopathy

● Severe untreated systemic infections can produce altered mental status, seizures, and shock

▶ *Localized infections* are limited to a specific body region and produce symptoms in only one or two body systems

● Presenting signs and symptoms include pain, warmth, swelling, erythema, and itching at the affected site

● Progression of infection is evidenced by increasing redness and induration and the development of exudate

◆ Diagnostic findings for both types of infection include elevated WBC counts and positive aerobic or anaerobic cultures

◆ Medical treatment for infections include antibiotic therapy, surgery to remove an infected body part, dead tissue debridement, and abscess drainage; these procedures remove the infection or reduce the number of organisms to be eliminated

◆ Nursing interventions for a patient with an infection consist primarily of monitoring and teaching

  ▶ Monitor the progression of infection
  - Take the patient's vital signs
  - Measure the extent of induration or visible erythema
  - Assess the patient's LOC
  - Administer oral, parenteral, or topical antibiotics
  - Apply heat to localized infections
  - Apply sterile dressings to draining or open wounds
  - Monitor drainage for amount, color, and odor
  - Maintain standard precautions
  - Document infection progression, treatments performed, and patient response
  - Encourage adequate nutrition for wound healing

  ▶ Teach the patient to prevent future infections
  - Instruct the patient to protect intact skin and mucous membranes by using precautions to prevent breakdown
  - Stress the importance of hand washing
  - Encourage nutritional maintenance of immune system responses
  - Discuss avoidance of pathogens transmitted by way of the respiratory or GI tract
  - Promote good hygiene
  - Teach about wound care and antibiotic therapy

❖ **Fluid imbalances**
  ■ General information
    ◆ Water accounts for 60% of the total body weight in adults and 80% in infants; the leaner the person, the greater the proportion of water to total body weight
    ◆ The *intracellular fluid (ICF) compartment* includes water in the cells; this compartment accounts for 70% of total body water, or about 25 L of fluid in an adult
    ◆ The *extracellular fluid (ECF) compartment* includes water outside the cells; this compartment accounts for 30% of total body water, or about 15 L of fluid (including 5 L of blood)
    ◆ Additional fluids are contained in other body compartments
      ▶ Interstitial fluid is found in the spaces between cells
      ▶ Plasma, an intravascular fluid, is found within arteries, veins, and capillaries
      ▶ Cerebrospinal fluid and intraocular fluid are found in the spinal cord and eyes, respectively
    ◆ Alterations in the amount or composition of body fluids can cause complications; a 10% fluid loss (4 L) is serious, and a 20% loss (8 L) is fatal

◆ Body fluids transport nutrients to and remove wastes from cells

■ Fluid movement

◆ Body compartments are separated by semipermeable membranes that control fluid movement through filtration, hydrostatic pressure, and osmosis

❱ Filtration is the passage of water and solutes across a semipermeable membrane

❱ Hydrostatic pressure is pressure caused by a fluid column in an enclosed area such as a blood vessel wall

❱ Osmosis is the passage of water through a semipermeable membrane from an area of low solute concentration to an area of high solute concentration

◆ A solution's osmolality, which is determined by the number of dissolved particles in the fluid, also influences fluid movement

❱ In an *isotonic solution,* the dissolved particle concentration equals that of ICF, causing no net water movement

❱ In a *hypertonic solution,* the dissolved particle concentration exceeds that of ICF, causing water to move out of the cell to the area of greater concentration; this movement causes cell shriveling

❱ In a *hypotonic solution,* the dissolved particle concentration is less than that of ICF, causing water to move into the cell; this movement causes cell swelling

■ Organs that regulate fluid movement

◆ The kidneys filter 170 L of plasma daily and excrete 1.5 L of urine daily (1 ml/kg/hour)

❱ They regulate ECF volume, osmolality, and electrolyte levels by selective retention and excretion of fluids and electrolytes

❱ They regulate the pH of ECF by influencing hydrogen ion excretion or retention and the excretion of metabolic wastes and toxic substances

◆ The heart and blood vessels affect fluid movement because adequate cardiac output is needed to maintain the renal perfusion pressure required for kidney function; decreased cardiac output decreases renal perfusion pressure

❱ Decreased renal perfusion pressure stimulates the stretch receptors in the atria and blood vessels to increase perfusion

❱ It also stimulates the release of aldosterone, which increases fluid retention

◆ The lungs expel water vapor at the rate of 300 to 400 ml/day

❱ Increased respiratory rate or depth increases vapor loss

❱ Vapor loss is considered insensible water loss because the actual loss can't be observed or measured

◆ Skin affects fluid movement by means of sweat (visible fluid loss) and evaporation

❱ The rate of fluid loss by means of sweat, which ranges from 0 to 1,000 ml/hour, is affected by body temperature; temperatures exceeding 101° F (38.3° C) increase the rate of loss, whereas temperatures below 101° F decrease the rate of loss

> ❱ Sweat is considered a sensible water loss because the actual loss can be observed and measured
> ❱ Evaporation of fluid from the skin also accounts for a water loss of 600 ml/day; it occurs as insensible perspiration
- ◆ The GI tract normally loses 100 to 200 ml of fluid daily; diarrhea and fistulas greatly increase this fluid loss
- ■ Hormonal influence
  - ◆ Antidiuretic hormone (ADH), or vasopressin, is a hormone synthesized in the hypothalamus and released by the posterior pituitary; it affects fluid balance by increasing water reabsorption in the renal tubules
    > ❱ Increased osmolality and water deficiency stimulate ADH release
    > ❱ Decreased osmolality and excess water intake inhibit ADH release
  - ◆ Aldosterone is a mineralocorticoid secreted by the adrenal cortex
    > ❱ Increased aldosterone levels increase sodium retention, thereby increasing water retention
    > ❱ Decreased sodium levels stimulate aldosterone secretion
    > ❱ Increased sodium levels inhibit aldosterone secretion
- ■ Thirst
  - ◆ The thirst center is located in the anterior hypothalamus; intracellular dehydration stimulates hypothalamus cells, causing a sensation of thirst
  - ◆ Thirst leads to increased water intake, which restores ECF volume
- ■ Fluid volume deficit
  - ◆ Description
    > ❱ Fluid volume deficit (FVD) results from loss of body fluids; isosmolar FVD occurs when equal proportions of water and sodium are lost; hyperosmolar FVD occurs when more water than sodium is lost, resulting in hypovolemia and hypernatremia
    > ❱ Isosmolar FVD can result from traumatic injury; rapid blood loss; and decreased fluid intake from nausea, anorexia, fatigue, depression, confusion, neurologic deficits that alter the ability to swallow or detect thirst, and oral or pharyngeal pain
    > ❱ Hyperosmolar FVD can result from loss of GI fluids through vomiting, diarrhea, GI suctioning, fistulas, drains, third-space fluid loss, and excessive use of tap water enemas; it also can result from polyuria or excessive urine formation, which is associated with diabetic ketoacidosis, hyperosmolar hyperglycemic nonketotic syndrome, nephritis, and diuretic use
    > ❱ Fever can increase fluid loss through diaphoresis and increased respiratory rate; a temperature more than 101° F (38.3° C) requires an extra 500 ml of fluid daily, and more than 103° F (39.4° C) requires an extra 1,000 ml of fluid daily
    > ❱ Sweating can contribute to FVD
  - ◆ Signs and symptoms
    > ❱ Weight loss may be rapid (1 L of fluid equals 2 lb)
    > ❱ Skin turgor and elasticity may be decreased
    > ❱ The oral cavity may be dry and have a smaller than normal tongue lined with visible longitudinal furrows

Understanding parenteral solutions

Type of parenteral solution	Examples	Indications
Hypertonic solution	● Dextrose 5% in normal saline solution ● 3% NaCl ● Dextrose 10% in water	● To treat severe hyponatremia ● To correct severe hyponatremia ● To treat hypoglycemia
Hypotonic solution	● Half-normal saline solution	● To expand the intracellular compartment; to replace free water; to replace sodium and chloride
Isotonic solution	● Normal saline solution ● Lactated Ringer's solution ● Dextrose 5% in water (D_5W) (Although D_5W is an isotonic solution, it's quickly metabolized to a hypotonic solution.)	● To increase extracellular fluid volume; to maintain fluid volume and treat hypovolemia; to replace sodium and chloride ● To treat hypovolemia and fluid lost from burns and GI tract; to provide electrolyte replacement ● To maintain fluid volume; to replace mild loss; to provide free water; to treat hypernatremia and hyperkalemia

⟩ Urine output may be decreased (less than 30 ml/hour for an adult), but specific gravity may be increased

⟩ Altered vital signs may include a subnormal body temperature, orthostatic hypotension, and increased heart rate

⟩ Signs of decreased volume may include decreased central venous pressure (CVP), flattened jugular veins, and slow-filling hand veins

⟩ Altered sensorium and cold extremities also may occur

⟩ Laboratory data may include elevated hematocrit, elevated blood urea nitrogen (BUN) level in relation to creatinine level, and serum sodium level greater than 150 mEq/L

◆ Medical management

⟩ Replace fluid loss orally, if possible, or by I.V. infusion (see *Understanding parenteral solutions*)

⟩ Correct the deficit's cause

◆ Nursing interventions

⟩ Encourage fluid intake, as appropriate, by providing adequate pain control, relieving nausea, offering fluids, performing frequent skin and mouth care, and consulting the practitioner if the patient can't ingest fluids orally

⟩ Maintain accurate input and output records to evaluate the effectiveness of interventions

⟩ Administer parenteral therapy as prescribed, and assess for complications

⟩ Teach the patient and family about preventing, recognizing, and treating FVD

■ Fluid volume excess

◆ Description

▶ Fluid volume excess (FVE) is the abnormal retention of water
  • When accompanied by altered sodium levels, the condition is referred to as hyperosmolar FVE
  • When water and sodium are retained in equal proportions, the condition is referred to as isosmolar FVE
▶ FVE results from compromised regulatory mechanisms, such as those seen in heart failure, renal failure, cirrhosis, and steroid excess
▶ It also can result from excessive administration of parenteral fluids (especially those with a high sodium content) and excessive ingestion of sodium chloride or sodium salts

◆ Signs and symptoms
  ▶ Rapid weight gain may be accompanied by peripheral edema
  ▶ Distended neck or peripheral veins and increased CVP
  ▶ Changes in breath sounds, pulmonary edema, ascites, and pleural effusion
  ▶ Bounding pulses
  ▶ Increased urine output
  ▶ Vital signs changes may include increased pulse rate and blood pressure
  ▶ Shortness of breath and orthopnea
  ▶ Laboratory data may include decreased BUN level, decreased hematocrit, and serum sodium level less than 135 mEq/L

◆ Medical management
  ▶ Reduce sodium intake through diet changes
  ▶ Reevaluate the need for I.V. therapy and the type of I.V. fluids administered

◆ Nursing interventions
  ▶ Monitor daily intake and output
  ▶ Encourage strict adherence to diet and fluid orders
  ▶ Administer a diuretic as prescribed, and prepare the patient for possible dialysis
  ▶ Assess the patient's need for an indwelling urinary catheter during diuresis
  ▶ Monitor patient for complications of diuretic therapy such as alterations in potassium levels
  ▶ Check weight daily; weight gain may reflect volume gain
  ▶ Check for signs of pitting edema in the extremities, and assess the patient for neck vein distention
  ▶ Monitor arterial blood gas (ABG) studies for respiratory alkalosis
  ▶ Monitor breath sounds for changes such as crackles, and administer a diuretic as ordered
  ▶ Encourage rest periods to relieve shortness of breath and fatigue
  ▶ Protect the patient's skin from breakdown caused by the pressure of pitting edema
  ▶ Encourage use of the semi-Fowler position to increase lung capacity
  ▶ Educate the patient and family about preventing, recognizing, and treating FVE

- Third-space fluid shift
  - ◆ Description
    - ▶ Third-space fluid shift occurs when body fluids move into the interstitial space from which these fluids aren't exchanged readily with ECF
    - ▶ It can result from acute intestinal obstruction, ascites, acute peritonitis, pancreatitis, acute gastric dilation, postoperative complications, fistulas, trauma, burns, fractures, hypoalbuminemia, lymphatic system blockage, and declamping phenomenon (which occurs when a clamp on the aorta is released during surgery)
  - ◆ Phases of third-space fluid shift
    - ▶ In the *fluid accumulation phase,* fluid shifts from the intravascular space to the interstitial space
      - • The clinical presentation is similar to that of FVD; fluid is lost from the intravascular space, thus decreasing perfusion
      - • Fluid losses can't be observed or measured
    - ▶ In the *fluid shifting phase,* interstitial fluid shifts back to the intravascular space; the clinical presentation is similar to that of FVE when fluid enters the intravascular space and enters the circulation
  - ◆ Medical management
    - ▶ Correct the fluid shift's cause
    - ▶ Treat the patient for symptoms of FVD or FVE as appropriate
  - ◆ Nursing interventions
    - ▶ For a patient with signs of FVD, see "Fluid volume deficit: Nursing interventions," page 71
    - ▶ For a patient with signs of FVE, see "Fluid volume excess: Nursing interventions," page 72

❖ Electrolyte imbalances

- General information
  - ◆ Electrolytes are substances that dissociate in solution and conduct a weak electrical current
  - ◆ Intracellular electrolytes include potassium, magnesium, and phosphate
    - ▶ *Potassium* is the principal intracellular cation; it controls cellular osmotic pressure, influences skeletal and cardiac muscle activity, and is dramatically affected by acid-base imbalance
    - ▶ *Magnesium,* which also is an intracellular cation, is contained mostly in bone; it activates intracellular enzymes, contributes to carbohydrate and protein metabolism, and acts to dilate vessels, decrease blood pressure, and trigger ventricular arrhythmias and cardiac arrest
    - ▶ *Phosphate* is the principal intracellular anion; it's essential for muscle, red blood cell (RBC), and nervous system functioning, and it plays a role in carbohydrate, protein, and fat metabolism
  - ◆ Extracellular electrolytes include sodium, calcium, bicarbonate, and chloride

▶ *Sodium* is the principal extracellular cation; it's responsible for the osmotic pressure of ECF, and it doesn't readily cross the cell membrane

▶ *Calcium,* an extracellular cation, is concentrated in the skeletal system; it acts as cell cement, has a sedative effect on nerve cells, regulates muscle contraction and relaxation (including heartbeat), activates enzymes that stimulate chemical reactions, and plays a role in blood coagulation

▶ *Bicarbonate,* an extracellular anion, plays a role in acid-base balance; it serves as a buffer to keep serum pH within normal limits and is regulated primarily by the kidneys

▶ *Chloride* is the principal extracellular anion; it helps maintain acid-base balance and works with sodium to help maintain osmotic pressure

◆ When the body can't maintain the normal level of an electrolyte, an imbalance can result (see *Understanding electrolyte imbalances*)

■ Electrolyte movement

◆ Electrolytes move in and out of cells through diffusion, osmosis, active transport, filtration, and plasma colloid osmotic pressure

◆ *Diffusion* is the movement of particles from an area of higher concentration to an area of lower concentration across a semipermeable membrane

▶ The number of particles diffused depends on permeability, or the relative size of cell membrane pores in relation to the particle's size

▶ The greater the difference in particle concentration, the greater the diffusion rate

▶ Cell membrane pores are lined with positively charged ions that repel other positive ions and attract negative ions

▶ The difference in electric potential helps diffusion occur even without a concentration difference

▶ The pressure increase intensifies the molecular forces striking the membrane, which increases the amount of diffusion

◆ *Osmosis* is the passive movement of fluid across a membrane from a region of low solute concentration to a region of high solute concentration in an effort to maintain homeostasis

▶ Osmolality refers to the specific gravity of body fluids; the higher the specific gravity, the greater the osmotic pressure, which attracts more water to the area

▶ Osmolality measures the number of dissolved particles per unit of water; normal osmolality of plasma is 280 to 294 mOsm/kg

◆ *Active transport* occurs when the cell membrane must move molecules against their concentration gradient; it requires energy (from cellular chemical reactions) and a carrier substance such as sodium

◆ *Filtration* is the movement of fluid through a permeable membrane from a region of high pressure to a region of low pressure

◆ *Plasma colloid osmotic pressure* is the osmotic pressure caused by plasma proteins; it results from the selective retention of colloids in plasma, which lowers the concentration of water and electrolytes

(*Text continues on page 79.*)

Understanding electrolyte imbalances

The following chart summarizes the etiology, signs and symptoms, and nursing care related to various electrolyte imbalances. For all imbalances, treatment goals include diagnosis and correction of the underlying cause, restoration of the normal electrolyte level, prevention of complications associated with the imbalance, and prevention of recurrence.

Cause	Signs and symptoms	Nursing care
Hypocalcemia • Hypoparathyroidism, infusion of citrated blood, acute pancreatitis, hyperphosphatemia, inadequate dietary intake of vitamin D, or continuous or long-term use of laxatives • Magnesium deficiency, medullary thyroid carcinoma, low serum albumin levels, or alkalosis • Use of aminoglycosides, caffeine, calcitonin, corticosteroids, loop diuretics, nicotine, phosphates, radiographic contrast media, or aluminum-containing antacids	• Ionized calcium level below 4.5 mEq/L; serum calcium levels below 8.5 mg/dl • Tingling around the mouth and in the fingertips and feet, numbness, painful muscle spasms, and tetany • Positive Trousseau's and Chvostek's signs • Bronchospasm, laryngospasm, and airway obstruction • Seizures • Changes in cardiac conduction • Hypotension • Depression, impaired memory, confusion, and hallucinations • Dry or scaling skin, brittle nails, dry hair, and cataracts • Skeletal fractures resulting from osteoporosis	• Identify patients at risk for hypocalcemia. • Assess the patient for signs and symptoms of hypocalcemia, especially changes in cardiovascular and neurologic status and in vital signs. • Administer I.V. calcium as prescribed. • Administer vitamin D supplementation as prescribed. • Administer a phosphate-binding antacid. • Review the procedure for eliciting Trousseau's and Chvostek's signs. • Take seizure or emergency precautions as needed. • Encourage a patient with osteoporosis to exercise regularly. • Encourage the patient to increase his intake of foods that are rich in calcium and vitamin D. • Teach the patient and family how to prevent, recognize, and treat hypocalcemia.
Hypercalcemia • Malignant neoplasms, metastatic bone cancer, hyperparathyroidism, immobilization and loss of bone mineral, or thiazide diuretic use • High calcium intake • Hyperthyroidism or hypothyroidism • Drugs, such as calcium-containing antacids, calcium preparations, lithium, vitamin A, and vitamin D	• Ionized calcium level above 5.5 mEq/L; serum calcium levels above 10.5 mg/dl • Muscle weakness and lack of coordination • Anorexia, constipation, abdominal pain, nausea, vomiting, peptic ulcers, and abdominal distention • Confusion, impaired memory, slurred speech, and coma • Polyuria and renal colic • Cardiac arrest	• Identify patients at risk for hypercalcemia. • If the patient is receiving digoxin, assess him for signs of digoxin toxicity. • Assess the patient for signs and symptoms of hypercalcemia. • Encourage ambulation. • Move the patient carefully to prevent fractures. • Take safety or seizure precautions as needed. • Have emergency equipment available. • Administer phosphate to inhibit GI absorption of calcium. • Administer a loop diuretic to promote calcium excretion. • Force fluids with a high acid-ash concentration, such as cranberry juice, to dilute and absorb calcium. • Reduce dietary calcium. • Teach the patient and family how to prevent, recognize, and treat hypercalcemia, especially if the patient has metastatic cancer.

(continued)

Understanding electrolyte imbalances *(continued)*

Cause	Signs and symptoms	Nursing care
Hypokalemia ● GI losses from diarrhea, laxative abuse, prolonged gastric suctioning, prolonged vomiting, ileostomy, or colostomy ● Renal losses related to diuretic use, renal tubular - acidosis, renal stenosis, or hyperaldosteronism ● Use of certain antibiotics, including penicillin G sodium, carbenicillin, or amphotericin B ● Steroid therapy ● Severe perspiration ● Hyperalimentation, alkalosis, or excessive blood insulin levels ● Poor nutrition ● Cushing's syndrome	● Potassium level under 3.5 mEq/L ● Fatigue, muscle weakness, and paresthesia ● Prolonged cardiac repolarization, decreased strength of myocardial contraction, orthostatic hypotension, reduced sensitivity to digoxin, increased resistance to antiarrhythmics, and cardiac arrest ● Flat ST segment and Q wave on electrocardiogram (ECG) ● Decreased bowel motility ● Suppressed insulin release and aldosterone secretion ● Inability to concentrate urine and increased renal phosphate excretion ● Respiratory muscle weakness ● Metabolic alkalosis, low urine osmolality, slightly elevated glucose level, and myoglobinuria	● Identify patients at risk for hypokalemia. ● Assess the patient's diet for a lack of potassium. ● Assess the patient for signs and symptoms of hypokalemia. ● Administer a potassium replacement as prescribed. ● Encourage intake of high-potassium foods, such as bananas, dried fruit, and orange juice. ● Monitor the patient for complications. ● Have emergency equipment available for cardiopulmonary resuscitation and cardiac defibrillation. ● Teach the patient and family how to prevent, recognize, and treat hypokalemia.
Hyperkalemia ● Decreased renal excretion related to oliguric renal failure, potassium-sparing diuretic use, or adrenal steroid deficiency ● High potassium intake related to the improper use of oral supplements, excessive use of salt substitutes, or rapid infusion of potassium solutions ● Acidosis, tissue damage, or malignant cell lysis after chemotherapy	● Potassium level above 5 mEq/L ● Cardiac conduction disturbances, ventricular arrhythmias, prolonged depolarization, decreased strength of contraction, and cardiac arrest ● Tall tented T wave, prolonged QRS complex and PR interval on ECG ● Muscle weakness and paralysis ● Nausea, vomiting, diarrhea, intestinal colic, uremic enteritis, decreased bowel sounds, abdominal distention, and paralytic ileus	● Identify patients at risk for hyperkalemia. ● Assess the patient's diet for excess use of salt substitutes. ● Assess patient for signs and symptoms of hyperkalemia. ● Assess arterial blood gas studies for metabolic alkalosis. ● Take precautions when drawing blood samples. A falsely elevated potassium level can result from hemolysis or prolonged tourniquet application. ● Have emergency equipment available. ● Administer calcium gluconate to decrease myocardial irritability. ● Administer insulin and I.V. glucose to move potassium back into cells. ● Administer sodium polystyrene sulfonate (Kayexalate) with 70% sorbitol to exchange sodium ions for potassium ions in the intestine. ● Perform hemodialysis or peritoneal dialysis to remove excess potassium. ● Teach the patient and family how to prevent, recognize, and treat hyperkalemia.

Understanding electrolyte imbalances *(continued)*

Cause	Signs and symptoms	Nursing care
Hypomagnesemia • Alcoholism, protein-calorie malnutrition, I.V. therapy without magnesium replacement, gastric suctioning, malabsorption syndromes, laxative abuse, bulimia, anorexia, intestinal bypass for obesity, diarrhea, or colonic neoplasms • Hyperaldosteronism or renal disease that impairs magnesium reabsorption • Use of osmotic diuretics or antibiotics (such as ticarcillin, gentamicin, carbenicillin, cyclosporine, and cisplatin) • Overdose of vitamin D or calcium, burns, pancreatitis, sepsis, hypothermia, exchange transfusion, hyperalimentation, or diabetic ketoacidosis	• Magnesium level under 1.5 mEq/L • Muscle weakness, tremors, tetany, and clonic or focal seizures • Laryngeal stridor • Decreased blood pressure, ventricular fibrillation, tachyarrhythmias, and increased susceptibility to digoxin toxicity • Apathy, depression, agitation, confusion, delirium, and hallucinations • Nausea, vomiting, and anorexia • Decreased calcium level • Positive Chvostek's and Trousseau's signs	• Identify patients at risk for hypomagnesemia. • Assess the patient for signs and symptoms of hypomagnesemia. • Administer I.V. magnesium as prescribed. • Encourage the patient to consume magnesium-rich foods. • If the patient is confused or agitated, take safety precautions. • Take seizure precautions as needed. • Have emergency equipment available. Calcium gluconate is used to treat tetany. • Teach the patient and family how to prevent, recognize, and treat hypomagnesemia.
Hypermagnesemia • Renal failure, excessive antacid use (especially in a patient with renal failure), adrenal insufficiency, or diuretic abuse • Excessive magnesium replacement or excessive use of milk of magnesia or other magnesium-containing laxative	• Magnesium level above 2.5 mEq/L • Peripheral vasodilation with decreased blood pressure, facial flushing, and sensations of warmth and thirst • Lethargy or drowsiness, apnea, and coma • Loss of deep tendon reflexes, paresis, and paralysis • Cardiac arrest	• Identify patients at risk for hypermagnesemia. • Review all medications for a patient with renal failure. • Assess the patient for signs and symptoms of hypermagnesemia. • Assess reflexes; if absent, notify the practitioner. • Administer calcium gluconate. • Have emergency equipment available. • Prepare the patient for hemodialysis if prescribed. • If the patient is taking an antacid, a laxative, or another drug that contains magnesium, instruct him to stop. • Teach the patient and family how to prevent, recognize, and treat hypermagnesemia.

(continued)

Understanding electrolyte imbalances *(continued)*

Cause	Signs and symptoms	Nursing care
Hyponatremia Dilutional • Excessive water gain caused by inappropriate administration of I.V. solutions, syndrome of inappropriate antidiuretic hormone secretion, oxytocin use for labor induction, water intoxication, heart failure, renal failure, or cirrhosis	• Sodium level under 136 mEq/L • Confusion • Nausea, vomiting • Weight gain • Edema • Muscle spasms, convulsions	• Identify patients at risk for hyponatremia. • Assess fluid intake and output. • Assess the patient for signs and symptoms of hyponatremia. • If patient has dilutional hyponatremia, restrict his fluid intake.
True • Excessive sodium loss due to GI losses, excessive sweating, diuretic use, adrenal insufficiency, burns, lithium use, or starvation	• Postural hypotension • Tachycardia • Dry mucous membranes • Weight loss • Nausea, vomiting • Oliguria • Muscle twitching and weakness	• If the patient has true hyponatremia, administer isotonic I.V. fluids, and observe for hypervolemia. • Teach the patient and family dietary measures that ensure appropriate fluid and sodium intake.
Hypernatremia • Sodium gain that exceeds water gain related to salt intoxication (resulting from sodium bicarbonate use in cardiac arrest), hyperaldosteronism, or use of diuretics, vasopressin, corticosteroids, or some antihypertensives • Water loss that exceeds sodium loss related to profuse sweating, diarrhea, polyuria resulting from diabetes insipidus or diabetes mellitus, high-protein tube feedings, inadequate water intake, or insensible water loss	• Sodium level above 145 mEq/L • Thirst; rough, dry tongue; dry, sticky mucous membranes; flushed skin; oliguria; and low grade fever that returns to normal when sodium levels return to normal • Restlessness, disorientation, hallucinations, lethargy, seizures, and coma • Muscle weakness and irritability • Serum osmolality above 295 mOsm/kg and urine specific gravity above 1.015	• If the patient is receiving lithium, teach him how to prevent alterations in his sodium levels. • If the patient has adrenal insufficiency, teach him how to prevent hyponatremia. • Teach the patient and family how to prevent, recognize, and treat hyponatremia.

Understanding electrolyte imbalances *(continued)*		
Cause	**Signs and symptoms**	**Nursing care**
Hypophosphatemia ● Glucose administration or insulin release, nutritional recovery syndrome, overzealous feeding with simple carbohydrates, respiratory alkalosis, alcohol withdrawal, diabetic ketoacidosis, or starvation ● Malabsorption syndromes, diarrhea, vomiting, aldosteronism, diuretic therapy, or use of drugs that bind with phosphate, such as aluminum hydroxide (Amphojel) or magnesium salts (milk of magnesia)	● Phosphorus level below 2.5 mg/dl or 0.97 mmol/L ● Irritability, apprehension, confusion, decreased level of consciousness, seizures, and coma ● Weakness, numbness, and paresthesia ● Congestive cardiomyopathy ● Respiratory muscle weakness ● Hemolytic anemia ● Impaired granulocyte function, elevated creatine phosphokinase level, hyperglycemia, and metabolic acidosis	● Identify patients at risk for hypophosphatemia. ● Assess the patient for signs and symptoms of hypophosphatemia, especially neurologic and hematologic ones. ● Administer phosphate supplements as prescribed. ● Note calcium and phosphorus levels because calcium and phosphorus have an inverse relationship. ● Gradually introduce hyperalimentation as prescribed. ● Teach the patient and family how to prevent, recognize, and treat hypophosphatemia.
Hyperphosphatemia ● Renal disease ● Hypoparathyroidism or hyperthyroidism ● Excessive vitamin D intake ● Muscle necrosis, excessive phosphate intake, or chemotherapy	● Phosphorus level above 4.5 mg/dl or 1.45 mmol/L ● Soft-tissue calcification (chronic hyperphosphatemia) ● Hypocalcemia, possibly with tetany ● Increased red blood cell count	● Identify patients at risk for hyperphosphatemia. ● Assess the patient for signs and symptoms of hyperphosphatemia and hypocalcemia, including tetany and muscle twitching. ● Advise the patient to avoid foods and medications that contain phosphorus. ● Administer phosphorus-binding antacids. ● Prepare the patient for possible dialysis. ● Teach the patient and family how to prevent, recognize, and treat hyperphosphatemia.

❖ Acid-base imbalances
- General information
  - ◆ An acid is any substance that can donate a hydrogen ion; a base is any substance that can accept or combine with a hydrogen ion
  - ◆ Acid-base balance optimizes enzymatic function, nerve conduction, synaptic transmission, and muscle contraction
  - ◆ Acids are generated by cellular metabolism of fats and carbohydrates; to maintain acid-base balance, acids must be excreted by the lungs and kidneys at the same rate they're generated
  - ◆ Acidemia is a condition in which the blood is too acidic (has a pH below 7.35); acidosis causes acidemia
  - ◆ Alkalemia is a condition in which the blood is too alkaline (has a pH above 7.45); alkalosis causes alkalemia (see *Understanding acid-base imbalances*, pages 80 to 82)

(Text continues on page 82.)

Understanding acid-base imbalances

The following chart summarizes the etiology, signs and symptoms, and nursing care related to various acid-base imbalances. Remember that in a mixed acid-base imbalance the etiology, signs and symptoms, and care will vary with the specific imbalances involved.

Description	Cause	Signs and symptoms	Nursing care
Metabolic acidosis Acid-base disturbance characterized by low pH, bicarbonate (HCO_3^-) ion deficit, and excess hydrogen ions in which the lungs compensate with hyperventilation to decrease the partial pressure of arterial carbon dioxide ($Paco_2$) concentration	• Conditions that increase acid production or absorption, such as impaired tissue perfusion, diabetes mellitus, salicylate poisoning, renal insufficiency, methanol or ethylene glycol toxicity, and starvation • Conditions that increase bicarbonate loss, such as diarrhea, intestinal or pancreatic fistula, adrenal insufficiency, ureterosigmoidostomy, renal tubular acidosis, and acetazolamide therapy	• Headache, confusion, drowsiness, stupor, and coma • Fruity breath • Nausea and vomiting • Increased respiratory rate and depth (classic Kussmaul's respirations) • Hyperkalemia • Warm, flushed skin • Cardiac arrhythmias • pH below 7.35, HCO_3^- under 22 mEq/L, and normal $Paco_2$ (34 to 44 mm Hg)	• Identify patients at risk for metabolic acidosis. • Assess the patient for signs and symptoms of metabolic acidosis, especially respiratory, neurologic, electrolyte, and arterial blood gas (ABG) changes. • Administer $NaHCO_3^-$ if necessary. • Evaluate and correct fluid and electrolyte imbalances. • Administer medications for nausea, vomiting, or diarrhea, as prescribed. • If the patient is confused, take safety precautions. • If the patient is diabetic, teach him and his family about blood glucose monitoring, diet, and drug administration. • Treat the underlying cause—for example, if diabetic ketoacidosis is the cause, administer insulin and fluids.
Metabolic alkalosis Acid-base disturbance characterized by high pH and excess HCO_3^- and base in which the lungs compensate through hypoventilation to increase $Paco_2$	• Excessive removal or vomiting of gastric acid, nasogastric suctioning, or pyloric stenosis • Hypokalemia • Steroid or diuretic therapy • Abrupt relief of chronic respiratory acidosis • Cushing's syndrome or aldosteronism • Excessive administration of sodium bicarbonate ($NaHCO_3$) (during code resuscitation) or bicarbonate-containing antacids	• Tingling in fingers and toes, dizziness, and hypertonicity • Compensatory hypoventilation with decreased respirations • Decreased chloride and potassium levels • Atrial tachycardia • Confusion, irritability • Diarrhea • Nausea, vomiting • Picking at bed clothes (carphology) • pH above 7.45 and HCO_3^- above 26 mEq/L	• Identify patients at risk for metabolic alkalosis. • Assess the patient for signs and symptoms of metabolic alkalosis, especially respiratory, electrolyte, and ABG changes. • Replace electrolytes, such as potassium and chloride, as prescribed, and monitor levels regularly. • Administer an acidifying agent, such as I.V. ammonium chloride. • Replace fluid volume, as prescribed. • Administer an antiemetic, as prescribed. • Prevent complications, such as hypoxemia caused by hypoventilation. • Teach the patient and family how to correctly administer an antacid.

Understanding acid-base imbalances *(continued)*

Description	Cause	Signs and symptoms	Nursing care
Respiratory acidosis Acid-base disturbance characterized by excessive carbonic acid (H_2CO_3), elevated $Paco_2$, and decreased serum pH that commonly is associated with decreased oxygenation resulting from hypoventilation	*Acute respiratory acidosis* • Pulmonary edema • Aspiration • Atelectasis • Pneumothorax • Sedative overdose • Pneumonia • Cardiac arrest • Laryngospasm • Improperly regulated mechanical ventilation *Chronic respiratory acidosis* • Bronchial asthma • Emphysema • Cystic fibrosis • Advanced multiple sclerosis • Bronchiectasis	*Acute respiratory acidosis* • Dulled sensorium, dizziness, feeling of fullness in head, and unconsciousness • Palpitations, tachycardia, and ventricular fibrillation • Muscle twitching and seizures • Warm, flushed skin, perspiration, and cyanosis • pH below 7.35, $Paco_2$ above 50 mm Hg, and normal or slightly elevated HCO_3^- *Chronic respiratory acidosis* • Weakness • Dull headache • pH below 7.35, $Paco_2$ above 42 mm Hg, and HCO_3^- above 26 mEq/L • Symptoms of underlying disease, such as barrel chest and productive cough caused by chronic obstructive pulmonary disease	• Identify patients at risk for respiratory acidosis. • Identify factors that increase the risk of hypoventilation, such as obesity, postoperative pain, tight dressings, and abdominal distention. • Assess the patient for signs and symptoms of respiratory acidosis, especially respiratory, pulse, and neurologic changes. • If the patient has a chronic condition, make sure he doesn't receive more than 2 L of oxygen without an order. • Relieve postoperative pain by administering the prescribed analgesic or teaching the patient relaxation techniques. • Maintain an open airway; use suction if the patient can't cough up secretions. • Encourage coughing, deep breathing, and ambulation in a postoperative patient. • Perform chest physiotherapy. • Maintain hydration to keep secretions loose. • Provide food appropriate for the patient's ability to chew and swallow. • If the patient has chronic respiratory acidosis, assist with routine pulmonary care. • If the patient requires ventilator assistance, intervene as needed.
Respiratory alkalosis Acid-base disturbance characterized by low H_2CO_3 and $Paco_2$ and caused by excessive "blowing off" of carbon dioxide during hyperventilation	• Extreme anxiety (most common cause) • Pulmonary emboli, pulmonary fibrosis, asthma, pneumonia, or injury to the respiratory center • Gram-negative bacteremia and sepsis • High fever • Hypoxemia • Early salicylate intoxication • High altitude	• Hyperventilation exceeding 40 breaths/minute • Cardiac arrhythmias that fail to respond to conventional treatment • Circumoral or peripheral paresthesia • Carpopedal spasms • Twitching (possibly progressing to tetany) • Seizures • Muscle weakness	• Identify patients at risk for respiratory alkalosis. • Assess the patient's anxiety level. • Assess the patient for signs of respiratory alkalosis, especially neurologic, electrolyte, and ABG changes. • If the patient is anxious, encourage him to breathe slowly. Have him breathe into a paper bag to increase $Paco_2$.

(continued)

	Understanding acid-base imbalances *(continued)*		
Description	**Cause**	**Signs and symptoms**	**Nursing care**
Respiratory alkalosis *(continued)*	● Hyperventilation caused by mechanical ventilation ● Pregnancy ● Hepatic failure ● Heart failure	● Light-headedness, inability to concentrate, dizziness, agitation ● pH above 7.45 and normal HCO_3^- level (during an acute episode); normal pH and HCO_3^- below 22 mEq/L (during compensation in an acute episode); and normal pH, HCO_3^- below 22 mEq/L, and $Paco_2$ below 32 mm Hg (during a chronic episode)	● Administer a sedative, as prescribed, and take safety measures. ● Intervene to decrease hyperthermia. ● Teach the patient and family how to perform relaxation techniques and prevent, recognize, and treat hyperventilation. ● Teach the patient and family about safety precautions for household medications, especially those containing aspirin.

■ Regulation of acid-base balance
  ◆ Most of the 12,000 to 20,000 mEq of carbon dioxide produced daily is excreted by the lungs
    ❱ Carbon dioxide is carried from peripheral tissues to the lungs by RBCs, plasma proteins, and plasma (as carbonic acid and bicarbonate)
    ❱ The acid-base balance is regulated by adjustments in ventilation
      ● In acidosis, an increased arterial carbon dioxide content or a decreased pH (below 7.35) stimulates hyperventilation; less carbon dioxide results in less carbonic acid and hydrogen ion in the blood, increasing the blood pH
      ● In alkalosis, a decreased arterial carbon dioxide content or an increased pH leads to hypoventilation; carbon dioxide retention increases the acid load, thus decreasing the blood pH
  ◆ The kidneys usually excrete 70 mEq of acid daily
    ❱ Renal tubular excretion occurs in several ways
      ● Hydrogen ions are directly excreted in exchange for sodium ions
      ● Hydrogen ions are indirectly excreted with urine buffers
      ● Hydrogen ions are indirectly excreted with the ammonia produced in the distal tubular cells
    ❱ Sodium and bicarbonate are absorbed, and hydrogen is secreted in the proximal tubule
    ❱ Carbonic acid is dissociated into hydrogen ions and bicarbonate in the distal tubule; hydrogen ions are excreted, and bicarbonate moves into the bloodstream
    ❱ Renal compensation for imbalances can take hours to days; in acidosis, the kidneys excrete hydrogen ions and conserve bicarbonate ions, but in alkalosis, the kidneys retain hydrogen ions and excrete bicarbonate ions

■ Buffering
   ◆ Buffering is a mechanism that corrects acid-base imbalances by removing or releasing hydrogen
   ◆ Buffers prevent significant pH changes when an acid or a base is added to a solution; they rapidly react with a strong acid or base by replacing it with a relatively weak acid or base
      ❯ Bicarbonate is a buffer for blood and interstitial fluid
         • The normal ratio of bicarbonate to carbonic acid is 20 to 1
         • Carbon dioxide mixed with water becomes carbonic acid
      ❯ Hemoglobin is a buffer for carbon dioxide
      ❯ Phosphates and plasma proteins are intracellular buffers
■ Evaluation of ABG studies
   ◆ *pH* is a measure of the acid-base balance in terms of the concentration of free hydrogen ions; the greater the concentration of hydrogen, the more acidic the solution, and the lower the pH
      ❯ A pH of 6.8 to 7.0 indicates severe, life-threatening acidosis
      ❯ A pH of 7.0 to 7.35 indicates acidosis
      ❯ A pH of 7.35 to 7.45 is normal
      ❯ A pH of 7.45 to 7.7 indicates alkalosis
      ❯ A pH of 7.7 to 7.8 indicates severe, life-threatening alkalosis
   ◆ Pa_{CO_2}, or the partial pressure of carbon dioxide in arterial blood, is the best measure of adequate alveolar ventilation
      ❯ A Pa_{CO_2} of 34 to 44 mm Hg is normal
      ❯ A Pa_{CO_2} above 44 mm Hg indicates hypercapnia resulting from hypoventilation; a Pa_{CO_2} below 34 mm Hg indicates hypocapnia resulting from hyperventilation
   ◆ Pa_{O_2}, or the partial pressure of oxygen in arterial blood, is a measure of the blood's oxygen content
      ❯ A Pa_{O_2} of 80 to 100 mm Hg is normal
      ❯ A Pa_{O_2} of 70 to 80 mm Hg is borderline hypoxemia; a Pa_{O_2} of 50 to 70 mm Hg indicates hypoxemia; a Pa_{O_2} below 50 mm Hg indicates severe hypoxemia
   ◆ HCO_3^- is the level of the buffer bicarbonate
      ❯ An HCO_3^- of 24 mEq/L is normal
      ❯ An HCO_3^- above 26 mEq/L indicates excess bicarbonate; an HCO_3^- below 22 mEq/L indicates inadequate bicarbonate
■ Compensation
   ◆ Compensation is the return of an abnormal pH to a normal pH
   ◆ The unaffected system (metabolic or respiratory) is responsible for returning the pH to normal
      ❯ In respiratory acidosis with a high Pa_{CO_2}, the kidneys compensate by retaining bicarbonate, which changes the HCO_3^-/Pa_{CO_2} ratio and returns the pH to normal
      ❯ In respiratory alkalosis with a low Pa_{CO_2}, the kidneys compensate by excreting bicarbonate, which changes the HCO_3^-/Pa_{CO_2} ratio and returns the pH to normal

Interpreting arterial blood gas levels

- Determine whether the pH value is normal or shows acidosis or alkalosis.
- Determine whether the partial pressure of arterial carbon dioxide ($Paco_2$) is normal or shows acidosis or alkalosis.
- Determine whether the bicarbonate (HCO_3^-) level is normal or shows acidosis or alkalosis.
- Determine whether the pH value matches the $Paco_2$ (respiratory) or the HCO_3^- (metabolic) value.
- If the pH value is abnormal and the $Paco_2$ value, the HCO_3^- value, or both are abnormal, the condition is uncompensated. If the pH value is normal and the $Paco_2$ value and the HCO_3^- value are abnormal, the condition is compensated.

▶ In metabolic acidosis with a low HCO_3^- or base excess, the lungs compensate through hyperventilation, which lowers $Paco_2$ and returns the pH to normal

▶ In metabolic alkalosis with high HCO_3^-, the lungs compensate through hypoventilation, which increases $Paco_2$ and returns the pH to normal

◆ Compensation can be assessed by examining the ABG values

▶ Look at the primary system affected ($Paco_2$ or HCO_3^-)

▶ Look at the system not affected ($Paco_2$ or HCO_3^-)

▶ If the ABGs in the unaffected system are moving in the same direction as those in the primary system, compensation is occurring (see *Interpreting arterial blood gas levels*)

❖ Pain
- General information
  ◆ Pain is a complex phenomenon that involves biological, psychological, cultural, and social factors; it's a primarily subjective experience
  ◆ McCaffery, a pain researcher, defines *pain* as "whatever the experiencing person says it is, existing whenever the experiencing person says it does"
  ◆ The International Association on Pain defines *pain* as unpleasant sensory and emotional experiences related to actual or potential tissue damage
- Pain theories
  ◆ All current pain control theories are hypothetical; none completely explain the pain experience and all its components
  ◆ The *specificity theory* holds that highly specific structures and pathways exist for pain transmission; this biologically oriented theory doesn't explain pain tolerance and ignores social, cultural, and empirical factors that influence pain
  ◆ The *pattern theory* holds that rapid and slow conduction pathways exist, which relay pain information through the spinal cord to the brain; although this theory addresses the brain's ability to determine the amount, intensity, and type of sensory input, it doesn't address nonbiological influences on pain perception and transmission

◆ The *gate control theory* describes a hypothetical gate mechanism in the spinal cord that allows nerve fibers to receive pain sensations; the gate can be closed to pain sensation by occupying the receptor sites with other stimuli

    ❚ This theory has encouraged a holistic approach to pain control and research by considering nonbiological components of pain

      ❚ Pain management techniques, such as cutaneous stimulation, distraction, and acupuncture, are partly based on this theory

■ Anatomic and physiologic basis of pain

◆ Stimulation of pain receptors in skin and soft tissues typically causes defined, localized pain

◆ Stimulation of pain receptors in deep tissues causes dull, poorly localized pain

◆ Stimulation of pain receptors in the viscera or organs causes diffuse, sometimes referred pain

◆ Pain can be stimulated by mechanical sources such as sharp objects; thermal sources such as fire; or chemical sources, such as stomach acids and battery acid

◆ Pain travels from the periphery to the spinal cord to the brain by way of a pathway composed of A (delta) fibers (intense pain) and C fibers (dull, aching pain)

◆ Pain is processed in the thalamus, midbrain, and cortex

◆ Certain neurotransmitters, such as histamine, serotonin, and prostaglandins, enhance pain impulse transmission

◆ Other neurotransmitters, such as endogenous opiates, endorphins, and enkephalins, inhibit pain impulse transmission; chronic pain syndrome may be related to a deficiency of these inhibitory neurotransmitters

■ Factors that affect pain response

◆ Pain is primarily a physical problem that has psychological effects

◆ The physical and psychological sources of pain are often complex and intertwined, with causative factors difficult to isolate

◆ Psychogenic pain is pain without a physiologic basis; this term isn't helpful because all physical causes of pain can't be diagnosed, and all pain is real to the patient

◆ Pain threshold is the point at which a patient experiences pain

◆ Pain tolerance is affected by individual, psychosocial, cultural, religious, and environmental factors; it influences pain duration and intensity

❖ Pain assessment

◆ Pain can be assessed with a subjective pain assessment tool

    ❚ *1 to 10 rating scale:* The patient is asked to rate pain on a scale of 1 to 10, with 1 being no pain and 10 being the worst pain imaginable

    ❚ *Face rating scale:* The patient is shown illustrations of five or more faces demonstrating varying levels of emotion, from happy to sad; by selecting the face that most closely approximates the pain sensation, the patient helps the nurse gauge the effectiveness of interventions

> ▶ *Visual analog scale:* The patient places a mark on the scale, ranging from no pain to pain as bad as it can be, to indicate current level of pain
>> ▶ *Body diagram:* The patient draws the location and radiation of pain on a paper illustration of the body
>>> ▶ *Questionnaire:* The patient answers questions about the pain's location, intensity, quality, onset, and relieving and aggravating factors
>>>> ▶ *Pain flow chart:* The nurse documents variations in pain, vital signs, and LOC in response to treatments; these forms are particularly useful for monitoring patient response to epidural opioid infusions and for titrating dosages

- ◆ Pain also can be assessed by observing for objective signs and symptoms such as facial grimacing; elevated blood pressure and increased pulse and respiratory rates; muscle tension; restlessness or an inability to concentrate; decreased interest in surroundings and increased focus on pain; perspiration and pallor; crying, moaning, or verbalizations of pain; and guarding the painful body part

■ Pain classification

- ◆ *Acute pain* is mild to severe pain that's rapid in onset and lasts less than 6 months; it can be intermittent or recurrent as in migraine and sinus headaches and gallbladder colic
- ◆ *Chronic pain* lasts beyond the expected healing time and may be difficult to relate to the original injury or tissue damage; it can be further classified as chronic benign pain (as in lower back pain), chronic cancer pain, or pain with ongoing peripheral pathology

■ Pharmacologic management of pain

- ◆ Nonopioid drugs, such as nonsteroidal anti-inflammatory drugs (NSAIDs) and acetaminophen, are used to treat acute pain caused by inflammation or tissue destruction and mild to moderate pain; they're useful adjuncts to opioid analgesics for controlling severe, acute pain
- ◆ Opioid analgesics such as narcotic agonist-antagonists relieve pain by occupying opioid receptor sites in the brain and spinal cord; they're used to treat moderate to severe acute pain (postoperative pain and fractures), recurrent acute pain (sickle cell crisis, angina, and renal colic), prolonged time-limited pain (cancer and burns), and pain that requires rapid, short-term relief (procedures such as bone marrow biopsy and thoracentesis)
- ◆ Sometimes small doses of antidepressants are used as adjuncts to pain control; they affect pain perception and reduce the accompanying anxiety
- ◆ The oral route of administration is the least expensive, easiest for patients to manage, and most widely accepted by patients; most NSAIDs and some opioids can be administered orally
- ◆ Parenteral routes (subcutaneous [SubQ], I.M., and I.V.) are widely used to administer opioids
- ◆ Intraspinal (epidural) routes are used for short-term acute pain, such as that caused by abdominal surgery; the opioid's systemic effect is reduced with the intraspinal route compared with other parenteral routes
- ◆ Topical patches, such as those containing fentanyl, are useful during the transition from epidural to oral opioids

◆ Rectal administration of opioids may be indicated when a patient can't tolerate oral medications temporarily because of nausea and vomiting

◆ Patient-controlled analgesia is the I.V., SubQ, or intraspinal administration of opioids by means of an electronic controller that's programmed to respond with small doses when the patient requests medication

◆ Scheduled dosing is preferred to "as needed"; around-the-clock dosing controls pain by avoiding the major peaks and valleys of the pain experience

■ Nonpharmacologic management of pain

◆ *Cutaneous stimulation* is a low-risk, inexpensive, noninvasive, readily available pain management technique that requires little skill to implement; examples include heat application, cold application, massage, pressure, vibration, and transcutaneous electrical nerve stimulation (the application of electric current through skin patches connected to a portable electrical source)

◆ *Therapeutic touch* unblocks congested areas of energy in the body; in this technique, the practitioner redirects energy by using touch to promote comfort, relaxation, healing, and a sense of well-being

◆ *Acupuncture* is the use of needles of various sizes to stimulate parts of the body to produce analgesia; this centuries-old technique originated in China and is gaining acceptance in Western medicine

◆ *Cognitive and behavioral pain management* uses imagery, distraction, relaxation techniques, and humor to help patients manage pain

◆ *Biofeedback* teaches patients to control involuntary body mechanisms, such as heart rate, muscle spasms, and circulation

■ Surgical management of pain

◆ Surgery seldom is used as a primary treatment for pain

◆ Nerve blocks involve the injection of phenol or alcohol to destroy nerve endings in a specific area

◆ Rhizotomy is the surgical destruction of sensory nerve roots where they enter the spinal cord; chordotomy is the transection of spinal cord nerves at the spinal cord's midline portion

◆ Spinal nerve blocks, rhizotomy, and chordotomy can impair bladder, bowel, and sexual functioning

■ Nursing care of the patient in pain

◆ Assess the pain's location, and ask the patient to rate the pain using a pain scale

◆ Ask the patient to describe the pain's quality and pattern, including any precipitating or relieving factors

◆ Monitor vital signs and note subjective responses to pain, such as facial grimacing and guarding of body part

◆ Administer pain medication around the clock

◆ Provide comfort measures, such as back massage, positioning, linen changes, and oral or skin care

◆ Teach the patient noninvasive techniques to control pain, such as relaxation, guided imagery, distraction, and cutaneous stimulation

◆ Teach the importance of taking prescribed analgesics before the pain becomes severe

◆ Instruct the patient on the need for adequate rest periods and sleep

■ Referral to a pain clinic or hospice
◆ Patients with chronic benign pain that can't be controlled by nonpharmacologic interventions may benefit from treatment at a pain clinic
◆ The clinic's interdisciplinary staff works with the patient to assess the pain and develops a pain-control regimen that helps the patient regain or maintain an acceptable level of functioning
◆ Hospice programs give care and support to dying patients and their families; pain control—one of the primary goals—provides the patient with adequate pain relief at home

Review questions

1. The nurse is teaching a group of patient-care attendants about infection-control measures. The nurse tells the group that the first line of intervention for preventing the spread of infection is:

○ **A.** wearing gloves.

○ **B.** administering antibiotics.

○ **C.** washing hands.

○ **D.** assigning private rooms for patients.

Correct answer: C Hand washing is the first line of intervention for preventing the spread of infection. Option B is incorrect because antibiotics should be initiated only when an organism is identified. Although wearing gloves (option A) and assigning private rooms (option D) can also decrease the spread of infection, they should be implemented according to standard precautions when indicated.

2. The nurse is caring for a patient who was given pain medication before leaving the recovery room. Upon returning to his room, the patient states that he's still experiencing pain and requests more pain medication. Of the following actions, which is the first for the nurse to take?

○ **A.** Tell the patient that he must wait 4 hours for more pain medication.

○ **B.** Give half of the ordered as-needed dose.

○ **C.** Document the patient's pain.

○ **D.** Notify the practitioner that the patient is still experiencing pain.

Correct answer: D The practitioner should be notified that the patient is still experiencing pain so that new medication orders can be established. Option A is incorrect because patients who have recently undergone surgery shouldn't have to wait 4 hours for pain relief. Option B is incorrect because a nurse can't alter a dose without first consulting the practitioner; doing so could result in a nurse being charged with practicing medicine without a license. Although the nurse should document the patient's pain, option C, it isn't the first action the nurse should take.

3. A patient is admitted to the hospital with a possible electrolyte imbalance. The patient is disoriented and weak, has an irregular pulse, and takes hydrochlorothiazide. The patient most likely suffers from:

○ **A.** hypernatremia.

○ **B.** hyponatremia.

○ **C.** hyperkalemia.

○ **D.** hypokalemia.

Correct answer: D Signs and symptoms of hypokalemia include GI, cardiac, renal, respiratory, and neurologic symptoms. Options A, B, and C are incorrect because the use of a potassium-wasting diuretic, such as hydrochlorothiazide, without potassium supplement therapy causes hypokalemia.

4. The nurse is assessing a patient who may be in the early stages of dehydration. Early signs and symptoms of dehydration include:

○ **A.** coma and seizures.

○ **B.** sunken eyeballs and poor skin turgor.

○ **C.** increased heart rate with hypotension.

○ **D.** thirst and confusion.

Correct answer: D Early signs and symptoms of dehydration include thirst, irritability, confusion, and dizziness. Options A, B, and C are incorrect because coma, seizures, sunken eyeballs, poor skin turgor, and increased heart rate with hypotension are all later signs and symptoms of dehydration.

5. The nurse is evaluating a postoperative patient for infection. Which sign or symptom would be most indicative of infection?

○ **A.** Presence of an indwelling urinary catheter

○ **B.** Rectal temperature of 100° F (37.8° C)

○ **C.** Redness, warmth, and tenderness at the incision site

○ **D.** WBC count of 8,000/μl

Correct answer: C Redness, warmth, and tenderness at the incision site would lead the nurse to suspect a postoperative infection. Option A is incorrect because the presence of an invasive device predisposes a patient to infection but alone doesn't indicate infection. Option B is incorrect because a rectal temperature of 100° F is a normal finding in a postoperative patient because of the inflammatory response. Option D is incorrect because a normal WBC count ranges from 4,000 to 10,000/µl.

CHAPTER 7

Cardiovascular disorders

❖ Introduction

- Proper functioning of the cardiovascular system ensures the adequate delivery of nutrients to and the removal of wastes from body cells
- Disruptions in the cardiovascular system can lead to alterations in organ function, disability, and death
- Nursing history
    - ◆ The nurse asks the patient about his *chief complaint*
        - ▶ The patient with a cardiovascular problem will likely cite a specific complaint, including chest pain; irregular heartbeat or palpitations; shortness of breath on exertion, lying down, or at night; cough; cyanosis or pallor; weakness; fatigue; unexplained weight change; swelling of the extremities; dizziness; high or low blood pressure
        - ▶ The patient with a cardiovascular problem may also report peripheral skin changes, such as decreased hair distribution, skin color changes, or a thin, shiny appearance to the skin; and pain in the extremities, such as leg pain or cramps
    - ◆ The nurse then questions the patient about his *present illness*
        - ▶ Ask the patient about his symptom, including when it started, associated signs and symptoms, location, radiation, intensity, duration, frequency, precipitating and alleviating factors, and if pain is the symptom, rate on a scale of 0 to 10 (with 0 being no pain and 10 worst pain experienced)
        - ▶ Ask about the use of prescription and over-the-counter drugs, herbal remedies, vitamin and nutritional supplements; and alternative or complementary therapies used
    - ◆ The nurse asks about *medical history*
        - ▶ Question the patient about other cardiac disorders, such as hypertension, diabetes mellitus, hyperlipidemia, stroke, scarlet fever, rheumatic fever, strep throat, anemia, and syncope
        - ▶ Ask the female patient about the use of oral contraceptives and hormones and whether she's premenopausal or postmenopausal
    - ◆ The nurse then assesses the *family history*
        - ▶ Ask about a family history of hypertension, coronary artery disease (CAD), vascular disease, congenital heart disease, or hyperlipidemia
        - ▶ Also ask the patient if he has a family history of diabetes mellitus
    - ◆ The nurse obtains a *social history*
        - ▶ Ask about work, exercise, diet, use of recreational drugs, alcohol use, and hobbies
        - ▶ Also ask about stress, support systems, and coping mechanisms

Auscultatory sequence

When auscultating for heart sounds, place the stethoscope over the four different valve sites and at Erb's point. Follow the same auscultation sequence during every cardiovascular assessment:

● First, place the stethoscope in the second intercostal space along the right sternal border, as shown. In the aortic area, blood moves from the left ventricle during systole, crossing the aortic valve and flowing through the aortic arch.

● Then move to the pulmonic area, located in the second intercostal space at the left sternal border. In the pulmonic area, blood ejected from the right ventricle during systole crosses the pulmonic valve and flows through the main pulmonary artery.

● Next, listen at Erb's point, located in the third intercostal space at the left sternal border. At Erb's point, you'll hear aortic and pulmonic sounds.

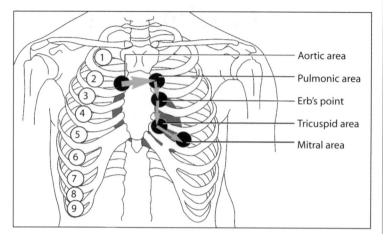

Aortic area
Pulmonic area
Erb's point
Tricuspid area
Mitral area

● At the fourth auscultation site, listen over the tricuspid area, which lies in the fifth intercostal space along the left sternal border. In the tricuspid area, sounds reflect blood movement from the right atrium across the tricuspid valve, filling the right ventricle during diastole.

● Finally, listen in the mitral area, located in the fifth intercostal space near the midclavicular line. (If the patient's heart is enlarged, the mitral area may be closer to the anterior axillary line.) In the mitral (apical) area, sounds represent blood flow across the mitral valve and left ventricular filling during diastole.

■ Physical assessment
  ◆ The nurse begins with *inspection*
    ▶ Observe the patient's general appearance: Is he thin, cachectic, or obese? Is he alert or anxious? Check his hair distribution
    ▶ Note the skin color: Is it pink, pale, or cyanotic?
    ▶ Note any clubbing, edema, and skin lesions
    ▶ Observe the chest and thorax: The lateral diameter should be twice the anteroposterior diameter; note any deviations from the typical chest shape
    ▶ Inspect the neck for visible pulsations and jugular vein distention
    ▶ Look for pulsations, symmetry of movement, retractions, or heaves; note the location of the apical impulse
  ◆ Next, the nurse uses *palpation*
    ▶ Palpate the precordium for heaves, thrills, and the point of maximum impulse; also palpate the sternoclavicular, aortic, pulmonic, tricuspid, and epigastric areas
    ▶ Palpate pulses in the extremities and neck for strength, rhythm, and equality
    ▶ Palpate the extremities for skin temperature, edema, capillary refill time, and turgor
  ◆ Then the nurse *percusses* the heart
    ▶ Percuss the left border of the heart, noting the sound change from resonance to dullness

> ❯ Try to percuss the right border of the heart; in most people, it's under the sternum and can't be percussed
- ◆ The nurse continues by *auscultating* the heart and vessels
  > ❯ Note heart rate and rhythm
  > ❯ Listen for first and second heart sounds (S_1 and S_2) as well as adventitious sounds, such as third and fourth heart sounds (S_3 and S_4), murmurs, clicks, snaps, and rubs (see *Auscultatory sequence*)
  > ❯ Auscultate for bruits over the abdominal aorta and the carotid and femoral arteries

❖ Acute coronary syndrome
- ■ Description
  - ◆ Acute coronary syndrome (ACS) includes three major thrombotic effects of CAD (see *Acute coronary syndrome,* pages 94 and 95)
    > ❯ Unstable angina
    > ❯ Non-ST-segment elevation myocardial infarction (non-STEMI)
    > ❯ STEMI
  - ◆ ACS requires prompt evaluation to differentiate noncardiac pain from cardiac pain, so proper treatment can be quickly initiated

❖ Aortic aneurysm
- ■ Description
  - ◆ An aortic aneurysm is a localized or diffuse dilation of the wall of the aorta, particularly the abdominal aorta below the renal arteries
  - ◆ Causes of aortic aneurysm include atherosclerosis, severe hypertension, pregnancy (when hormonal changes affect the smooth muscle and media of the aorta), trauma, congenital abnormalities, infectious arteritis, syphilis, and Marfan syndrome (which increases aortic wall elasticity)
- ■ Signs and symptoms
  - ◆ An abdominal aortic aneurysm may cause abdominal pulsations, abdominal aortic bruit, abdominal aching, dull lower back pain with radiation to flank and groin, nausea, and vomiting; if it ruptures, it may produce severe abdominal or lower back pain with nausea and vomiting
  - ◆ A thoracic aortic aneurysm (most common site of dissecting aneurysm) may cause cough, hoarseness, dysphagia (from pressure on the esophagus), abrupt loss of radial and femoral pulses and right and left carotid pulses, and dyspnea (from pressure on the trachea); if it ruptures, it may produce sudden, tearing pain in the chest and back
- ■ Diagnosis and treatment
  - ◆ Diagnostic tests may include chest or abdominal X-rays, aortography, duplex ultrasonic imaging, computed tomography (CT) scan, and magnetic resonance imaging (MRI)
  - ◆ Laboratory tests may include complete blood count (CBC) and blood urea nitrogen (BUN) and creatinine levels
  - ◆ If the aneurysm is chronic and small, an antihypertensive and a negative inotropic agent may be prescribed to decrease the force of muscle contractions
  - ◆ If the aneurysm is at risk to rupture or cause damage to other organs, surgical repair may be required

Acute coronary syndrome

Thrombotic effect	Description	Signs & Symptoms	Diagnosis	Treatment	Nursing Considerations
Unstable Angina	• Angina increasing in frequency and severity from patient's baseline • Easily induced • Lasts 5 to 15 minutes	• Burning, squeezing, substernal or retrosternal pain spreading across chest; may radiate to inside of arm, neck, jaw, or shoulder blade • Associated symptoms may include shortness of breath, dizziness, nausea, palpitations, weakness, and cold sweats • Associated signs may include hypertension or hypotension, tachycardia or bradycardia • Most often occurs with physical activity • Often relieved by rest or nitrates	• ECG may show ischemia • Cardiac biomarkers usually remain within normal limits	• Rest • Nitrates to reduce myocardial oxygen consumption • Beta-adrenergic blockers to reduce the workload and oxygen demand • Calcium channel blockers if caused by coronary artery spasm • Oxygen to increase oxygenation of the blood • Antiplatelet drugs to minimize platelet aggregation • Coronary angiography to determine stenosis or obstruction with possible angioplasty or stent placement	• During acute anginal episode, monitor blood pressure and heart rate. • Obtain an ECG before administering nitrates. • Record duration of pain, amount of medication required to relieve pain, and accompanying symptoms. • Obtain cardiac enzyme levels. • Administer oxygen. • Administer medications as ordered.
Non-ST-segment elevation myocardial infarction	• MI that usually occurs due to occlusion of coronary vessel • Occlusion may be complete or partial	• Burning, squeezing, substernal or retrosternal pain spreading across chest; may radiate to inside of arm, neck, jaw, or shoulder blade; pain more intense than that of angina • Associated symptoms: shortness of breath, dizziness, nausea, palpitations, weakness, and cold sweats	• Positive cardiac markers • ECG shows ST-segment depression or may be normal • ECG may have ST-segment elevation for less than 20 minutes	• Oxygen to increase oxygenation of the blood • Nonenteric coated aspirin for antiplatelet effect • Beta-adrenergic blockers to reduce the workload and oxygen demand • ACE inhibitor to reduce afterload and preload	• Administer oxygen. • Administer medications as ordered. • Monitor ECG, vital signs, and LOC. • Obtain cardiac markers. . • Monitor cardiopulmonary status frequently and notify practitioner of changes.

Acute coronary syndrome *(continued)*

Thrombotic effect	Description	Signs & Symptoms	Diagnosis	Treatment	Nursing Considerations
Non-ST-segment elevation myocardial infarction (continued)		• Associated signs: hypertension or hypotension, tachycardia or bradycardia • Pain not relieved with rest • Difficult to distinguish from angina • S_3 and S_4 may be present			
ST-segment elevation myocardial infarction	• MI that usually occurs due to complete occlusion of coronary vessel	• Burning, squeezing, substernal or retrosternal pain spreading across chest; may radiate to inside of arm, neck, jaw, or shoulder blade. Pain more intense than that of angina • Associated symptoms: shortness of breath, dizziness, nausea, palpitations, weakness, and cold sweats • Associated signs: hypertension or hypotension, tachycardia or bradycardia • Pain not relieved with rest • S_3 and S_4 may be present	• Positive cardiac markers • ECG shows ST-segment elevation or new left bundle branch block	• Oxygen to increase oxygenation of the blood • Nonenteric coated aspirin for antiplatelet effect • Fibrinolytic therapy for eligible patients • Coronary angioplasty with percutaneous coronary intervention • Beta-adrenergic blockers to reduce the workload and oxygen demand • ACE inhibitor to reduce afterload and preload	• Administer oxygen. • Administer medications as ordered. • Monitor ECG, vital signs, and LOC. • Obtain cardiac markers as ordered. • If patient received fibrinolytic, monitor for bleeding. • Monitor cardiopulmonary status frequently and notify practitioner of changes.

■ Nursing interventions
   ◆ Monitor vital signs
   ◆ Monitor hemodynamic variables
   ◆ Reduce anxiety by encouraging the patient to verbalize concerns and by providing emotional support
   ◆ Relieve pain by pharmacologic and nonpharmacologic methods

◆ Prepare the patient and family for surgery, if needed; discuss the procedure and their concerns about it

❖ Arrhythmias
- ■ Description
  - ◆ During a cardiac arrhythmia, abnormal electrical conduction or automaticity changes heart rate and rhythm
  - ◆ Arrhythmias vary in severity, from mild and asymptomatic ones that require no treatment (such as sinus arrhythmia, in which heart rate increases and decreases with respirations) to catastrophic ventricular fibrillation, which necessitates immediate resuscitation
  - ◆ Arrhythmias are generally classified according to their origin (atrial or ventricular); their effect on cardiac output and blood pressure, partially influenced by the site of origin, determines their clinical significance (see *The 8-step method of rhythm strip analysis*)
  - ◆ Causes of arrhythmias include congenital heart disease, degeneration of the conduction system, drug effects or toxicity, heart disease, myocardial ischemia, stress, alcohol, electrolyte imbalance, acid-base imbalances, cellular hypoxia, and conditions such as anemia, anorexia, thyroid dysfunction, adrenal insufficiency, and pulmonary disease (see *Cardiac arrhythmias*, pages 99 to 101)
- ■ Signs and symptoms
  - ◆ The patient with an arrhythmia may be asymptomatic or may report palpitations, chest pain, dizziness, weakness, fatigue, and feelings of impending doom
  - ◆ Other signs and symptoms include an irregular heart rhythm, bradycardia or tachycardia, hypotension, syncope, reduced level of consciousness, diaphoresis, pallor, nausea, vomiting, and cold, clammy skin
  - ◆ Life-threatening arrhythmias may result in pulselessness, absence of respirations, and no palpable blood pressure
- ■ Nursing interventions
  - ◆ Monitor the pulse for an irregular pattern or an abnormally rapid or slow rate; if the patient is receiving continuous cardiac monitoring, observe him for arrhythmias
  - ◆ Assess the patient for signs and symptoms of hemodynamic compromise
  - ◆ If the patient has an arrhythmia, promptly assess his airway, breathing, and circulation
  - ◆ Initiate ,, if indicated, until other advanced cardiac life support measures are available and successful
  - ◆ Perform defibrillation early for ventricular tachycardia and ventricular fibrillation
  - ◆ Administer medications as needed, and prepare for medical procedures (for example, cardioversion or pacemaker insertion) if indicated
  - ◆ Monitor patient for fluid and electrolyte imbalance and signs of drug toxicity, especially digoxin; correct the underlying cause—for example, if the patient has a toxic reaction to a drug, withhold the next dose
  - ◆ Provide adequate oxygen and reduce the heart's workload, while carefully maintaining metabolic, neurologic, respiratory, and hemodynamic status

The 8-step method of rhythm strip analysis

Rhythm strip analysis requires a sequential and systematic approach. The following eight steps provide a good outline for you to follow.

Step 1: Determine rhythm

To determine the heart's atrial and ventricular rhythms, use either the pen-and-pencil method or the caliper method.

To determine the atrial rhythm, measure the P-P intervals, the intervals between consecutive P waves. These intervals should occur regularly, with only small variations associated with respirations. Then compare the P-P intervals in several cycles. Consistently similar P-P intervals indicate regular atrial rhythm; dissimilar P-P intervals indicate irregular atrial rhythm.

To determine the ventricular rhythm, measure the intervals between two consecutive R waves in the QRS complexes. If an R wave isn't present, use either Q waves or S waves of consecutive QRS complexes. The R-R intervals should occur regularly. Then compare the R-R intervals in several cycles. As with atrial rhythms, consistently similar intervals mean a regular rhythm; dissimilar intervals point to an irregular rhythm.

After completing your measurements, ask yourself:
● Is the rhythm regular or irregular? Consider a rhythm with only slight variations (up to 0.04 second) to be regular.
● If the rhythm is irregular, is it slightly irregular or markedly irregular? Does the irregularity occur in a pattern (a regularly irregular pattern)?

Step 2: Calculate rate

You can use one of three methods to determine the atrial and ventricular heart rates from an electrocardiogram (ECG) waveform. Although these methods can provide accurate information, you shouldn't rely solely on them when assessing your patient. Keep in mind that the ECG waveform represents electrical, not mechanical, activity. Therefore, although an ECG can show that ventricular depolarization has occurred, it doesn't mean that ventricular contraction has occurred. To determine this, you must assess the patient's pulse.
● *Times-ten method.* The simplest, quickest, and most common way to calculate rate is the times-ten method, especially if the rhythm is irregular. ECG paper is marked in increments of 3 seconds, or 15 large boxes. To calculate the atrial rate, obtain a 6-second strip, count the number of P waves that appear on it, and multiply this number by 10. Ten 6-second strips equal 1 minute. Calculate the ventricular rate the same way, using the R waves.
● *1,500 method.* If the heart rhythm is regular, use the 1,500 method, so named because 1,500 small squares equal 1 minute. Count the number of small squares between identical points on two consecutive P waves,

and then divide 1,500 by that number to determine the atrial rate. To obtain the ventricular rate, use the same method with two consecutive R waves.
● *Sequence method.* The third method of estimating heart rate is the sequence method, which requires memorizing a sequence of numbers. For the atrial rate, find a P wave that peaks on a heavy black line, and assign the following numbers to the next six heavy black lines: 300, 150, 100, 75, 60, and 50. Then find the next P-wave peak, and estimate the atrial rate, based on the number assigned to the nearest heavy black line. Estimate the ventricular rate the same way, using the R wave.

Step 3: Evaluate P waves

When examining a rhythm strip for P waves, ask yourself:
● Are P waves present?
● Do the P waves have a normal configuration?
● Do all of the P waves have a similar size and shape?
● Is there one P wave for every QRS complex?

Step 4: Determine PR interval duration

To measure the PR interval, count the small squares between the start of the P wave and the start of the QRS complex; then multiply the number of squares by 0.04 second. After you perform this calculation, ask yourself:
● Does the duration of the PR interval fall within normal limits, 0.12 to 0.20 second (or 3 to 5 small squares)?
● Is the PR interval constant?

Step 5: Determine QRS complex duration

When determining QRS complex duration, make sure to measure straight across from the end of the PR interval to the end of the S wave, not just to the peak. Remember, the QRS complex has no horizontal components. To calculate duration, count the number of small squares between the beginning and the end of the QRS complex, and multiply this number by 0.04 second. Then ask yourself the following questions:
● Does the duration of the QRS complex fall within normal limits, 0.06 to 0.10 second?
● Are all QRS complexes the same size and shape? (If not, measure each one and describe them individually.)
● Does a QRS complex appear after every P wave?

Step 6: Evaluate T wave

Examine the T waves on the ECG strip. Then ask yourself:

(continued)

The 8-step method of rhythm strip analysis *(continued)*

- Are T waves present?
- Do all of the T waves have a normal shape?
- Could a P wave be hidden in a T wave?
- Do all of the T waves have a normal amplitude?
- Do the T waves have the same deflection as the QRS complexes?

Step 7: Determine QT interval duration

Count the number of small squares between the beginning of the QRS complex and the end of the T wave, where the T wave returns to the baseline. Multiply this number by 0.04 second. Ask yourself:
- Does the duration of the QT interval fall within normal limits, 0.36 to 0.44 second?

Step 8: Evaluate other components

Note the presence of ectopic or aberrantly conducted beats or other abnormalities. Also, check the ST segment for abnormalities, and look for the presence of a U wave.

Next, interpret your findings by classifying the rhythm strip according to one or all of the following features:
- *Site of origin of the rhythm.* For example, sinus node, atria, atrioventricular node, or ventricles.
- *Rate.* Normal (60 to 100 beats/minute), bradycardia (less than 60 beats/minute), or tachycardia (greater than 100 beats/minute).
- *Rhythm.* Normal or abnormal; for example, flutter, fibrillation, heart block, escape rhythm, or other arrhythmias.

◆ Provide support to the patient and family

◆ Tell the patient signs and symptoms of an arrhythmia to report, and teach him how to take his pulse

◆ Explain all procedures such as pacemaker insertion to the patient

❖ **Arteriosclerosis obliterans**
  ■ Description
    ◆ Arteriosclerosis obliterans is an obstructive, degenerative arterial disorder representing a late stage of atherosclerosis; it's the most common form of obstructive disease after age 30
    ◆ It may result from atherosclerosis and is associated with diabetes and cigarette smoking
    ◆ In arteriosclerosis obliterans, atheromas partially or completely occlude arteries; the femoral artery is most commonly affected, but the carotid arteries also may be involved
    ◆ This disorder produces symptoms when the arteries can no longer provide enough blood to supply oxygen and nutrients to the limbs and remove the waste products of metabolism
  ■ Signs and symptoms
    ◆ Characteristic symptoms of arteriosclerosis obliterans include intermittent claudication and pain in the affected limb that occurs with exercise and is relieved with rest
    ◆ Other signs and symptoms include cool feet and hands with poor hair growth, differences in the color and size of the lower legs, and altered arterial pulsations and bruits over the affected area, and ischemic ulcers
  ■ Diagnosis and treatment
    ◆ Diagnostic tests may include arteriography, Doppler ultrasonography, CT scan, and MRI
    ◆ Treatment aims to prevent circulatory compromise
      ▶ Patients are encouraged to stop smoking

Cardiac arrhythmias

Normal sinus rhythm

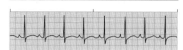

- Ventricular and atrial rates of 60 to 100 beats/minute (BPM)
- QRS complexes and P waves regular and uniform
- PR interval 0.12 to 0.2 second
- Duration of QRS complex < 0.12 second
- Identical atrial and ventricular rates, with constant PR interval

Sinus tachycardia

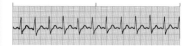

Description
- Rate > 100 BPM; rarely > 160 BPM
- Every QRS complex follows a P wave

Treatment
- Correction of underlying cause; a beta-adrenergic blocker or calcium channel blocker, if symptomatic or cardiac related

Sinus bradycardia

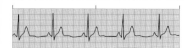

Description
- Rate < 60 BPM
- QRS complex follows each P wave

Treatment
- For low cardiac output, dizziness, weakness, altered level of consciousness, or low blood pressure, advanced cardiac life support (ACLS) protocol for administration of atropine I.V.
- Dopamine, epinephrine, if atropine fails
- Transcutaneous pacemaker (TCP)

Paroxysmal atrial tachycardia or paroxysmal supraventricular tachycardia

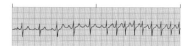

Description
- Heart rate > 140 BPM; rarely exceeds 250 BPM
- P waves regular but aberrant; difficult to differentiate from preceding T wave
- Sudden onset and termination of arrhythmia
- May cause palpitations and lightheadedness

Treatment
- Vagal maneuvers
- Adenosine by rapid I.V. push
- Other treatments: beta-adrenergic blockers, verapamil, diltiazem, and digoxin (if it isn't the cause of arrhythmia) to alter atrioventricular (AV) node conduction
- Elective cardioversion, if patient symptomatic and unresponsive to drugs
- Radiofrequency catheter ablation

Atrial flutter

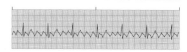

Description
- Ventricular rate depends on degree of AV block (may be 60 to 100 BPM, however, 150 BPM isn't uncommon)
- Atrial rate 250 to 400 BPM and regular
- QRS complexes uniform in shape, but typically irregular in rate
- P waves may have sawtooth configuration (F waves)

Treatment
- If patient is stable, ACLS protocol for cardioversion and drug therapy including calcium channel blockers, beta-adrenergic blockers, or antiarrhythmics
- If patient is unstable with a ventricular rate > 150 BPM, immediate cardioversion
- Radiofrequency ablation to control rhythm
- Possible anticoagulation therapy

Atrial fibrillation

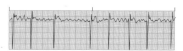

Description
- Atrial rate > 400 BPM, ventricular rate varies
- QRS complexes uniform in shape but at irregular intervals
- PR interval indiscernible
- No P waves, or P waves appear as erratic, irregular baseline F waves

Treatment
- If patient is unstable with a ventricular rate > 150 BPM, immediate cardioversion
- If patient is stable, ACLS protocol and drug therapy including calcium channel blockers, beta-adrenergic blockers, or antiarrhythmics
- In some patients uncontrolled by drugs, radiofrequency ablation
- Anticoagulation therapy to reduce risk of thromboemboli

AV junctional rhythm (nodal rhythm)

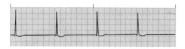

Description
- Ventricular rate usually 40 to 60 BPM (60 to 100 BPM is accelerated junctional rhythm)
- P waves may precede, hidden within, or follow a QRS complex; if visible, they're altered
- Duration of QRS complex normal, except in aberrant conduction
- Patient may be asymptomatic unless ventricular rate very slow

(continued)

Cardiac arrhythmias *(continued)*

Treatment
- Correction of underlying cause
- Atropine or pacemaker for slow rate
- If patient taking digoxin, it's discontinued

First-degree AV block

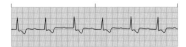

Description
- PR interval prolonged > 0.20 second
- QRS complex normal

Treatment
- Digoxin (cautiously)
- Correction of underlying cause; otherwise, monitoring for increasing block
- Possibly atropine, if severe symptomatic bradycardia develops

Second-degree AV block Mobitz Type I (Wenckebach)

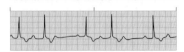

Description
- PR interval becomes progressively longer with each cycle until QRS complex disappears (dropped beat); after a dropped beat, PR interval shorter
- Ventricular rate irregular; atrial rhythm regular

Treatment
- Atropine, if patient symptomatic
- May discontinue digoxin
- Temporary pacing, if ventricular rate slow

Second-degree AV block Mobitz Type II

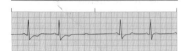

Description
- PR interval constant, with QRS complexes dropped
- Ventricular rhythm may be irregular, with varying degree of block
- Atrial rate regular

Treatment
- Temporary pacemaker, sometimes followed by permanent pacemaker
- If patient taking digoxin, it's discontinued
- Atropine, dopamine, or epinephrine for symptomatic bradycardia

Third-degree AV block (complete heart block)

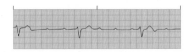

Description
- Atrial rate regular; ventricular rate slow and regular
- No relationship between P waves and QRS complexes
- No constant PR interval
- QRS interval normal (nodal pacemaker); wide and bizarre (ventricular pacemaker)

Treatment
- Usually requires TCP, followed by permanent pacemaker
- Dopamine and epinephrine to maintain blood pressure
- Atropine for symptomatic bradycardia
- Cardiopulmonary resuscitation (CPR), until pacing initiated

Premature ventricular contraction (PVC)

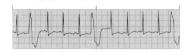

Description
- Beat occurs prematurely, usually followed by complete compensatory pause after a PVC; irregular pulse
- QRS complex wide and distorted

- Can occur singly, in pairs, or in threes; can alternate with normal beats; focus can be from one or more sites
- PVCs most ominous when clustered, multifocal, with R wave on T pattern

Treatment
- May not be treated if patient's condition is stable
- If warranted, lidocaine, amiodarone, or procainamide I.V.
- If induced by digoxin, cessation of drug; if induced by hypokalemia, potassium chloride I.V.; if induced by hypomagnesemia, magnesium sulfate I.V.
- An oral type III agent (such as amiodarone or sotalol), if maintenance therapy necessary

Ventricular tachycardia

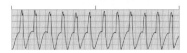

Description
- Ventricular rate 100 to 220 BPM; may be regular
- Three or more PVCs in a row
- QRS complexes wide, bizarre, and independent of P waves
- Usually no visible P waves
- Can produce chest pain, anxiety, palpitations, dyspnea, shock, coma, and death

Treatment
- If pulses are absent, CPR, following ACLS protocol for defibrillation and administration of epinephrine I.V. or vasopressin; followed by amniodarone, lidocaine, magnesium, or procainamide
- If pulse present with polymorphic QRS complexes and normal QT interval, beta-adrenergic blockers, lidocaine, amiodarone, procainamide, or sotalol (following ACLS protocol); if drug unsuccessful, cardioversion
- If pulse present with polymorphic QRS and prolonged QT inter-

Cardiac arrhythmias *(continued)*

val, magnesium I.V., then overdrive pacing if rhythm persists
- If pulse present and patient's condition stable with monomorphic QRS compleses, procainamide, sotalol, amiodarone, or lidocaine (follow ACLS protocol); if drugs ineffective, cardioversion
- Correction of underlying cause
- Maintenance therapy with drugs, such as amiodarone and sotalol
- Implanted cardioverter defibrillator if recurrent ventricular tacycardia

Ventricular fibrillation

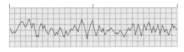

Description
- Ventricular rhythm rapid and chaotic
- No QRS complexes; no visible P waves
- Loss of consciousness, with no peripheral pulses, blood pressure, or respirations; possible seizures; sudden death

Treatment
- CPR, following ACLS protocol for defibrillation and administration of epinephrine, vasopressin, amiodarone, or lidocaine and, if ineffective, magnesium sulfate or procainamide
- Implanted cardioverter defibrillator if risk for recurrent ventricular fibrillation

Pulseless electrical activity (electromechanical dissociation)

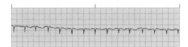

Description
- Organized electrical activity without pulse or other evidence of effective myocardial contraction

Treatment
- CPR
- Epinephrine
- Atropine for bradycardia
- Correction of underlying cause

Ventricular standstill (asystole)

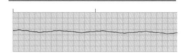

Description
- *Primary ventricular standstill:* regular P waves, no QRS complexes
- *Secondary ventricular standstill:* QRS complexes wide and slurred, occurring at irregular intervals; agonal heart rhythm
- Loss of consciousness, no peripheral pulses, blood pressure, or respirations

Treatment
- CPR
- ACLS protocol for endotracheal intubation, transcutaneous pacing, and epinephrine and atropine administration

- ▶ They're encouraged to exercise, eat a proper diet, and lose weight, if necessary
- ▶ They're advised on proper posture and the need to wear nonconstrictive clothing
- ▶ Pentoxifylline may be prescribed to improve blood flow through the capillaries
- ▶ Hypertension is controlled through drug therapy and lifestyle modifications
- ▶ An antilipemic may be necessary to lower elevated cholesterol levels
- ◆ Surgery is used to correct the obstruction if the disease progresses rapidly and the patient otherwise is in good health
  - ▶ Angioplasty and laser therapy may be performed to reestablish blood flow
- ◆ Bypass grafting may use an artificial or autologous graft
  - ▶ Patch grafting replaces a damaged segment of the artery with a vein patch
  - ▶ Endarterectomy strips plaques from the intimal lining
- ■ Nursing interventions
  - ◆ Check arterial pulses frequently

◆ Have the patient sleep with the head of the bed slightly elevated to aid perfusion to the lower extremities

◆ Don't massage the affected extremities because massage could further damage tissue

◆ Tell the patient to dress warmly and to avoid constrictive clothing

◆ Discuss gradual exercise programs, proper diet, and skin care

◆ Perform appropriate postoperative care

▶ Assess the affected extremity

▶ Maintain bed rest for 12 to 24 hours after surgery

▶ Avoid sharp flexion of the affected extremity

▶ Assess for signs and symptoms of infection

❖ Buerger's disease

■ Description

◆ Buerger's disease, also called thromboangiitis obliterans, is an inflammatory, nonatheromatous occlusive condition that causes segmental lesions and subsequent thrombus formation in the small and medium arteries (and sometimes the veins), resulting in decreased blood flow to the feet and legs

◆ It usually occurs in men between ages 20 and 30 and in heavy smokers

■ Signs and symptoms

◆ Buerger's disease typically causes intermittent claudication of the instep or legs, which is aggravated by exercise and relieved by rest

◆ Pulses are diminished or absent, and patient may experience coldness, numbness, tingling, or burning in the affected extremity

◆ As the disease progresses, redness, heat, tingling, or cyanosis may appear when the extremity is in a dependent position, and ulcers and gangrene may appear

■ Diagnosis and treatment

◆ Diagnostic tests may include Doppler ultrasonography, plethysmography, arteriography, venography, and digital subtraction angiography

◆ For patients with severe disease, lumbar sympathectomy may improve blood flow through vasodilation

◆ Amputation may be necessary for nonhealing ulcers, intractable pain, or gangrene

◆ Vasodilator therapy hasn't proved to be effective, but pentoxifylline, calcium channel blockers, and thromboxane inhibitors may be helpful, especially if vasospasm is present

■ Nursing interventions

◆ Encourage the patient to stop smoking and avoid cold to reduce vasoconstriction

◆ Avoid the use of vasoconstricting medications

◆ Teach the patient to take measures to protect the extremities from trauma and infection

◆ Encourage the patient to participate in progressive exercise

❖ Cardiomyopathy

■ Description

◆ Cardiomyopathy is a disease of the heart muscle, reducing cardiac output and eventually resulting in heart failure

◆ Three types of cardiomyopathy exist: dilated, or congestive (most common form; dilated cardiac chambers contract poorly, causing blood to pool and thrombi to form); hypertrophic obstructive (hypertrophied left ventricle is small, unable to relax and fill properly); and restrictive (rare form; stiff ventricles are resistant to filling)

◆ Causes of dilated cardiomyopathy include chronic alcoholism, viral or bacterial infection, metabolic and immunologic disorders, and pregnancy and postpartum disorders; causes of hypertrophic cardiomyopathy include congenital disorders and hypertension; causes of restrictive cardiomyopathy include amyloidosis, cancer, heart transplant, or idiopathic

■ Signs and symptoms

◆ Signs and symptoms of heart failure are present, including tachycardia, S_3 and S_4 heart sounds, exertional dyspnea, paroxysmal nocturnal dyspnea, cough, fatigue, jugular venous distention, dependent pitting edema, and hepatomegaly

◆ Heart murmurs and arrhythmias may also occur

■ Diagnosis and treatment

◆ Diagnostic tests include ECG, echocardiogram, cardiac catheterization, radionuclide studies, and chest X-ray

◆ Medications for dilated cardiomyopathy include an ACE inhibitor or hydralazine plus a nitrate (the mainstay of therapy), a beta-adrenergic blocker, digoxin, a diuretic, and an anticoagulant

◆ Medications for hypertrophic cardiomyopathy include a beta-adrenergic blocker and a calcium channel blocker

◆ No specific medications are used to treat restrictive cardiomyopathy; however, diuretics, digoxin, nitrates, and other vasodilators can worsen the condition and should be avoided

◆ An antiarrhythmic, a pacemaker, or an implantable cardiac defibrillator may be necessary to control arrhythmias

◆ Surgery, such as heart transplantation or cardiomyoplasty (for dilated cardiomyopathy) or ventricular myotomy or myectomy (for hypertrophic obstructive cardiomyopathy) may be indicated if medications fail

■ Nursing interventions

◆ Monitor ECG results, cardiovascular status, vital signs, and hemodynamic variables to detect heart failure and arrhythmias and assess response to medications

◆ If the patient is receiving a diuretic, monitor his serum electrolyte levels to detect abnormalities such as hypokalemia

◆ Administer oxygen and keep the patient in semi-Fowler's position to promote oxygenation

◆ Make sure the patient maintains bed rest to reduce oxygen demands on the heart

◆ Teach the patient the signs and symptoms of heart failure he should report to the practitioner

◆ Explain the importance of checking his weight daily and reporting an increase of 3 lb (1.4 kg) or more (1 liter of fluid equals 1 kg or 2.2 lb)

◆ Encourage the patient to express his feelings such as a fear of dying

❖ Coronary artery disease

- ■ Description
  - ◆ In CAD, plaques partially or totally occlude the coronary artery vasculature; it's the leading cause of death and disease in the United States
  - ◆ Some risk factors for CAD can't be modified: old age, male gender, and family history of heart disease
  - ◆ Other risk factors can be modified: increased levels of triglycerides, low-density lipoprotein, and very-low-density lipoprotein; high-fat diet; hypertension; obesity; diabetes; cigarette smoking; sedentary lifestyle; and high stress level
  - ◆ CAD begins when endothelial cells in the arterial lining are injured, making them permeable to lipoproteins
    - ❯ Clot-forming platelets adhere to the injury site, and lipoproteins build up around smooth-muscle cells, causing fatty streaks
    - ❯ Fibrofatty plaques form from repeated injury to the endothelial cells; as the process is repeated, the vessel progressively narrows
    - ❯ Plaques can rupture, causing emboli, or can worsen and compromise myocardial oxygenation and blood flow, thus precipitating angina or MI
- ■ Signs and symptoms
  - ◆ Anginal pain is a classic symptom of CAD (see *Angina*)
  - ◆ Others include the secondary effects of CAD, such as MI, heart failure, sudden cardiac death, cardiomegaly, valvular insufficiencies, cardiogenic shock, and stroke
- ■ Diagnosis and treatment
  - ◆ Diagnostic tests may include ECG, exercise ECG (stress test), cardiac catheterization, coronary angiography, intravascular ultrasound, myocardial perfusion imaging, and echocardiography
  - ◆ Laboratory tests for cardiac isoenzymes (CK-MB and LD_1), troponin, myoglobin, cholesterol, lipoproteins, and triglycerides also may be performed
  - ◆ Treatment aims to modify risk factors for CAD to prevent acute myocardial events (for example, smoking cessation, decreased intake of dietary fat, and increased activity level); treatment may also include medication for anginal pain as well as beta-adrenergic blockers, calcium channel blockers, antiplatelet, antilipemic, and antihypertensive drugs
  - ◆ Surgical treatment such as angioplasty, rotational atherectomy or stent placement, PTCA, or coronary artery bypass grafting (CABG) may be required to prevent progression to MI (see *Nursing care of the cardiac surgical patient requiring CABG*, page 106)
- ■ Nursing interventions
  - ◆ Increase the patient's knowledge of the relationship between risk factors and the development of CAD
  - ◆ Teach the patient and family how to modify risk factors
  - ◆ Encourage the patient to establish healthful habits, such as regular exercise and low-fat diet
  - ◆ Encourage participation in a smoking cessation program
  - ◆ Emphasize the importance of prevention in treating heart disease
  - ◆ Administer medication for anginal pain as ordered

Angina

Description

- Four types of angina: stable (angina that hasn't increased in severity or frequency over several months), unstable (angina that has increased in frequency, severity, or duration or has changed in quality and occurs with minimal exertion and rest), Prinzmetal's or variant (angina that occurs at rest, long after exercise, or during sleep), and microvascular (angina-like chest pain due to impairment of vasodilator reserve in patient with normal coronary arteries)
- Angina may result from atherosclerosis of coronary arteries, vasospasm, or from hypotension that decreases blood flow through these arteries

Signs and symptoms

- The major symptom is substernal or anterior chest pain that may radiate to the arms, neck, jaw, and shoulders; it may be described as mild-to-moderate pressure, tightness, squeezing, burning, smothering, indigestion, choking, or mild soreness; the patient may exhibit Levine's sign (clenched fist over sternum)
- Atypical chest pain, such as arm or shoulder pain; jaw, neck, or throat pain; toothache; back pain; or pain under the breastbone or in the stomach is likely to be seen in women
- Related signs and symptoms include shortness of breath, diaphoresis, nausea, increased heart rate, pallor, weak or numb feelings in the arms and hands, and unexplained anxiety

Diagnosis and treatment

- Diagnostic tests may include electrocardiogram (ECG) (a patient with stable or unstable angina may have ST-segment depression; a patient with Prinzmetal's angina, ST-segment elevation), exercise ECG (stress test), cardiac catheterization, radioisotope imaging, and echocardiogram
- Laboratory tests may include levels of cardiac isoenzymes (creatine kinase [CK], CK-MB, and lactate dehydrogenase [LD]), troponin, myoglobin, cholesterol, lipoproteins, triglycerides, high-sensitivity C-reactive protein, and homocysteine
- Treatment aims to decrease myocardial oxygen demand and increase myocardial oxygen supply
- Precipitating factors — such as exercise, overexertion, emotional upset, cold weather, and large meals — are identified and avoided if possible
- Exercise programs are prescribed to build collateral circulation and increase myocardial efficiency

- A nitrate (for example, nitroglycerin in oral, sublingual, spray, ointment, or patch forms; isosorbide dinitrate; or isosorbide mononitrate), a beta-adrenergic blocker, a calcium channel blocker, or an antiplatelet drug (for example, aspirin, clopidogrel (Plavix), or ticlopidine [Ticlid]) also may be prescribed to relieve symptoms
- A calcium channel blocker may be useful for a patient with Prinzmetal's or variant angina (see Nursing implications in clinical pharmacology, page 359)
- Angioplasty, stent placement, laser therapy, or atherectomy may be necessary to treat stable but debilitating anginal pain

Nursing interventions

- Tell the patient to call an ambulance and seek medical attention immediately if the angina persists or changes in quality or severity or if other symptoms develop
- Inform the patient and family that angina is more easily evoked in cold weather and in times of emotional upset or extreme stress; these conditions should be avoided if possible
- Discuss structured exercise regimens, and encourage family support
- Instruct the patient to plan rest periods between activities to prevent fatigue
- Tell the patient to take medications exactly as prescribed and not to change the medications without first consulting the practitioner
- Educate the patient about nitroglycerin
- Teach the patient how to take nitroglycerin before certain activities to prevent angina and how to take it for acute anginal episodes (for example, to sit down when taking the tablet; to take one tablet at 5-minute intervals but not to exceed three tablets; and to be aware that a burning sensation will be felt under the tongue)
- Tell the patient to dispose of nitroglycerin that has been open for more than 6 months and to keep the tablets in a container protected from heat, light, and moisture
- Tell the patient and family to carry antianginal medications and nitroglycerin when traveling, even on short trips
- Emphasize to the family the importance of learning cardiopulmonary resuscitation and basic life support
- Prepare the patient and family for surgery (if indicated), and offer psychological and emotional support
- Reinforce the importance of lifestyle modifications, such as diet, exercise, stress reduction, and smoking cessation

Nursing care of the cardiac surgical patient requiring CABG

The medical-surgical nurse is an integral part of the multidisciplinary team caring for the patient undergoing coronary artery bypass grafting (CABG). The nurse's astute assessments and prompt interventions can affect the patient's experience of and recovery from CABG.

Preoperative care

- Obtain an accurate and complete medical history. The degree of cardiac impairment is demonstrated by the patient's lifestyle limitations.
- Assess the patient's physiologic status before surgery. Baseline vital signs, integrity of pulses and extremities, neurologic status, respiratory status, height, weight, nutritional status, elimination patterns, and psychological status should be assessed and recorded.
- Teach the patient and family about the surgery and the immediate postoperative period in the intensive care unit. Prepare them for postoperative equipment that will be used, such as pulmonary artery lines, chest tubes, I.V. lines, indwelling urinary catheters, and equipment for mechanical ventilation and cardiac monitoring.
- Discuss specific issues with the patient and family. For example, the patient should always report pain. (Reassure a patient who will be intubated and unable to speak that pain will be detected by facial grimaces and other physiologic measures.) Bloody drainage in the chest tube is normal, as is feeling the need to void while the urinary catheter is in place. The tubes and lines may restrict patient movement, but the nurse should help the patient to prevent injury.

Intraoperative procedure

- The patient is placed on a cardiopulmonary bypass machine, which drains blood from the left ventricle and atrium and passes it through a pulsatile or roller pump to the femoral artery or descending aorta. Pulmonary circulation isn't interrupted.
- Myocardial tissue is preserved during surgery by arresting the heart with a cardioplegic solution, which usually is cold (39.4° F [4.1° C]). External cooling also may be achieved with a slush saline solution administered into the pericardium.
- After the patient is cooled sufficiently, bypass grafts, which are usually harvested from saphenous veins in the legs, are placed surgically from the aorta to sites distal to the occlusions on coronary arteries. The internal mammary artery may also be rerouted to bypass an occlusion.
- After the procedure is completed, the blood in the bypass machine is slowly warmed, and the patient's body temperature is returned to normal. While the incisions are closed, epicardial pacing wires are placed and grounded, and chest tubes are inserted.

Postoperative care

- Achieve and maintain body temperature. Monitor cardiovascular function with serial blood pressure, hemodynamic monitoring (cardiac output, central venous pressure, pulmonary artery wedge pressure, systemic vascular resistance), and electrocardiogram evaluations, and maintain it with various medications. Monitor drainage from chest tubes in the mediastinal area, and assess peripheral pulses.
- Turn the patient every 2 hours to promote drainage. A sudden change in drainage color to bright red, hemorrhaging that lasts more than 1 minute, or cessation of drainage are abnormal; report them to the practitioner immediately.
- Monitor respiratory status. Maintain an open airway at all times. Promote aggressive pulmonary hygiene.
- Inform the practitioner if the patient doesn't awaken 1 to 3 hours after surgery. Report any neurologic change from the baseline value.
- Maintain adequate renal circulation. Postoperative renal insufficiency is caused by complications of extracorporeal circulation during surgery and can lead to hemodialysis if permanent damage occurs.
- Document daily weight and fluid intake and output. Monitor serum electrolytes frequently.
- Make the patient as comfortable as possible; for example, by administering an opioid analgesic or positioning for comfort.
- Organize activities so that the patient can rest frequently. A structured program of early, progressive ambulation and activity can be helpful, but must allow for individual differences.
- Provide a program of cardiac risk modification. Encourage participation in a cardiac rehabilitation program.

❖ Endocarditis

■ Description

◆ Endocarditis is an infection of the lining of the endocardium, heart valves, or a cardiac prosthesis resulting from bacterial (particularly streptococci, staphylococci, or enterococci) or fungal invasion

◆ Conditions that increase the risk of endocarditis are having a prosthetic heart valve or having a damaged heart valve—for example, from rheumatic fever, a congenital heart or heart valve defect, mitral valve prolapse with a murmur, hypertrophic cardiomyopathy, Marfan syndrome, or I.V. drug abuse

■ Signs and symptoms

◆ Nonspecific signs and symptoms include chills, diaphoresis, fatigue, anorexia, weight loss, pleuritic pain, and arthralgia (intermittent fever and night sweats may recur for weeks)

◆ The classic physical sign of endocarditis is a loud, regurgitant heart murmur, or sudden change in an existing murmur, or the discovery of a new murmur along with fever

◆ Other signs include petechiae of the skin and mucous membranes and splinter hemorrhages under the nails

◆ Rarely, endocarditis produces Osler's nodes (tender, raised subcutaneous lesions on the fingers or toes), Roth's spots (hemorrhagic areas with white centers on the retina), and Janeway lesions (purplish macules on the palms or soles)

◆ Embolization from vegetating lesions or diseased valve tissues may produce specific signs and symptoms of infarction of splenic, renal, cerebral, pulmonary, or peripheral vascular infarction

■ Diagnosis and treatment

◆ Diagnostic tests may include echocardiogram and ECG

◆ Laboratory tests may include white blood cell count, erythrocyte sedimentation rate, and serum rheumatoid factor

◆ Three or more blood cultures in a 24- to 48-hour period identify the causative organism in up to 90% of organisms

◆ An antibiotic is prescribed, based on the infecting organism

◆ Surgery may be necessary to repair or replace a defective heart valve

■ Nursing interventions

◆ Make sure the patient maintains bed rest to reduce myocardial oxygen demands

◆ Encourage adequate fluid intake

◆ Watch for signs and symptoms of embolization (such as hematuria, flank pain, pleuritic chest pain, dyspnea, left upper quadrant pain, neurologic deficits, and numbness and tingling of the extremities)

◆ Assess patient for signs and symptoms of heart failure, such as dyspnea, tachycardia, tachypnea, crackles, neck vein distention, edema, and weight gain

◆ Suggest quiet diversionary activities to prevent excessive physical exertion

◆ Teach the patient about the need for prophylactic antibiotics when undergoing invasive procedures, such as dental work; genitourinary, GI, or gynecologic procedures; or childbirth

◆ Tell the patient about signs and symptoms of endocarditis that should immediately be reported to the practitioner

❖ Heart failure

■ Description

◆ Heart failure is a condition in which the heart can no longer pump enough blood to meet the body's demands

◆ Left-sided heart failure may be caused by anterior MI, ventricular septal defect, cardiomyopathy, cardiac tamponade, constrictive pericarditis, increased circulating blood volume, aortic stenosis and insufficiency, or mitral stenosis and insufficiency

◆ Right-sided heart failure may be caused by left-sided heart failure, a right ventricular MI, atrial septal defect, fluid overload and sodium retention, mitral stenosis, pulmonary embolism, pulmonary outflow stenosis, chronic obstructive pulmonary disease, pulmonary hypertension (cor pulmonale), or thyrotoxicosis

◆ With left-sided heart failure, the diseased left ventricle can't pump effectively because of decreased cardiac output, decreased contractility, increased volume, and increased left ventricular pressure

❭ The left atrium can't empty into the left ventricle, causing increased pressure in the left atrium; this pressure increase affects the lungs, causing pulmonary congestion that leads to decreased oxygenation

❭ Increased pressure in the lungs causes increased right-sided heart pressure; the right ventricle can't relieve the pressure by emptying into the lungs, which impairs venous return to the right side of the heart

❭ As systemic pressure builds, body organs become congested with venous blood

◆ Heart failure may also be classified as systolic or diastolic dysfunction

❭ With systolic dysfunction, poor ventricular contraction results in inadequate emptying of the ventricle

❭ With diastolic dysfunction, reduced ventricular compliance results in increased resistance to ventricular filling

◆ High-output failure may occur in high output states, such as anemia, pregnancy, thyrotoxicosis, beriberi, and arteriovenous fistula

❭ High-output failure results in high cardiac output and leads to ventricular dysfunction

❭ Despite increased cardiac output, the heart is unable to meet the body's increased metabolic needs

■ Signs and symptoms

◆ Both types of heart failure may cause chest discomfort, shortness of breath, paroxysmal nocturnal dyspnea, bloating, edema in the extremities, and decreased urine output

◆ Left-sided heart failure also may produce anxiety, orthopnea, dyspnea on exertion and at night, Cheyne-Stokes respirations, cough with frothy sputum, diaphoresis, crackles, rhonchi, cyanosis of extremities, respiratory acidosis, hypoxia, increased pulmonary artery pressures (determined with a pulmonary artery catheter), mental confusion, abnormal heart sounds (S_3 and S_4), fatigue, lethargy, mitral insufficiency murmur, oliguria, edema, anoxia, and nausea

◆ Right-sided heart failure also may produce hepatomegaly, splenomegaly, dependent edema, hepatojugular reflex, bounding peripheral pulses, oliguria, arrhythmias, increased right- and left-sided heart pressures (determined with a pulmonary artery catheter), Kussmaul's respirations, abnormal heart sounds (S_3 and S_4), fatigue, lethargy, abdominal pain, and recent weight gain

■ Diagnosis and treatment

◆ Diagnostic tests may include ECG, chest X-ray, echocardiography, pulmonary artery catheter insertion, and arterial blood gas studies

◆ Laboratory tests may include CBC, liver function tests, serum creatinine, BUN, electrolyte, glucose, albumin levels (patients with atrial fibrillation should have thyroid function tests performed), and B-type natriuretic peptide

◆ The goals of treatment are to decrease cardiac workload, increase cardiac output and contractility, decrease fluid and sodium retention, and decrease venous congestion

◆ Activity is restricted to decrease cardiac workload

◆ Oxygen may be administered to counteract desaturation

◆ Drug therapy includes an ACE inhibitor (the cornerstone of therapy) to decrease afterload; a diuretic to decrease preload and afterload; digoxin to increase contractility and cardiac efficiency and decrease heart rate; and a beta-adrenergic blocker to reduce heart rate and myocardial oxygen consumption

◗ Diuretics and vasodilators should be avoided in patients with diastolic dysfunction because they may not be able to tolerate reduced blood pressure or reduced volume

◗ Other drugs that may be useful in treating heart failure include vasodilators (such as hydralazine) combined with a nitrate (such as isosorbide), angiotensin II receptor blockers in patients who can't tolerate ACE inhibitors, or nesiritide (a human B-type natriuretic peptide) to augment diuresis and decrease afterload

◆ Patients with acute pulmonary edema may also be treated with nitroglycerin I.V., morphine sulfate, oxygen, and mechanical ventilation

◆ If the patient has high-output failure, correct the underlying cause

■ Nursing interventions

◆ Monitor the patient for common signs and symptoms of heart failure, such as chest discomfort, shortness of breath, and paroxysmal nocturnal dyspnea

◆ Monitor the patient for signs and symptoms of left-sided heart failure, such as anxiety, orthopnea, and abnormal breath sounds

◆ Monitor the patient for signs and symptoms of right-sided heart failure, such as jugular venous distension, hepatomegaly, splenomegaly, peripheral edema, and bounding peripheral pulses

◆ Encourage bed rest in semi-Fowler's position for ease of breathing

◆ Provide rest intervals between periods of activity

◆ Restrict fluids as prescribed

◆ Administer medications as prescribed, and monitor for their therapeutic and adverse effects (see Nursing implications in clinical pharmacology, page 359)

◆ Monitor fluid intake and output

◆ Administer oxygen as prescribed

◆ Monitor vital signs carefully, especially when administering vasoactive drugs

◆ Check the patient's weight daily

◆ Frequently assess for cardiac and respiratory signs of heart failure

◆ Note changes that suggest worsening of heart failure or fluid imbalance

◆ Explain procedures and provide reassurance to decrease patient and family anxiety

◆ Teach the patient and family about medications and the importance of careful management of fluids, sodium intake, and weight

❖ Hypertension

■ Description

◆ Hypertension is persistent high blood pressure, usually defined as a systolic pressure above 140 mm Hg or a diastolic pressure above 90 mm Hg based on two or more consecutive readings over a 2-week period (see *Classifying blood pressure readings*)

◆ Three types of hypertension exist: essential or idiopathic (elevated blood pressure of unknown cause); secondary (elevated blood pressure of known cause, such as renovascular disease, pregnancy, and coarctation of the aorta); and malignant (severe, fulminant form with a diastolic pressure above 140 mm Hg)

◆ Hypertension may result from poor compliance with an antihypertensive regimen, renovascular disease, toxemia of pregnancy, pheochromocytoma, pituitary tumor, coarctation of the aorta, adrenocortical hyperfunction, Cushing's syndrome, polycythemia, atherosclerosis, and some medications; a genetic predisposition, smoking, and obesity increase the risk of developing hypertension

■ Signs and symptoms

◆ The cardinal sign is consistently elevated blood pressure

◆ Related signs and symptoms may include headache (usually in the morning), dizziness, bruits, flushed face, epistaxis, blurred vision, retinopathy, retinal hemorrhages, restlessness, crackles, and dyspnea (if the lungs are involved)

■ Diagnosis and treatment

◆ Diagnostic tests depend on the suspected cause or effects of hypertension

▶ For example, kidney function tests, such as urinalysis and creatinine and BUN levels, may be performed because renal damage can cause hypertension

▶ ECG, chest X-ray, and echocardiography may be done to determine if hypertension has affected cardiac function

▶ Ophthalmic examination may affect retinal damage

◆ Diet, exercise, and lifestyle modifications (such as smoking cessation, reducing alcohol intake, stress management, and weight reduction) are recommended first

◆ If nonpharmacologic measures fail to maintain blood pressure within normal limits, antihypertensives, such as diuretics, ACE inhibitors, beta-adrenergic blockers, calcium channel blockers, angiotensin II receptor

Classifying blood pressure readings

In 2003, the National Institutes of Health issued the Seventh Report of the Joint National Committee on Prevention, Detection, Evaluation, and Treatment of High Blood Pressure. Categories now are normal, prehypertension, and stages 1 and 2 hypertension.

The revised categories are based on the average of two or more readings taken on separate visits after an initial screening. They apply to adults age 18 and older. (If the systolic and diastolic pressures fall into different categories, use the higher of the two readings to classify the readings.)

Patients with prehypertension are at increased risk of developing hypertension and should follow health-promoting lifestyle modifications to prevent cardiovascular disease.

Category	Systolic		Diastolic
Normal	< 120 mm Hg	*and*	< 80 mm Hg
Prehypertension	120 to 139 mm Hg	*or*	80 to 89 mm Hg
Hypertension Stage 1	140 to 159 mm Hg	*or*	90 to 99 mm Hg
Stage 2	160 mm Hg	*or*	100 mm Hg

blockers, alpha-adrenergic blockers, and combined alpha- and beta-adrenergic blockers, are prescribed
- Nursing interventions
  - ◆ Monitor the patient's blood pressure regularly, and assess for other signs and symptoms of hypertension, such as headache and retinal hemorrhages
  - ◆ Provide a calm, quiet environment
  - ◆ Teach the patient and family about weight control, stress reduction, and smoking cessation
  - ◆ Discuss the importance of a low-sodium diet; include the dietitian in teaching low-sodium recipes and recipe modification for the patient and the person who does the cooking
  - ◆ Teach the patient how to take his blood pressure
  - ◆ Administer antihypertensive medications as prescribed
  - ◆ Emphasize the importance of adhering to the medication regimen
  - ◆ Advise the patient to avoid alcohol during antihypertensive therapy

❖ Raynaud's disease
- Description
  - ◆ Raynaud's *disease* is characterized by episodic vasospasm in the small peripheral arteries and arterioles, precipitated by exposure to cold or stress
  - ◆ This disease is most prevalent in women, particularly between puberty and age 40
  - ◆ Raynaud's *phenomenon*, however, a condition commonly associated with connective tissue disorders—such as scleroderma, systemic lupus erythematosus, and polymyositis—has a progressive course, leading to ischemia, gangrene, and amputation
- Signs and symptoms

◆ After exposure to cold or stress, the skin of the fingers typically blanches, then becomes cyanotic before changing to red; numbness and tingling may also occur

◆ In long-standing disease, trophic changes, such as sclerodactyly, ulcerations, or chronic paronychia may result (ulceration and gangrene are rare)

■ Diagnosis and treatment

◆ Diagnostic tests may include Doppler studies, arteriography, plethysmography, and antinuclear antibody titer

◆ Vasodilators, such as phenoxybenzamine, calcium channel blockers, and adrenergic blockers

) Pentoxifylline may also be effective

) Sympathectomy may be performed if conservative measures fail to prevent ischemic ulcers

■ Nursing interventions

◆ Teach the patient to avoid exposure to the cold

◆ Advise the patient to avoid stressful situations and to stop smoking; teach the patient biofeedback and relaxation exercises

◆ Teach the patient to inspect the skin and to seek immediate treatment for signs of skin breakdown or infection

❖ Thrombophlebitis

■ Description

◆ Thrombophlebitis is marked by inflammation of the venous wall and thrombus formation of the deep or superficial veins

◆ Deep vein thrombophlebitis may lead to occlusion of the vessels or systemic embolization such as pulmonary embolism

◆ Three conditions may lead to thrombophlebitis: hypercoagulability (such as from cancer, blood dyscrasias, or oral contraceptives); injury to the venous wall (such as from I.V. injections, fractures, or antibiotics); and venous stasis (such as from varicose veins, pregnancy, heart failure, or prolonged bed rest)

■ Signs and symptoms

◆ Signs and symptoms of deep vein thrombophlebitis include cramping pain, edema, positive Homans' sign, tenderness to touch, fever, chills, and malaise

◆ Superficial thrombophlebitis produces visible and palpable signs, such as heat, pain, swelling, rubor, tenderness, and induration along the affected vein's length

■ Diagnosis and treatment

◆ Diagnostic tests may include photoplethysmography, Doppler ultrasonography, and venography; laboratory tests include a CBC

◆ Superficial thrombophlebitis requires no specific therapy other than treatment for symptoms

◆ An anticoagulant (initially I.V. heparin or low-molecular-weight heparin followed by oral warfarin) is administered to prolong clotting time

◆ Thrombolytic therapy (such as streptokinase) is indicated for acute, extensive deep vein thrombophlebitis

◆ Embolectomy, venous ligation, or insertion of a vena caval umbrella or filter may also be indicated

■ Nursing interventions

◆ If the patient is receiving a thrombolytic, heparin, or warfarin (Coumadin), monitor him for signs and symptoms of bleeding

◆ If the patient is receiving heparin, measure partial thromboplastin time (PTT) regularly; if patient is receiving warfarin, measure prothrombin time (PT) and international normalized ratio (INR) (therapeutic values for PTT and PT are 1½ to 2 times control values; for INR, between 2 and 3)

◆ Assess patient for signs and symptoms of pulmonary embolism, such as crackles, dyspnea, tachypnea, hemoptysis, tachycardia, and chest pain

◆ Make sure the patient maintains bed rest and elevates the affected extremity

◆ Apply moist, warm compresses to improve circulation to the affected area and relieve pain

◆ Tell the patient to avoid prolonged sitting and standing to help prevent recurrence

◆ Teach the patient how to properly apply and use antiembolism stockings

◆ To prevent thrombophlebitis in high-risk patients, perform range-of-motion exercises while the patient is on bed rest, use intermittent pneumatic calf massage during lengthy surgical or diagnostic procedures, apply antiembolism stockings or pneumatic compression devices postoperatively, and encourage early ambulation

❖ Valvular heart disease

■ Description

◆ Three types of mechanical disruption can occur in patients with valvular heart disease: narrowing (stenosis) of the valve opening, incomplete closure of the valve (insufficiency), or prolapse of the valve

◆ Valvular heart disease may result from conditions such as endocarditis (most common), congenital defects, or inflammation and can lead to heart failure

◆ The most common forms of valvular heart disease include mitral stenosis, mitral insufficiency, mitral valve prolapse, aortic stenosis, aortic insufficiency, and tricuspid insufficiency (see *Types of valvular heart disease,* pages 114 to 116)

■ Treatment

◆ Medications are administered to treat heart failure and arrhythmias

◆ An anticoagulant may be prescribed to prevent thrombus formation around diseased or replaced valves

◆ Surgery to repair or replace valves is indicated when medical management can no longer control symptoms

■ Nursing interventions

◆ Offer a low-sodium diet, and maintain fluid restrictions

◆ Place the patient in an upright position to relieve dyspnea

◆ Instruct the patient on the use of anticoagulants, including signs and symptoms of bleeding to report, the need for frequent monitoring, and precautions to take while taking the drug

◆ Explain that he'll need to take a prophylactic antibiotic if he undergoes dental work, surgery, or another invasive procedure

Types of valvular heart disease

Causes and incidence	Clinical features	Diagnostic measures
Aortic insufficiency • Results from rheumatic fever, syphilis, hypertension, endocarditis, or may be idiopathic • Associated with Marfan syndrome • Most common in males • Associated with ventricular septal defect, even after surgical closure	• Dyspnea, cough, fatigue, palpitations, angina, syncope • Pulmonary vein congestion, heart failure, pulmonary edema (left-sided heart failure), "pulsating" nail beds (Quincke's sign) • Rapidly rising and collapsing pulses (pulsus biferiens), cardiac arrhythmias, wide pulse pressure in severe insufficiency • Auscultation reveals a third heart sound (S$_3$) and a diastolic blowing murmur at left sternal border • Palpation and visualization of apical impulse in chronic disease	• Cardiac catheterization: reduction in arterial diastolic pressures, aortic insufficiency, other valvular abnormalities, and increased left ventricular end-diastolic pressure • X-ray: left ventricular enlargement, pulmonary vein congestion • Echocardiography: left ventricular enlargement, alterations in mitral valve movement (indirect indication of aortic valve disease), and mitral thickening • Electrocardiography (ECG): sinus tachycardia, left ventricular hypertrophy, and left atrial hypertrophy in severe disease
Aortic stenosis • Results from congenital aortic bicuspid valve (associated with coarctation of the aorta), congenital stenosis of valve cusps, rheumatic fever, or atherosclerosis in the elderly • Most common in males	• Exertional dyspnea, paroxysmal nocturnal dyspnea, fatigue, syncope, angina, palpitations • Pulmonary vein congestion, heart failure, pulmonary edema • Diminished carotid pulses, decreased cardiac output, cardiac arrhythmias; may have pulsus alternans • Auscultation reveals systolic murmur at base or in carotids and, possibly, a fourth heart sound (S$_4$)	• Cardiac catheterization: pressure gradient across valve (indicating obstruction), increased left ventricular end-diastolic pressures • X-ray: valvular calcification, left ventricular enlargement, and pulmonary venous congestion • Echocardiography: thickened aortic valve and left ventricular wall • ECG: left ventricular hypertrophy
Mitral insufficiency • Results from rheumatic fever, hypertrophic cardiomyopathy, mitral valve prolapse, myocardial infarction, severe left-sided heart failure, or ruptured chordae tendineae • Associated with other congenital anomalies such as transposition of the great arteries • Rare in children without other congenital anomalies	• Orthopnea, dyspnea, fatigue, angina, palpitations • Peripheral edema, jugular vein distention, hepatomegaly (right-sided heart failure) • Tachycardia, crackles, pulmonary edema • Auscultation reveals a holosystolic murmur at apex, possible split second heart sound (S$_2$), and an S$_3$	• Cardiac catheterization: mitral insufficiency with increased left ventricular end-diastolic volume and pressure, increased atrial pressure and pulmonary artery wedge pressure (PAWP); and decreased cardiac output • X-ray: left atrial and ventricular enlargement, pulmonary venous congestion • Echocardiography: abnormal valve leaflet motion, left atrial enlargement • ECG: may show left atrial and ventricular hypertrophy, sinus tachycardia, and atrial fibrillation.

Types of valvular heart disease *(continued)*

Causes and incidence	Clinical features	Diagnostic measures
Mitral stenosis ● Results from rheumatic fever (most common cause), atrial myxoma, or endocarditis ● Most common in females ● May be associated with other congenital anomalies	● Exertional dyspnea, paroxysmal nocturnal dyspnea, orthopnea, weakness, fatigue, palpitations ● Peripheral edema, jugular vein distention, ascites, hepatomegaly (right-sided heart failure in severe pulmonary hypertension) ● Crackles, cardiac arrhythmias (atrial fibrillation), signs of systemic emboli ● Auscultation reveals a loud first heart sound (S_1) or opening snap and a diastolic murmur at the apex	● Cardiac catheterization: diastolic pressure gradient across valve; elevated left atrial pressure and PAWP with severe pulmonary hypertension and pulmonary artery pressures; elevated right-sided heart pressure; decreased cardiac output; and abnormal contraction of the left ventricle ● X-ray: left atrial and ventricular enlargement, enlarged pulmonary arteries, and mitral valve calcification ● Echocardiography: thickened mitral valve leaflets, left atrial enlargement ● ECG: left atrial hypertrophy, atrial fibrillation, right ventricular hypertrophy, and right axis deviation
Mitral valve prolapse syndrome ● Cause unknown; researchers speculate that metabolic or neuroendocrine factors cause constellation of signs and symptoms ● Most commonly affects young women but may occur in both sexes and in all age-groups	● May produce no signs ● Chest pain, palpitations, headache, fatigue, exercise intolerance, dyspnea, syncope, light-headedness, mood swings, anxiety, panic attacks ● Auscultation typically reveals a mobile, midsystolic click, with or without a mid-to-late systolic murmur	● Two-dimensional echocardiography: prolapse of mitral valve leaflets into left atrium ● Color-flow Doppler studies: mitral insufficiency ● Resting ECG: ST-segment changes, biphasic or inverted T waves in leads II, III, or A_V ● Exercise ECG: evaluates chest pain and arrhythmias
Pulmonic insufficiency ● May be congenital or may result from pulmonary hypertension ● May rarely result from prolonged use of pressure monitoring catheter in the pulmonary artery	● Dyspnea, weakness, fatigue, chest pain ● Peripheral edema, jugular vein distention, hepatomegaly (right-sided heart failure) ● Auscultation reveals diastolic murmur in pulmonic area	● Cardiac catheterization: pulmonic insufficiency, increased right ventricular pressure, and associated cardiac defects ● X-ray: right ventricular and pulmonary arterial enlargement ● ECG: right ventricular or right atrial enlargement
Pulmonic stenosis ● Results from congenital stenosis of valve cusp or rheumatic heart disease (infrequent) ● Associated with other congenital heart defects such as tetralogy of Fallot	● Asymptomatic or symptomatic with exertional dyspnea, fatigue, chest pain, syncope ● May lead to peripheral edema, jugular vein distention, hepatomegaly (right-sided heart failure) ● Auscultation reveals a systolic murmur at the left sternal border, a split S_2 with a delayed or absent pulmonic component	● Cardiac catheterization: increased right ventricular pressure, decreased pulmonary artery pressure, and abnormal valve orifice ● ECG: may show right ventricular hypertrophy, right axis deviation, right atrial hypertrophy, and atrial fibrillation

(continued)

Causes and incidence	Clinical features	Diagnostic measures
Tricuspid insufficiency • Results from right-sided heart failure, rheumatic fever and, rarely, trauma and endocarditis • Associated with congenital disorders	• Dyspnea and fatigue • May lead to peripheral edema, jugular vein distention, hepatomegaly, and ascites (right-sided heart failure) • Auscultation reveals possible S_3 and systolic murmur at lower left sternal border that increases with inspiration	• Right-sided heart catheterization: high atrial pressure, tricuspid insufficiency, decreased or normal cardiac output • X-ray: right atrial dilation, right ventricular enlargement • Echocardiography: shows systolic prolapse of tricuspid valve, right atrial enlargement • ECG: right atrial or right ventricular hypertrophy, atrial fibrillation
Tricuspid stenosis • Results from rheumatic fever • May be congenital • Associated with mitral or aortic valve disease • Most common in females	• May be symptomatic with dyspnea, fatigue, syncope • Possibly peripheral edema, jugular vein distention, hepatomegaly, and ascites (right-sided heart failure) • Auscultation reveals diastolic murmur at lower left sternal border that increases with inspiration	• Cardiac catheterization: increased pressure gradient across valve, increased right atrial pressure, decreased cardiac output • X-ray: right atrial enlargement • Echocardiography: leaflet abnormality, right atrial enlargement • ECG: right atrial hypertrophy, right or left ventricular hypertrophy, and atrial fibrillation

Types of valvular heart disease *(continued)*

Review questions

1. While auscultating the heart sounds of a patient with mitral insufficiency, the nurse hears an extra heart sound immediately after the second heart sound (S_2). The nurse should document this extra heart sound as:

○ **A.** a first heart sound (S_1).

○ **B.** a third heart sound (S_3).

○ **C.** a fourth heart sound (S_4).

○ **D.** a mitral murmur.

Correct answer: B An S_3 is heard following an S_2, indicating that the patient is experiencing heart failure and results from increased filling pressures. Option A (S_1) is a normal heart sound made by the closing of the mitral and tricuspid valves. Option C (S_4) is heard before S_1 and is caused by resistance to ventricular filling. Option D (murmur of mitral insufficiency) occurs during systole and is heard when there's turbulent blood flow across the valve.

2. A 55-year-old black male is found to have a blood pressure of 150/90 mm Hg during a work site health screening. What should the nurse do?

○ **A.** Consider this to be a normal finding for his age and race.

○ **B.** Recommend he have his blood pressure rechecked in 1 year.

○ **C.** Recommend he have his blood pressure rechecked within 2 weeks.

○ **D.** Recommend he see his practitioner immediately for further evaluation.

Correct answer: C A blood pressure of 150/90 mm Hg should be rechecked within 2 weeks according to current recommendations. If confirmed, assessment and treatment should be initiated by the practitioner. Option A is incorrect because although hypertension is more prevalent among blacks, a blood pressure of 150/90 mm Hg isn't considered normal. Option B is incorrect because a person with a blood pressure of 150/90 mm Hg shouldn't wait as long as 1 year to have it rechecked. Option D is incorrect because he need not see his practitioner immediately, but he should have his blood pressure monitored.

3. The nurse is administering warfarin (Coumadin) to a patient with deep vein thrombophlebitis. Which laboratory value indicates warfarin is at therapeutic levels?

○ **A.** PTT 1½ to 2 times the control

○ **B.** PT 1½ to 2 times the control

○ **C.** INR of 3 to 4

○ **D.** Hematocrit of 32%

Correct answer: B Warfarin is at therapeutic levels when the patient's PT is 1½ to 2 times the control. Higher values indicate increased risk of bleeding and hemorrhage, and lower values indicate increased risk of blood clot formation. Option A is incorrect because heparin, not warfarin, prolongs PTT. Option C is incorrect because although the INR may also be used to determine if warfarin is at a therapeutic level, an INR of 2 to 3 is considered therapeutic. Option D is incorrect because HCT doesn't provide information on the effectiveness of warfarin; however, a falling HCT in a patient taking warfarin may be a sign of hemorrhage.

4. A patient is receiving captopril for heart failure. The nurse should notify the practitioner that the medication therapy is ineffective if an assessment reveals:

○ **A.** a skin rash.

○ **B.** peripheral edema.

○ **C.** a dry cough.

○ **D.** postural hypotension.

Correct answer: B Peripheral edema is a sign of fluid volume overload and worsening heart failure. The other options (a skin rash, dry cough, and postural hypotension) are adverse reactions to captopril, but they don't indicate that therapy isn't effective.

Hematologic disorders

❖ Introduction

- Blood circulates in the cardiovascular system, carrying oxygen to the cells and removing wastes from them
- The continuous movement of blood also provides a defense against pathogens and injury, which are more likely to occur with stasis
- The cellular components of red blood cells (RBCs), white blood cells (WBCs), and platelets are subject to pathologic alterations that can cause severe disruptions in homeostasis
- Nursing history
  - ◆ The nurse asks the patient about his *chief complaint*
  - ◆ A patient with a hematologic disorder may report any of the following signs or symptoms, including aching bones, anorexia, bleeding gums, bruising, dyspnea, fatigue, infection, lethargy, malaise, nausea, numbness, paresthesia, swollen and tender lymph nodes, tarry stools, tingling, vomiting, nosebleeds, and in women, heavy menses
  - ◆ The nurse then questions the patient about his *present illness*
    - ❫ Ask the patient about his symptoms, including when they started, associated symptoms, location, radiation, intensity, duration, and frequency
    - ❫ Question the patient about what factors make the symptoms feel better or worse
  - ◆ The nurse asks about *medical history*
    - ❫ Ask about the present and past use of prescription and over-the-counter drugs, herbal remedies, and vitamin and nutritional supplements because many of these products can interfere with hematologic function
    - ❫ Ask the patient about previous problems, such as anemia, leukemia, enlarged lymph nodes, malabsorption, spleen or liver disorders
    - ❫ Ask about previous treatments, such as blood transfusions and radiation treatments
    - ❫ Question him about his diet, and look for deficiencies—for example, in folic acid, iron, or vitamin B_{12}
  - ◆ The nurse then assesses the *family history*
    - ❫ Ask about a family history of blood and lymph disorders, acquired and genetic
    - ❫ Ask about a family history of cancers involving the blood or lymph systems
  - ◆ The nurse obtains a *social history*

> ◗ Ask about ethnic background and race
> ◗ Question the patient about use of cigarettes, alcohol, and recreational drugs
> ◗ Ask him about occupational or household exposure to radiation or chemicals

■ Physical assessment
  ◆ The nurse begins with *inspection*
    ◗ Observe the patient's general appearance; does he appear alert, confused, tired, or irritable?
    ◗ Note the patient's skin color; look for bruising, diaphoresis, dyspnea, lesions, petechiae, and swelling of lymph nodes
    ◗ Note the size and color of his tongue
    ◗ Ask the patient whether his abdominal girth is enlarged
  ◆ The nurse uses *auscultation*
    ◗ Listen to heart sounds, noting abnormal sounds, rhythms, or tachycardia
    ◗ Auscultate the abdomen, noting bowel sounds, bruits, friction rubs, or venous hums
  ◆ Next, the nurse uses *palpation*
    ◗ Palpate the lymph nodes, noting consistency, mobility, shape, size, and tenderness; compare nodes on one side of the body with those on the other side
    ◗ Palpate the abdomen, noting ascites, enlarged organs, or tenderness
  ◆ The nurse then uses *percussion*
    ◗ Percuss the liver and spleen to estimate size
    ◗ Note the size and location of other abdominal organs

❖ Anemias

■ Anemia exists when the number of RBCs in a designated volume of blood is less than normal
■ Anemias include those from blood loss or hemolysis and aplastic, iron deficiency, and megaloblastic anemias (see *Types of anemia,* pages 120 to 122)

❖ Hodgkin's disease

■ Description
  ◆ Hodgkin's disease is a malignant B lymphocyte cell line disease of the lymph system that primarily affects those between ages 15 and 30 and those older than age 55
  ◆ Although the cause is unknown, this cancer is associated with viral infections and sustained immunosuppression; a genetic and environmental association may also exist
  ◆ It's among the most treatable of adult cancers and has a better prognosis than malignant, or non-Hodgkin's disease
■ Signs and symptoms
  ◆ This cancer is characterized by greatly enlarged, painless, movable lymph nodes in the cervical or supraclavicular area
  ◆ The patient may also experience fever, malaise, night sweats, pruritus, and weight loss (referred to as "B" symptoms)

(Text continues on page 122.)

Types of anemia

This chart summarizes the etiology, signs and symptoms, medical management, and nursing interventions for each type of anemia, which is defined as a decreased number of red blood cells (RBCs).

Description and etiology	Signs and symptoms	Medical management	Nursing interventions
Anemia from blood loss Anemia resulting from the loss of more than 500 ml of blood ● Acute blood loss, as in trauma or surgery ● Chronic blood loss, as in menstrual or GI bleeding	● RBC indices below normal on serum blood tests ● *With acute blood loss:* sudden onset of symptoms, such as hypovolemia, hypotension, hypoxemia, irritability, stupor, weakness, tachycardia; and cool, moist skin ● *With chronic blood loss:* gradual and vague symptoms, such as exertional dyspnea, increased fatigue, and pallor	● The source of the bleeding is identified and controlled through medical or surgical means. ● Transfusion and iron supplementation may be needed. Whole blood is transfused if the total blood volume has dropped; packed RBCs are transfused if it hasn't dropped. ● Shock must be treated if it occurs.	● Help determine the cause of bleeding by testing stool, urine, vomitus, or sputum for blood. ● Help control blood loss by applying pressure to obvious bleeding sites, assessing the patient for internal bleeding, and performing dressing changes as needed to assess blood loss.
Aplastic anemia Anemia characterized by a decreased hemoglobin level and pancytopenia ● Unknown etiology or an autoimmune disturbance (50% of cases) ● Drug therapy with a chemotherapeutic drug, chloramphenicol, mephenytoin, phenylbutazone, or a sulfonamide ● Exposure to environmental or occupational hazards, such as benzene, insecticides, or radiation ● Infection, such as cytomegalovirus, Epstein-Barr virus, hepatitis, or miliary tuberculosis ● Congenital causes	● Exertional dyspnea, fatigue, infections, pallor, and palpitations ● Hemorrhage — for example, bleeding (nasal, oral, rectal, or vaginal), ecchymosis, petechiae, or purpura ● Low platelet, RBC, and white blood cell counts ● Dry bone marrow (on aspiration)	● Initial treatment involves removing the causative agent, if possible, and administering transfusions. ● Medications such as antithymocyte globulin (ATG), cyclosporine, granulocyte-colony stimulating factors, and granulocyte monocyte CSF may be administered. ● Treat the idiopathic form of the disease with steroids. ● If the anemia can't be reversed or if it results from an autoimmune disturbance, bone marrow transplantation is recommended; this treatment is more effective if the patient doesn't receive blood products first and is younger than age 30.	● Help identify the causative agent. ● Assist a weak patient with daily activities. ● If the patient has pancytopenia, take safety precautions and steps to control infection because his ability to fight infection and sustain clotting are decreased. ● Help the patient and family cope with the severity of the illness and its prognosis. (Death may result from infection or hemorrhage.) ● If the patient is receiving ATG, perform skin testing, and monitor him for allergic reaction.

Types of anemia *(continued)*

Description and etiology	Signs and symptoms	Medical management	Nursing interventions
Congenital hemolytic anemia: Sickle cell anemia Anemia characterized by RBC destruction beyond the bone marrow's ability to produce these cells and misshapen hemoglobin and RBCs • Inherited (primarily affects blacks)	• Painful vaso-occlusive events in the extremities or affected organs (sickle cell crisis) • Other symptoms similar to other chronic anemias	• No cure or prevention is available. • Supportive interventions are used to prevent infection, relieve pain, and provide fluid and oxygen during a sickle cell crisis, which can cause massive organ damage.	• If the patient has sickle cell anemia, provide genetic counseling and possible gene replacement therapy. • Teach the patient to avoid factors that may precipitate sickle cell crisis, such as cold exposure, dehydration, excessive exercise, high altitudes, and smoking.
Congenital hemolytic anemia: Thalassemia Anemia characterized by RBC destruction beyond the bone marrow's ability to produce these cells and mutated hemoglobin • Inherited (primarily affects Blacks, Asians, and people of Mediterranean origin)	• Cardiac problems, such as cardiomegaly, heart failure, and murmurs • Excessive hematopoiesis and iron overload • Other symptoms similar to other chronic anemias	• Transfusions are the primary treatment. Chelating agents are used to remove excess iron from the blood after multiple transfusions have been administered. • Splenectomy may be required for severe thalassemia. • Bone marrow transplant also is an option.	• If the patient has thalassemia, provide genetic counseling.
Iron-deficiency anemia Anemia caused by inadequate iron supplies • Chronic blood loss without iron replacement • Poor nutrition • Decreased iron absorption from the intestines • Increased need for iron, such as during childhood or pregnancy	• Possibly asymptomatic • Possible sense of being cold due to iron's role in regulating body temperature • Brittle, spoon-shaped nails with longitudinal ridges; cheilosis (painful mouth cracks or sores); exertional dyspnea; insidious development of fatigue; and red, shiny tongue • Hypochromic, microcytic anemia (on blood smears); low serum iron level; and elevated serum iron-binding capacities	• The cause of blood loss or nutritional deficits is identified and corrected. • An oral iron supplement may be prescribed. If the patient is unable to tolerate it, a parenteral iron formulation may be administered I.M. via the Z-track method or I.V.	• Help determine the cause of bleeding by testing stool, urine, vomitus, and sputum for blood. • Teach the patient how to take oral iron. Advise the patient to take iron pills with meals to reduce GI irritation and to continue therapy until the underlying problem is corrected. • Teach the patient about adverse reactions to oral iron therapy, such as black stools, constipation or diarrhea, and GI disturbances. • Educate the patient about nutrition, including the need for iron-rich foods and adequate vitamin C to enhance iron absorption.

(continued)

Types of anemia (continued)

Description and etiology	Signs and symptoms	Medical management	Nursing interventions
Megaloblastic anemia Anemia characterized by a predominance of megaloblasts and a relative lack of normoblasts; it includes pernicious, vitamin B_{12} deficiency, and folic acid deficiency anemias • Gastric surgery, particularly of the terminal ileum where vitamin B_{12} is absorbed; strict vegetarian diets; and prolonged exposure to nitrous oxide • Aging and long-term gastritis (pernicious anemia) • Alcoholic malnutrition and malabsorption (folic acid deficiency anemia)	• Epithelial atrophy, loss of coordination, neuropathy, and paresthesia of the extremities • Gastritis, glossitis (red, beefy tongue), and malabsorption with anorexia and weight loss • Decreased RBC and platelet counts	• Monthly administration of parenteral vitamin B_{12} typically is required for pernicious and vitamin B_{12} deficiency anemias. • An oral folic acid supplement and dietary improvement typically are required for a patient with folic acid deficiency, which commonly results from nutritional deficits.	• Provide care for oral mucous membranes to help relieve glossitis. • Teach the patient how to increase dietary intake of folic acid and vitamin B_{12}. • Refer the patient with anemia related to alcohol abuse to an alcohol rehabilitation clinic. • If the patient has a vitamin B_{12} deficiency, teach him about long-term treatment with an oral or parenteral vitamin B_{12} supplement. Treatment typically calls for monthly I.M. administration of cyanocobalamin.

◆ Symptoms resulting from compression by the enlarged lymph nodes depend on the area involved

■ Diagnosis and treatment

◆ Lymph node biopsy showing Reed-Sternberg cells supports the diagnosis

◆ Staging is done after the initial diagnosis of Hodgkin's disease is confirmed

▶ The stage of disease is determined by biopsies of distant lymph nodes, bilateral bone marrow biopsies, lymphangiography, computed tomography scan or magnetic resonance imaging (MRI) of the thorax and abdomen, gallium scan, positron emission tomography (PET), chest X-ray, a complete blood count (CBC), and serum alkaline phosphatase

▶ A splenectomy is traditionally done during staging

◆ Hodgkin's disease has four stages (see *Staging lymphomas*)

◆ Early stages of Hodgkin's disease are treated with external radiation of the affected lymph nodes

◆ More advanced stages require a combination of chemotherapy and radiation therapy

Staging lymphomas

Hodgkin's disease and non-Hodgkin's lymphoma are classified into stages so that treatment protocols can be established and outcomes predicted. The Ann Arbor classification system is used.

Stages

Stage I
- Involvement of a single lymph node region

or

- Localized involvement of a single extranodal organ or site

Stage II
- Involvement of two or more lymph node regions on the same side of the diaphragm

or

- Localized involvement to a single associated extranodal organ or site and its regional lymph nodes with or without other lymph node regions on the same side of the diaphragm

Stage III
- Involvement of lymph node regions on both sides of the diaphragm that may also be accompanied by localized involvement of an extranodal organ or site, by involvement of the spleen, or by both

Stage IV
- Disseminated involvement of one or more extralymphatic sites with or without associated lymph node involvement

or

- Isolated extralymphatic organ involvement with distant (nonregional) nodal involvement

  Extralymphatic sites include the liver, lungs, bone marrow, pleurae, bone, and skin as well as tissues separate from but near to major lymphatic clusters. The spleen is considered a lymphatic site.

Letter designation

The stages are also accompanied by a letter designation that refers to patient symptoms as follows:
- **A** means absence of the specific symptoms listed in **B** but may include other common symptoms such as pruritus.
- **B** includes the presence of at least one of the following three symptoms:
  - temperature greater than 100.4° F (38° C)
  - unexplained loss of more than 10% of body weight in the preceding 6 months
  - drenching night sweats

- ◆ Autologous bone marrow transplantation or autologous peripheral blood sternal transfusions and immunotherapy for disease resistant to standard treatment
- ■ Nursing interventions
  - ◆ Provide supportive care related to the adverse effects of radiation therapy and chemotherapy (see Nursing implications in oncology care, page 351)
  - ◆ Provide psychological support to help the patient cope with the diagnosis, treatment, and effects of treatment
  - ◆ Provide education to the patient and his family regarding the diagnosis of Hodgkin's disease and its treatment

❖ Leukemia
- ■ Description
  - ◆ Leukemia is a group of malignant disorders of the hematopoietic system that involves the bone marrow and lymph nodes and is characterized by the uncontrolled proliferation of immature WBCs

Types of leukemia

The following chart compares the incidence and signs and symptoms for various types of leukemia.

Leukemia	Incidence	Signs and symptoms
Acute leukemias Acute lymphocytic leukemia (ALL)	• Primarily affects children ages 2 to 4. Incidence declines dramatically after age 10. Survival rates are higher in children than adults, and the prognosis for ALL is better than that of acute myeloblastic leukemia.	• Anemia with fatigue and pallor • Bleeding — such as ecchymosis, gingival or rectal bleeding, and petechiae — particularly in a patient with AML • Decreased hematocrit, hemoglobin level, and platelet count
Acute myelogenous leukemia (AML), also known as acute nonlymphocytic leukemia	• Primarily affects those between ages 12 and 20 and those older than age 55. Survival rates for AML have improved with the use of autologous and allogenic bone marrow transplants.	• Infections, particularly those of the mucous membranes, respiratory tract, and skin • Normal, decreased, or increased white blood cell (WBC) count • Bone or joint pain, fever without infection, hepatosplenomegaly, lymphadenopathy, and weight loss, particularly in patients with ALL
Chronic leukemias Chronic lymphocytic leukemia (CLL)	• Primarily affects men between ages 50 and 70. CLL runs a long course (4 to 10 years) and rarely progresses to acute leukemia.	• Elevated WBC count • Enlarged spleen • Hepatomegaly in patients with CML; lymphadenopathy in patients with CLL
Chronic myelogenous leukemia (CML), or chronic granulocytic leukemia	• Primarily affects those between ages 30 and 50.	• Mild anemia

◆ Leukemias are classified by onset and severity of symptoms (acute or chronic) and by the precursor cell (myeloid or lymphoid) involved in the formation of the abnormal cells (see *Types of leukemia*)

◆ Although the cause of leukemia is unknown, it has been linked to genetic damage to cells, which transforms normal cells into malignant cells; it's associated with Down syndrome and other chromosomal abnormalities, chronic exposure to chemicals such as benzene, use of drugs that cause aplastic anemia, radiation exposure, and chemotherapy

◆ In leukemia, WBC (leukocyte) proliferation interferes with the production of other cells, leading to thrombocytopenia and anemia; the immature leukocytes decrease immunocompetence and increase susceptibility to infection

■ Signs and symptoms

◆ A patient with either acute or chronic leukemia may report vague signs and symptoms, such as fatigue, malaise, petechiae, night sweats, bone or joint pain, and weight loss

◆ Acute leukemia produces anemia, bleeding, and symptoms of infection such as sudden onset of high fever; hepatosplenomegaly and lymphadenopathy may also be present

◆ Chronic leukemia causes milder anemia and splenomegaly; however, many patients are asymptomatic at the time of diagnosis

◆ Additional signs and symptoms depend on the organ or tissue involved — for example, central nervous system involvement may cause headache and vomiting

■ Diagnosis and treatment

◆ Diagnosis is usually based on bone marrow examination that reveals leukemic blast cells and on CBC

◆ Chemotherapy, with or without stem cell transplantation, is standard treatment for leukemia (see Nursing implications in oncology care, page 351)

◆ Patients with low-risk chronic lymphocytic leukemia may not receive treatment if they're asymptomatic

◆ Stem cell transplantation is used to treat leukemia

  ❯ In *allogenic transplantation,* donor stem cells are transplanted into the patient

    ● Before transplantation, the patient undergoes chemotherapy and total body radiation to eliminate the leukemic cells; these procedures destroy all the patient's bone marrow in preparation for grafting from the donor

    ● The principal complication of this type of transplantation is graft-versus-host disease (GVHD), a type of organ rejection in which the transplanted cells reject the patient

  ❯ An alternative method is to harvest the patient's own stem cells during remission, treat the cells to remove residual tumor cells, and reinfuse them after the patient undergoes immunosuppressant chemotherapy and radiation therapy; this method, called *autologous stem cell transplantation,* avoids GVHD because the patient receives his own cells

◆ Transfusion therapy may be necessary to treat severe thrombocytopenia, leukopenia, and anemia resulting from the disease process or from treatment

  ❯ Most RBC transfusions involve 250 to 300 ml/unit of packed RBCs; whole blood is seldom transfused to treat leukemia

    ● The blood must be refrigerated until it's used

    ● The nurse must take baseline vital signs before transfusion, monitor cardiac status before and during transfusion, confirm blood product compatibility with the patient's blood type, administer blood through a filter (only with normal saline solution), check the blood according to facility policy with another professional nurse, infuse it slowly (2 to 4 hours/unit), observe for reactions, and record vital signs at least hourly and at the end of the transfusion

  ❯ Platelet transfusions may be prescribed; a 6-unit I.V. bolus of platelets should be infused over 20 to 30 minutes

    ● Platelets shouldn't be refrigerated

    ● The nurse must take baseline vital signs before transfusion, premedicate with steroids or antihistamines, as prescribed, to prevent reactions, and administer platelets through a filter (only with normal saline solution)

> ▶ WBC transfusions must be infused within 24 hours of collection; the process for WBC transfusions is similar to that for RBC transfusions

■ Nursing interventions

◆ Follow infection-control procedures if the WBC count is low — for example, place a severely neutropenic patient in a private room, with no flowers, plants, or fresh fruits; avoid unnecessary invasive procedures; limit patient contact with infected personnel or visitors; and teach handwashing techniques to the patient, family, and visitors

◆ If the patient has a low platelet count, monitor blood counts and take precautions to prevent bleeding — for example, avoid parenteral injections, limit the number of venipunctures, and advise the patient to use an electric razor for shaving

◆ Prevent or manage stomatitis by inspecting the oral cavity daily and encouraging oral care with peroxide or saline solution on a regular basis

◆ Teach the patient how to care for an indwelling vascular access device and how to detect infection in the line

◆ Educate patients undergoing chemotherapy about the effects, adverse effects, and length of treatment

◆ Provide supplemental feedings as prescribed

◆ Conserve the patient's energy, but promote his independence

◆ Provide emotional support to the patient and his family, and encourage the patient and his family to verbalize feelings

❖ Multiple myeloma

■ Description

◆ Multiple myeloma is a malignancy of plasma cells that invades the bone marrow, lymph nodes, liver, spleen, and kidneys and leads to bone destruction throughout the body

◆ Usually occurs in black men between ages 50 and 70; men are 50% more likely to develop the disease than women

◆ Other risks include radiation exposure, family history, obesity, and occupational exposure in petroleum-related industries

■ Signs and symptoms

◆ Confusion, weakness, dizziness, weight loss, fractures, renal failure, skeletal deformities, and constant, severe bone pain may occur

◆ Anemia, leukopenia, and thrombocytopenia — with resulting bleeding, infection, shortness of breath, weakness, and protein in blood and urine — may also occur

■ Diagnosis and treatment

◆ Serum and urine protein electrophoresis showing immunoglobulin or beta$_2$-microglobulin are indicative of multiple myeloma; urine studies may show Bence Jones proteins and hypercalciuria

◆ Bone X-rays or MRI may show bone destruction

◆ Bone marrow aspiration and biopsy may show an increased number of immature plasma cells

◆ Chemotherapy suppresses plasma cell growth, and radiation therapy may be used to treat bone lesions and relieve pain

◆ Radiation therapy to damage myeloma cells and stop growth

◆ Patients with multiple myeloma may also receive interferon to slow the growth of the myeloma cells and thalidomide to inhibit angiogenesis

◆ Autologous bone marrow transplantation isn't a cure but may put the patient into remission for a period; allogenic transplant carries a higher risk of serious complications but produces longer-lasting remissions

◆ Plasmapheresis is sometimes used to temporarily remove the high-myeloma protein and thereby improve symptoms

◆ Hypercalcemia may be managed with a diuretic, hydration, or a phosphate

◆ Other therapies: bortezomib (Velcade) for resistant forms and thaliclomide (Thalomid)

■ Nursing interventions

◆ Educate the patient and his family about diagnostic and treatment procedures and adverse effects

◆ Assess the patient for pain, and administer an analgesic regularly

◆ Instruct the patient on safety measures to prevent fractures of affected bones; direct the patient not to walk without assistance; have the patient use devices, such as splints or braces, to prevent injury and reduce pain

◆ Encourage the patient to drink plenty of fluids, or administer I.V. fluids, to dilute calcium, prevent dehydration, and prevent renal precipitates

◆ Assess the patient for symptoms of infection and bleeding, and take measures to prevent their occurrence

❖ Non-Hodgkin's lymphoma

■ Description

◆ Non-Hodgkin's lymphoma describes a group of malignant neoplasms arising from abnormal lymphocytes that affect the immune system; this disease is usually disseminated when diagnosed and produces systemic symptoms

◆ It may be associated with viral infection, congenital immunodeficiency, or immunosuppression after organ transplantation

◆ The prognosis is poor but depends on the histologic type and progression of the disease

■ Signs and symptoms

◆ Non-Hodgkin's lymphoma can affect any organ or tissue and produces a wide range of symptoms

◆ Signs and symptoms resemble those of Hodgkin's disease

◆ Fever, painless lymphadenopathy, profuse sweating (especially at night), severe pruritus, abdominal pain or swelling, and weight loss are common signs and symptoms

■ Diagnosis and treatment

◆ Diagnostic procedures are similar to those for Hodgkin's disease; however, no Reed-Sternberg cells are present

◆ Staging is similar to Hodgkin's disease (see *Staging lymphomas,* page 123)

◆ Radiation therapy, chemotherapy, and stem cell transplantation are the principal treatments

◆ Biological response modifiers, such as interferon and monoclonal antibodies, also may be used to change the tumor-host relationship

◆ Radioimmunotherapy

■ Nursing interventions

◆ Educate the patient and his family about transfusions, chemotherapy, and stem cell transplantation

◆ Initiate interventions similar to those for leukemia

◆ Prevent infection

◆ Support nutritional status

❖ **Thrombocytopenia**

■ Description

◆ Thrombocytopenia is an abnormally low level of circulating platelets (less than 100,000/mm^3) due to decreased production, decreased survival, increased destruction, or increased sequestration of platelets in the spleen

◆ It may result from antibody production (idiopathic thrombocytopenic purpura [ITP]), bone marrow radiation, excessive alcohol use, or a disease, such as aplastic anemia or leukemia, disseminated intravascular coagulation, hypothermia, or an autoimmune disorder

◆ It also may result from drug therapy with an analgesic, an antibiotic (resulting in idiopathic thrombocytopenic purpura), a chemotherapeutic drug, an anti-inflammatory, or a thiazide diuretic; although the platelet count may return to normal 1 to 2 weeks after the drug is withdrawn, more than 90% of adults don't go into spontaneous remission

■ Signs and symptoms

◆ Ecchymoses, petechiae, and purpura may affect the skin

◆ Epistaxis, gingival bleeding, severe hemorrhage, and menorrhagia also may occur

■ Diagnosis and treatment

◆ The diagnosis is made by examining the platelet count, blood smear, bleeding time, and bone marrow to determine whether the platelet loss is caused by lack of production or increased destruction

◆ Treatment focuses on correcting the underlying cause

◆ For ITP, the principal treatment is corticosteroid therapy; for severe or resistant cases, immunosuppressant therapy or splenectomy may be used; platelet transfusions aren't helpful because of continued platelet destruction

◆ For other types of thrombocytopenias, platelet transfusions are indicated and can increase the platelet count for 1 to 3 days

■ Nursing interventions

◆ Monitor platelet counts; the patient is more susceptible to injury and bleeding when the platelet count falls below 60,000/mm^3 and may develop spontaneous hemorrhage, particularly cerebral hemorrhage when the platelet count drops below 20,000/mm³

◆ Test all stools and urine for blood
◆ Avoid taking the patient's temperature rectally and giving injections I.M.
◆ Apply pressure to venipuncture and arterial puncture sites
◆ Provide meticulous oral care to prevent stomatitis
◆ Tell the patient to use only electric shavers and to avoid contact sports, elective surgery, tooth extraction, and the use of aspirin and ibuprofen

Review questions

1. When assessing a patient with anemia from acute blood loss, the nurse would expect to find which of the following?

○ **A.** Sudden onset of symptoms, hypotension, and tachycardia

○ **B.** Exertional dyspnea, poor nutrition, and hypotension

○ **C.** Sudden onset of symptoms, glossitis, and tachycardia

○ **D.** Fatigue, neuropathy, and tachycardia

Correct answer: A Acute blood loss occurs suddenly. Hypotension and tachycardia are compensatory mechanisms in response to rapid loss of blood volume. Although anemia may produce exertional dyspnea and hypotension, option B is incorrect because poor nutrition is neither a symptom nor a cause of anemia due to blood loss. Options C and D are incorrect because anemia due to acute blood loss neither produces glossitis nor neuropathy.

2. When teaching safety precautions to a patient with thrombocytopenia, the nurse should include which of the following directives?

○ **A.** Eat foods high in iron.

○ **B.** Avoid products that contain aspirin.

○ **C.** Avoid people with respiratory tract infections.

○ **D.** Eat only cooked vegetables.

Correct answer: B Patients with a low platelet count should avoid products that contain aspirin because they increase the tendency to bleed. Option A would be important to teach the patient with anemia. Options C and D are correct for the patient with leukopenia.

3. When assessing the patient, the nurse knows the body system that's least affected by multiple myeloma is:

○ **A.** Skeletal system

○ **B.** Renal system

○ **C.** Nervous system

○ **D.** Cardiovascular system

Correct answer: D Multiple myeloma usually doesn't have a direct effect on the heart. Options A, B, and C are incorrect because multiple myeloma usually affects the skeletal, renal, and nervous systems.

4. The nurse is reviewing assessment data for a patient with a diagnosis of stage III Hodgkin's disease. This diagnosis is most strongly supported by lymphatic involvement on both sides of the:

○ **A.** blood-brain barrier.

○ **B.** diaphragm.

○ **C.** descending aorta.

○ **D.** spinal column.

Correct answer: B With stage III Hodgkin's disease, malignant cells are widely disseminated to lymph nodes on both sides of the diaphragm. Options A, B, and D are incorrect because these structures aren't involved in the staging of Hodgkin's disease.

5. A 50-year-old male with a diagnosis of leukemia is responding poorly to treatment. He's tearful and trying to express his feelings, but he's having difficulty. The nurse should first:

○ **A.** tell him that she'll leave for now but she'll be back.

○ **B.** offer to call pastoral care.

○ **C.** ask if he would like her to sit with him while he collects his thoughts.

○ **D.** tell him that she can understand how he's feeling.

Correct answer: C The patient needs to feel that people are concerned with his situation. Option A is incorrect because leaving the patient doesn't show acceptance of his feelings. Option B is incorrect because offering to call pastoral care may be helpful for some patients but should be done after the nurse has spent time with the patient. Option D is incorrect because telling the patient that she understands how he's feeling is inappropriate because it doesn't help him express his feelings.

Respiratory disorders

CHAPTER 9

❖ Introduction

- ■ The function of the respiratory system is to exchange gases (oxygen and carbon dioxide) with the external environment; the respiratory system maintains the level of these gases within a narrow range, regardless of the demand for oxygen
- ■ Respiration, which the central nervous system controls, is regulated by metabolic demands and cardiac output
- ■ Nursing history
  - ◆ The nurse asks the patient about his *chief complaint*
    - ▶ A patient with a respiratory disorder may report the following signs or symptoms: chest pain, cough, dyspnea, orthopnea, shortness of breath, or wheezing
    - ▶ The patient may also report hemoptysis, increased sputum production, or a change in the characteristics of his sputum
  - ◆ The nurse then questions the patient about his *present illness*
    - ▶ Ask the patient about his symptom, including when it started, associated symptoms, location, duration, frequency, and precipitating and alleviating factors
    - ▶ If the patient has dyspnea, ask him to rate it on a scale of 0 to 10, in which 0 means no dyspnea and 10 means the worst dyspnea experienced
    - ▶ If the patient has orthopnea, ask him how many pillows he uses to sleep
    - ▶ Ask if the patient's cough is productive or nonproductive. Is the cough recent? If not recent, how long experienced? Has it changed recently?
    - ▶ When a patient produces sputum, ask him to estimate the amount produced in teaspoons or another common measurement; ask him at what time of day he coughs the most; question him about the color and consistency of his sputum; ask whether its character has changed recently. If so, how? Does he cough up blood?
    - ▶ If a patient wheezes, ask when the wheezing occurs. What makes the patient wheeze? Does he wheeze loudly enough for others to hear it? What helps stop the wheezing?
    - ▶ If the patient has chest pain, ask him where the pain is located, what it feels like, what characteristics it has, whether it moves or radiates, how long it lasts, what causes it to occur, and what makes it better;

rate the pain on a scale of 0 to 10 (with 0 being no pain and 10 worst pain experienced)

▶ Ask about the use of prescription and over-the-counter drugs, herbal remedies, and vitamin and nutritional supplements, alternative or complementary therapies used

◆ The nurse asks about *medical history*

▶ Question the patient about other respiratory disorders — such as allergies, asthma, cystic fibrosis, pneumonia, tuberculosis, and upper respiratory tract infections

▶ Ask the patient if he has undergone chest or lung surgery

◆ The nurse then assesses the *family history*

▶ Ask about a family history of chronic obstructive pulmonary disease (COPD), pneumonia, or tuberculosis

▶ Determine if there's a family history of lung cancer

◆ The nurse obtains a *social history*

▶ Ask about smoking habits and environmental exposure to irritants such as asbestos

▶ Question the patient about his tolerance for exercise

■ Physical assessment

◆ Nurse begins with *inspection*

▶ Observe the patient's general appearance; note the patient's position. Is he sitting upright? Leaning forward? In a tripod position?

▶ Take note of his level of awareness and general appearance. Does he appear relaxed? Anxious? Uncomfortable? Is he having trouble breathing?

▶ Note deformities, masses, or scars of the chest; look for chest wall symmetry at rest and with inspiration; note the anterior-posterior chest diameter; observe chest wall movement. Is it paradoxical, or uneven?

▶ Note tracheal deviation; look for spinal abnormalities such as kyphosis; note whether the costal angle is enlarged

▶ Observe the patient's respirations, noting rate, depth, rhythm, and inspiratory-expiratory ratio; look for the use of accessory muscles with breathing, pursed lip breathing, and nostril flaring

▶ Observe the color of the patient's skin, lips, mucous membranes, and nail beds; check nails for clubbing

◆ Next, the nurse uses *palpation*

▶ Palpate the chest for temperature, dryness, crepitus, pain, and tactile fremitus

▶ Check for respiratory excursion

◆ Then the nurse *percusses* the heart

▶ Percuss the anterior and posterior chests, noting lung boundaries and movement of the diaphragm

▶ Also note percussion sounds; describe any abnormal ones, including the location and size of the area

◆ The nurse continues by *auscultating* the chest

◗ Classify each sound according to its intensity, location, pitch, duration, and characteristic; note whether the sound occurs during inhalation, exhalation, or both

◗ Auscultate for vocal fremitus, noting bronchophony, egophony, and whispered pectoriloquy

❖ Acute respiratory distress syndrome
  ■ Description
    ◆ Acute respiratory distress syndrome (ARDS) occurs when the lungs can't maintain the oxygen–carbon dioxide balance
    ◆ Although its exact cause is unknown, ARDS may occur as a complication of a systemic disorder and may result in acute lung injury; its mortality rate is 50% or higher; death is usually due to a multisystem failure or an infection
    ◆ Risk factors for ARDS include aspiration pneumonia, drug overdose, fat or amniotic emboli, head injury, hemorrhagic shock, massive blood transfusions or transfusion reactions, near drowning, pulmonary contusion, sepsis, smoke inhalation, and trauma
    ◆ With ARDS, capillaries leak, causing interstitial edema; this decreases blood flow to the lungs and causes platelet aggregation
      ◗ The respiratory membrane becomes inflamed; alveolar edema develops, leading to pulmonary edema
      ◗ Lung compliance decreases, and patches of atelectasis develop; the patient hyperventilates, thereby causing hypocapnia and hypoxemia, and leads to multisystem organ dysfunction syndrome
  ■ Signs and symptoms
    ◆ Vital sign measurements reveal increased blood pressure, tachycardia, and tachypnea (along with increased respiratory effort and accessory muscle use)
    ◆ Other signs and symptoms may include barotrauma symptoms, bibasilar crackles, crepitus, cyanosis, decreased breath sounds, diaphoresis, dyspnea, progressive hypoxemia despite oxygen therapy, restlessness, and thick, frothy sputum
  ■ Diagnosis and treatment
    ◆ Early diagnosis and prompt treatment allow for successful management of ARDS
    ◆ Arterial blood gas (ABG) studies reveal decreased partial pressure of arterial carbon dioxide and partial pressure of arterial oxygen (Pao_2), and respiratory and metabolic acidosis
    ◆ A pulmonary artery (PA) catheter inserted to measure pressures reveals pulmonary artery wedge pressure (PAWP) less than 18 mm Hg
    ◆ Chest X-ray shows bilateral infiltrates (in early stages) and lung fields with ground-glass appearance, irreversible hypoxemia, and massive consolidation seen as "white lung" (in later stages)
    ◆ Mechanical ventilation may be necessary
      ◗ Raising the fraction of inspired oxygen (Fio_2) with a ventilator helps to reverse hypoxemia but may increase the risk of oxygen toxicity and pulmonary fibrosis

▶ Supplementing mechanical ventilation with positive end–expiratory pressure (PEEP) provides a constant pressure that prevents the alveoli from collapsing

 ▶ PEEP allows the use of a lower FIO_2 to obtain an adequate PaO_2

 ▶ Pressure control ventilation that prevents overdistention of the alveoli and inverse ratio ventilation in which inspiration is longer than expiration may also be used

◆ A diuretic may be administered to reduce pulmonary edema

◆ An antibiotic is used to treat any respiratory tract infection or underlying systemic infection

◆ Pharmacologic paralysis is used to decrease oxygen consumption; the patient must be sedated for this treatment

◆ Vasopressors to maintain blood pressure

◆ Correction of electrolyte and acid-base imbalances to maintain cellular integrity

■ Nursing interventions

◆ Make sure the patient maintains bed rest with prone positioning, if possible, to improve oxygenation

◆ Provide oxygen therapy (and mechanical ventilation, if indicated) to maintain PaO_2 above 60 mm Hg; this will maintain oxygenation and help to reverse hypoxemia

◆ Implement chest physiotherapy to loosen secretions

◆ If the patient isn't on mechanical ventilation, teach him effective coughing and deep-breathing exercises to maximize lung expansion and reexpand collapsed alveoli

◆ Suction the patient's airway as needed to maintain patency and to clear secretions; sterile technique prevents bacterial contamination of lower airways

◆ Administer drugs to relieve pain and discomfort as needed

◆ If the patient is on mechanical ventilation, administer a paralyzant and a sedative as necessary

◆ Monitor fluid intake and output to determine the effectiveness of diuretic therapy

◆ Frequently reposition the patient to prevent complications of immobility, help loosen secretions, and promote lung perfusion

◆ Provide 2,500 calories daily to prevent weakness and increase immune response; use enteral or parenteral feeding if needed

◆ Teach relaxation techniques, and encourage the patient not to fight the ventilator

◆ Because a mechanically ventilated patient can't speak, provide communication alternatives, such as letter and picture boards

❖ Atelectasis

■ Description

◆ Atelectasis is the partial or total collapse of the functioning alveoli

◆ Airway obstruction, COPD, ascites, and lung compression resulting from hemothorax, pneumothorax, or tumor can cause atelectasis; atelec-

tasis also is a common complication of thoracic and upper abdominal surgery and occurs 24 to 48 hours postoperatively
   ◆ General anesthesia, immobility, lung disease, obesity, opioid use, pain, and smoking increase the risk of atelectasis
   ◆ A patient with atelectasis has normal pulmonary perfusion but decreased ventilation because the collapsed alveoli can't exchange gases; this decreased ventilation leads to hypoxemia
   ◆ Stasis of mucus leads to bacterial growth and pneumonia
- Signs and symptoms
   ◆ Vital sign assessment typically reveals fever (which may occur 24 to 48 hours postoperatively), tachycardia, and tachypnea
   ◆ Auscultation may reveal crackles and decreased breath sounds over the affected area
   ◆ Other effects may include cyanosis, dyspnea, and increased sputum production
- Diagnosis and treatment
   ◆ The patient should undergo ABG studies, chest X-ray, and sputum culture
   ◆ A bronchodilator is administered to open the collapsed alveoli
   ◆ An antibiotic is administered to treat infection
   ◆ If present, tumors are removed surgically or treated with radiation therapy
   ◆ A chest tube is inserted for a patient with hemothorax (to drain blood) or pneumothorax (to reinflate the lung)
- Nursing interventions
   ◆ Encourage the patient to cough and breathe deeply to maximize lung expansion and reexpand collapsed alveoli; use an incentive spirometer hourly after surgery
   ◆ Provide adequate hydration to liquefy secretions; thin secretions are easier to expectorate
   ◆ Implement chest physiotherapy to help clear secretions; postural drainage uses gravity to clear secretions, whereas percussion and vibration loosen secretions, making them easier to cough up
   ◆ Suction the patient's airway to maintain patency and to clear secretions
   ◆ Provide oxygen therapy to improve Pao_2 and maintain adequate oxygenation
   ◆ Medicate for pain or discomfort as needed, which will allow the patient to cough and deep-breathe effectively
   ◆ Teach the patient to use a pillow to splint abdominal and chest incisions during coughing exercises
   ◆ Encourage early ambulation and frequent position changes to prevent complications of immobility and promote lung expansion

❖ Avian influenza
- Description
   ◆ Avian influenza, also known as "bird flu," is an infection caused by avian (bird) influenza viruses

◆ Infected migratory and domestic birds shed the virus in their saliva, nasal secretions, and feces

◆ The strain is known as H5N1

◆ Transmission has been limited to people, and some animals such as cats, in contact with infected birds

◆ Should this virus become more easily transmissible person-to-person, it may lead to a pandemic

■ Signs and symptoms

◆ Symptoms range from typical human influenza-like symptoms, such as fever, cough, sore throat, and muscle aches, to eye infections, pneumonia, and acute respiratory distress

◆ Diarrhea, vomiting, and abdominal pain may occur

■ Diagnosis and treatment

◆ Chest X-ray may show pneumonia, infiltrates, or consolidations

◆ Sputum Gram stains and culture to isolate virus

◆ Neuraminidase inhibitor class drugs, such as oseltamivir and zanamivir, can reduce the severity and duration of illness caused by seasonal influenza; efficacy depends on early administration

◆ M2 inhibitors amantadine and rimantadine could possibly be used for pandemic infuenza, but resistance to these drugs may develop

◆ Maintain fluid and electrolyte balance

◆ Mechanical ventilation for acute respiratory distress

■ Nursing interventions

◆ Follow standard and contact precautions, and wear a fit-tested ventilator

◆ Wear eye protection within 3 feet of patient

◆ Maintain patent airway, suctioning patient when necessary

◆ Notify National Respiratory and Enteric Virus Surveillance System

❖ Chest trauma

■ Description

◆ *Rib fracture* can result from a blunt or penetrating injury; fractures commonly involve multiple ribs

◆ *Flail chest* is usually caused by blunt trauma; it results when two or more ribs are fractured at two different places on each rib, leaving a rib section that isn't connected at either end

◆ *Pneumothorax,* which can be caused by blunt or penetrating trauma, means that air has entered the pleural cavity; the air causes complete or partial collapse of the lung

◆ *Tension pneumothorax* can be caused by blunt trauma and is life-threatening if untreated because of its effects on respiratory and cardiac function

◆ *Cardiac tamponade* is the accumulation of blood in the pericardial sac, resulting from blunt or penetrating injury to the pericardium or heart; it's life-threatening if untreated (see *Comparing types of chest trauma*)

■ Pathophysiology

◆ With a rib fracture, pain may cause hypoventilation that leads to atelectasis

Comparing types of chest trauma

Each type of chest trauma produces characteristic signs and symptoms and requires specific treatment and nursing care.

Signs and symptoms	Diagnosis and treatment	Nursing care
Cardiac tamponade • Varied symptoms, depending on speed of blood accumulation • Chest pain, hypotension, muffled heart sounds, and tachycardia • Cyanosis, diaphoresis, dyspnea, and restlessness • Distended neck veins • Narrowed pulse pressure and paradoxical pulse • When tamponade develops more slowly: ascites, edema in arms and legs, liver enlargement	• Echocardiography can be used to diagnose cardiac tamponade. • Central venous pressure, which is elevated in patients with cardiac tamponade, is monitored. • Pericardiocentesis is used to remove fluid from the pericardial sac. • The injured area is repaired surgically. • I.V. fluids are rapidly infused. • Inotropic drugs are given to improve myocardial contractility.	• Administer oxygen to maintain adequate oxygenation, improve partial pressure of arterial oxygen (Pao_2), and reverse the hypoxemia. • Watch for complications, such as ventricular fibrillation, vasovagal response, or cardiac compression.
Flail chest • Cyanosis and dyspnea • Hypercapnia and hypoxemia • Increased respiratory effort • Pain on inspiration and on palpation of the injured area • Paradoxical movement of the flail segment	• Chest X-ray and arterial blood gas (ABG) studies typically are ordered. • Several types of analgesia may be used to relieve pain: patient-controlled analgesia, transcutaneous electrical nerve stimulation, or intercostal nerve block. • A chest tube may be inserted to treat hemothorax or pneumothorax. • Endotracheal intubation and mechanical ventilation may be used to stabilize the chest wall. • The flail segment may need to be repaired surgically.	• Teach the patient techniques for effective coughing and deep breathing to improve airway clearance. • Medicate for pain to promote effective coughing and deep breathing. • Provide hydration to liquefy secretions; thin secretions are easier to cough up. • Administer oxygen to improve Pao_2 and reverse hypoxemia. • Suction the patient's airway as needed to maintain patency and to clear secretions. • Provide pillows and teach the patient to support and splint the flail segment to minimize pain and to allow maximum lung expansion.
Pneumothorax • Asymmetrical lung expansion • Chest pain, crepitus, and dyspnea • Decreased or absent breath sounds on the affected side • Restlessness • Signs of mediastinal shift and tension pneumothorax	• Chest X-ray and ABG studies typically are ordered. • Analgesia is provided to relieve pain. • A chest tube may be inserted and attached to a suction device. In a three-chamber device, the first chamber allows for fluid drainage, the second one is a water seal that acts as a one-way valve to prevent air from entering the pleural cavity, and the third one controls the amount of suction, which is needed to remove air from the pleural cavity.	• Administer oxygen to improve Pao_2 and reverse hypoxemia. • Teach the patient techniques for effective coughing and deep breathing to prevent atelectasis and promote lung expansion. • Maintain the integrity of the chest tube system to facilitate air drainage from around the lung and promote lung expansion. Crepitus near the tube insertion site reflects air leakage into tissue and a possible leak in the chest tube system. When an air leak is no longer evident, the lung has healed itself and sealed off the injured

(continued)

Comparing types of chest trauma *(continued)*

Signs and symptoms	Diagnosis and treatment	Nursing care
Pneumothorax (continued)	• In an emergency, a Cook catheter with a Heimlich valve may be used to prevent air from entering the pleural cavity.	area. If the chest drainage system is impaired and loses its seal, place the end of the chest tube in a container of sterile water. • Encourage frequent position changes to prevent complications of immobility and promote lung expansion and perfusion. • Provide an analgesic as needed to reduce anxiety and encourage coughing and deep breathing.
Rib fractures • Pain on inspiration • Pain and tenderness of injured area upon palpation • Ineffective ventilation and retention of secretions • Signs of other injury such as soft-tissue injury	• Chest X-ray and ABG studies typically are ordered. • Analgesia is given to relieve pain. • An epidural catheter may be inserted for administration of narcotic analgesia. • A nerve block into the intercostal nerves above and below the fractured ribs may be used to relieve severe pain.	• Tell the patient not to wear tight or constrictive clothing, which can inhibit lung expansion and decrease effective ventilation. • Encourage the patient to breathe deeply and use an incentive spirometer hourly to maximize lung expansion and reexpand collapsed alveoli. • Medicate for pain or discomfort as needed, which will allow the patient to deep-breathe effectively. • Implement chest physiotherapy, unless contraindicated, to loosen secretions, which makes them easier to expectorate. • Provide adequate hydration to liquefy secretions; thin secretions are easier to cough up.
Tension pneumothorax • Asymmetrical lung expansion and tracheal deviation to affected side • Cyanosis, hypotension, and tachycardia • Decreased or absent breath sounds on the affected side • Distended neck veins • Severe chest pain and respiratory distress • Subcutaneous emphysema	• Chest X-ray and ABG studies typically are ordered. • Needle decompression is used for emergency air removal. • A chest tube may be inserted and attached to a suction device, such as a three-chamber device.	• Administer oxygen to improve Pao_2, reverse hypoxemia, and promote lung expansion. • Teach the patient techniques for effective coughing and deep breathing to prevent atelectasis and promote lung expansion. • Maintain the integrity of the chest tube system to facilitate air drainage from around the lung and promote lung expansion, as in pneumothorax. • Encourage frequent position changes to prevent complications of immobility and promote lung expansion and perfusion. • Provide an analgesic as needed to reduce anxiety and encourage coughing and deep breathing.

◆ With a flail chest, the flail segment moves in a manner opposite that of normal rib movement during respirations; as a result, the lungs can't fully expand

◆ Pneumothorax can result when a fractured rib or penetrating trauma perforates a lung

  ▶ Air escapes from the lung into the pleural cavity

  ▶ The lung can't fully expand, gas exchange is compromised, normal intrathoracic pressure is disturbed, and the lung may collapse

◆ With tension pneumothorax, trauma causes air to escape from the lung into the pleural cavity, where the air becomes trapped

  ▶ Pressure builds in the thoracic cavity, causing lung collapse

  ▶ The mediastinum shifts to the opposite side, compromising the other lung, and the vena cava becomes depressed, causing impaired venous return

◆ With cardiac tamponade, intrapericardial pressure increases, compressing the heart; cardiac output decreases, and cardiogenic shock occurs

❖ Chronic obstructive pulmonary disease

- ■ Description
  - ◆ COPD is a group of disorders that blocks the normal flow of air through the lungs, thereby trapping air in the alveoli
  - ◆ Included in this group are asthma, chronic bronchitis, and emphysema (see *Comparing chronic obstructive pulmonary diseases*, pages 140 and 141)
- ■ Asthma
  - ◆ Asthma is a heightened response to various stimuli, causing widespread airway constriction
  - ◆ This response may last for a few minutes to several hours; chronic obstruction may be mild or severe and last for days or weeks
  - ◆ Asthma results from allergens, drugs, endocrine changes, environmental changes, exercise, fatigue, genetic factors, irritants, stress, and viral infections
  - ◆ With asthma, spasm of smooth muscle in the airways and edema of the bronchial mucosa narrows the airways and traps air; as the airways become occluded by thick secretions, the lungs hyperinflate
- ■ Chronic bronchitis
  - ◆ Chronic bronchitis affects the lung parenchyma; it's characterized by a productive cough for at least 3 months a year for 2 or more consecutive years
  - ◆ It results from lung irritants, such as air pollution and smoking as well as from genetic factors
  - ◆ With chronic bronchitis, increased bronchial mucus gland production and goblet cell hyperplasia result in increased sputum production; ciliary damage and epithelial metaplasia may occur
  - ◆ Bronchial irritants or infection may cause bronchial edema, bronchospasm, impaired mucociliary clearance, impaired ventilation (especially during expiration), increased secretions, and small-airway blockage

(Text continues on page 142.)

Comparing chronic obstructive pulmonary diseases

Asthma, chronic bronchitis, and emphysema have distinctive signs and symptoms and require specific treatments and nursing care.

Signs and symptoms	Diagnosis and treatments	Nursing care
Asthma • Accessory muscle use, increased anterior-posterior diameter, reduced chest excursion, and lowered diaphragm • Clear, viscous sputum • Cough (typically non-productive) • Cyanosis or pallor (during serious attacks) • Decreased activity tolerance • Distended neck veins • Dyspnea and hyperventilation • Heart failure, hyponatremia, and renal failure caused by fluid overload • Lung hyperresonance, decreased breath sounds at bases, wheezing (especially during expiration), crackles, prolonged expiration, distant breath sounds during inspiration, and audible breath sounds during expiration	• Chest X-ray, arterial blood gas (ABG) studies, serum gamma E immunoglobulin and eosinophil counts, sputum analysis, and pulmonary function tests typically are ordered. • A bronchodilator — such as a $beta_2$–adrenergic agonist, an anticholinergic, or a methylxanthine — is used to control chronic symptoms. • A mast cell stabilizer or a corticosteroid may be used to reduce the inflammatory reaction to allergens and stabilize mast-cell membranes. • A leukotriene receptor modifier may be used to reduce airway inflammation and produce bronchodilation. • Treatment for exacerbations includes short-acting inhaled and subcutaneous $beta_2$-adrenergic agonists, an anticholinergic by nebulizer or metered-dose inhaler (MDI), and a systemic corticosteroid. • Flu and pneumonia immunizations are given to prevent infection. If infection occurs, an antibiotic is the treatment of choice.	• Provide adequate hydration to liquefy secretions. Thin secretions are easier to expectorate. • Monitor electrolyte levels to detect hyponatremia, and monitor ABG studies to assess oxygenation. • Teach pursed-lip breathing, which decreases the respiratory rate to improve gas exchange. • Teach effective coughing techniques to help clear secretions. • Teach relaxation and stress reduction techniques to prevent anxiety, which can exacerbate the disease. • Advise the patient to use high Fowler's position, which allows easier descent of the diaphragm to facilitate breathing. • Instruct the patient to take his medications exactly as prescribed; explain the difference between maintenance drugs and rescue drugs. • Instruct the patient to avoid aspirin and aspirin-containing products (which may increase bronchospasms), and sedatives and opioids (which increase respiratory depression). • Advise the patient to remove allergens and other causative agents from the home.
Chronic bronchitis • Accessory muscle use, slight increase in antero-posterior chest diameter • Anxiety and depression • Bronchospasm • Chronic productive cough for thick, tenacious sputum that isn't clear and may have mucus plugs • Cyanosis and dyspnea • Decreased activity tolerance • Heart failure, hyponatremia, and renal failure caused by fluid overload late in disease	• Chest X-ray, pulmonary function tests, ABG studies, complete blood count, electrolyte levels, electrocardiogram, and sputum analysis typically are ordered. • An inhaled anticholinergic and an inhaled $beta_2$-adrenergic agonist are the mainstay of therapy; they're delivered by MDI or nebulizer to enlarge the airways. • Aminophylline or another methylxanthine is given orally or I.V. to relax bronchial spasms. • An antibiotic is used to prevent or treat infection.	• Administer oxygen to maintain a partial pressure of arterial oxygen (Pao_2) of 60 mm Hg or an arterial oxygen saturation of 90%. • Provide adequate hydration to liquefy secretions. Thin secretions are easier to expectorate. • Implement chest physical therapy. Postural drainage uses gravity to clear secretions; percussion and vibration loosen secretions, making them easier to cough up. • Teach the patient how to cough effectively to help clear secretions and to use diaphragmatic and pursed-lip breathing. • Teach the patient how to use an MDI with spacer correctly to ensure delivery of accurate doses to the small airways and to prevent overuse.

Comparing chronic obstructive pulmonary diseases *(continued)*

Signs and symptoms	Diagnosis and treatments	Nursing care
Chronic bronchitis (continued) ● Lung hyperresonance, decreased breath sounds, diffuse wheezes, crackles and rhonchi, and prolonged expiration ● Signs of right-sided heart failure (cor pulmonale)	● An inhaled or oral steroid is used to decrease the inflammatory response, thus decreasing bronchial edema during acute exacerbations.	● Educate the patient about the signs of respiratory tract infections, such as fever, change in sputum color or amount, and increased shortness of breath. Untreated infections may lead to acute respiratory failure. ● Teach about proper and safe use of home oxygen equipment. ● Teach the patient about the effects of smoking, and help the patient quit. ● Recommend yearly influenza vaccine and pneumococcal vaccine every 5 years to reduce the risk of these infections.
Emphysema ● Accessory muscle use, increased anteroposterior diameter (barrel chest), lowered diaphragm, and reduced chest excursion ● Anxiety and depression ● Characteristic patient positioning — that is, leaning slightly forward with arms resting on the sides of the chair ● Decreased activity tolerance ● Dyspnea ● Fatigue from increased work of breathing ● Pursed-lip breathing and hyperventilation ● Lung hyperresonance, decreased breath sounds, expiratory wheezes, and prolonged expiration	● Chest X-ray, pulmonary function tests, ABG studies, and sputum analysis typically are ordered. ● The patient is immunized against the flu to prevent infection. If infection occurs, an antibiotic is the treatment of choice. ● Smoking cessation is encouraged to prevent continued alveolar damage. ● See "Chronic bronchitis: Diagnosis and treatments" pages 140 and 141, for specific therapies.	● Administer oxygen to a hypoxemic patient to maintain a Pao_2 of 60 mm Hg. Be aware that excessive oxygenation may cause loss of the incentive to breathe. ● Teach about pursed-lip and abdominal breathing, which prevent small airway collapse during exhalation by slowing respiration and increasing bronchiole pressure. ● Encourage activity to help prevent muscle wasting, but schedule frequent rest periods to avoid tiring the patient. ● Teach the patient to conserve energy by sitting for activities when possible and alternating hard and easy tasks. ● Teach relaxation and stress reduction techniques to prevent anxiety, which can exacerbate the disease. ● Provide information about prescribed drugs. ● Explain the importance of adequate fluid intake, which liquefies secretions, and a balanced diet, which prevents muscle wasting. ● Instruct the patient to eat frequent small meals to prevent constipation and avoid gas-forming foods to prevent pressure on the diaphragm and increased shortness of breath. ● Help prevent infections by telling the patient to avoid crowds, small children, and exposure to persons with respiratory tract infections. ● Teach the patient about the symptoms of respiratory tract infections. Untreated infections can lead to acute respiratory failure. ● Teach the patient about the effects of smoking, and help the patient quit. ● Recommend yearly influenza vaccines and a pneumococcal vaccine every 5 years. ● Arrange for home oxygen therapy if needed.

◆ Impaired diffusion is caused by decreased airflow, mucus plugs, and secondary infection; cyanosis and polycythemia develop as a result of hypoxemia

◆ Signs of emphysema may be present, and as the disease progresses, cor pulmonale and pulmonary hypertension may develop

■ Emphysema

◆ Emphysema is a disease of the lung parenchyma characterized by changes in the alveolar wall and enlarged alveoli distal to the nonrespiratory bronchioles

◆ It results from alpha$_1$-antitrypsin deficiency and is associated with smoking and air pollution

◆ Emphysema impairs ventilation by decreasing lung elasticity, collapsing small airways during exhalation, trapping air, and causing poor gas exchange in the alveoli

◆ It impairs diffusion by enlarging distal air spaces (which increases the distance for diffusion) and causing loss of capillary membranes and pulmonary vasoconstriction

◆ It impairs perfusion by causing loss of pulmonary vasculature, pulmonary hypertension, and cor pulmonale

❖ Hemothorax

■ Description

◆ Hemothorax is the presence of blood in the pleural cavity; it typically accompanies pneumothorax

◆ It may result from chest trauma, lacerated liver, penetrating trauma, perforated blood vessels, perforated diaphragm, pleural damage that causes bleeding, or rib fracture

◆ In hemothorax, blood collects in the pleural layer, compressing the lung on the affected side; this lung compression compromises gas exchange

■ Signs and symptoms

◆ Chest pain, cyanosis, dyspnea, and tachypnea commonly occur

◆ With marked blood loss, hypertension and shock may occur

◆ Asymmetrical lung expansion is accompanied by decreased breath sounds on the affected side

■ Diagnosis and treatment

◆ Chest X-ray and ABG studies are commonly prescribed

◆ A chest tube is inserted, and a water seal or suction is used to facilitate drainage

◆ Thoracotomy may be indicated if blood loss is severe

◆ If total blood loss is severe, treat with I.V. fluids and transfusion

■ Nursing interventions

◆ Administer oxygen to maintain adequate oxygenation, improve Pao$_2$, and reverse hypoxemia

◆ Teach techniques for effective coughing and deep breathing to prevent atelectasis and promote lung expansion

◆ Maintain the integrity of the chest tube system to facilitate blood drainage from around the lung and promote lung expansion

◆ Check the chest tube insertion site for crepitus, which indicates air leakage into tissue and may indicate a leak in the chest tube system

  ❭ An air leak in the system may indicate that the lung is damaged, causing air to leak from the lung into the pleural space

  ❭ If the air leak is outside the chest cavity (such as from the chest tube), air entering the system may increase air accumulation in the pleural space

◆ Encourage frequent position changes to prevent complications of immobility and promote lung expansion

◆ Provide an analgesic as needed to reduce anxiety, relieve pain, and ease coughing and deep breathing

❖ Laryngeal cancer

■ Description

◆ Laryngeal cancer affects the epithelial lining of the mucous membrane of the larynx, most commonly as squamous cell carcinoma; it usually affects men in their 60s and 70s

◆ Although laryngeal cancer has no proven cause, it's associated with cigarette smoking and alcohol consumption; workplace exposure to asbestos or wood dust is another predisposing factor

■ Signs and symptoms

◆ Hoarseness for more than 2 weeks, an early warning sign, may become progressively worse

◆ Dysphagia, dyspnea, and hemoptysis may be present

◆ Pain may be referred to the ear or throat if ulceration occurs

◆ Cervical lymph nodes may be enlarged

■ Diagnosis and treatment

◆ Laryngoscopy shows nodules on the vocal cords, and nodule biopsy reveals cancer cells

◆ Radiation therapy and surgery may be used alone or together

  ❭ Partial laryngectomy changes the voice and preserves the respiratory tract

  ❭ Total laryngectomy produces a complete loss of voice and creates a permanent tracheostomy opening

■ Nursing interventions

◆ Encourage deep breathing to maintain respiratory function

◆ Suction the patient's airway as needed to maintain patency and to clear secretions

◆ Administer oxygen to improve PaO_2 and maintain adequate oxygenation

◆ Provide tracheostomy care to prevent infection and maintain the airway

◆ Ensure adequate hydration and nutrition while preventing aspiration and aspiration-induced infection

  ❭ Have the patient eat slowly and in sitting position only

  ❭ Provide frequent small meals, and advance the diet as tolerated

  ❭ Have suction equipment readily available

◆ Provide pain relief as needed to reduce anxiety, and encourage deep breathing and activity

◆ If needed, teach the patient and family alternative methods of communication, such as an alphabet board or gesturing

◆ Discuss and initiate speech therapy, if appropriate, to maximize remaining vocal function

❖ Lung cancer

■ Description

◆ Four major types of malignant tumors can affect the lungs: adenocarcinoma, large-cell carcinoma, small-cell carcinoma (oat cell), and squamous cell carcinoma

◆ Up to 40% of lung cancers are metastatic; breast, GI, prostate, and renal cancers commonly metastasize to the lungs

◆ Risk factors for lung cancer include cigarette smoking, environmental factors such as air pollution, genetic factors, and occupational exposure to carcinogens

◆ Adenocarcinoma tends to grow slowly and is peripherally located; this well-circumscribed tumor seldom cavitates but spreads early to regional lymph nodes

◆ Large-cell carcinoma produces large necrotic masses that tend to grow rapidly and are peripherally located; it tends to cavitate, metastasizes early, and spreads extensively

◆ Small-cell carcinoma, the most aggressive lung cancer, tends to grow rapidly and is centrally located; it rapidly metastasizes through lymph and blood systems but responds to chemotherapy

◆ Squamous cell carcinoma, the most common lung cancer, tends to grow slowly and is centrally located; it produces early local symptoms, tends to cavitate, and metastasizes to intrathoracic sites first

■ Signs and symptoms

◆ Some lung cancers are asymptomatic; symptoms arise from metastasis to other body areas

◆ Dyspnea may range from mild dyspnea during extreme exertion to severe dyspnea at rest

◆ Auscultation may reveal decreased breath sounds, localized wheezing, and pleural rub (with pleural effusion)

◆ A chronic cough may be nonproductive; however, hemoptysis is common

◆ Enlarged lymph nodes and fatigue may occur

◆ Finger clubbing may be a late sign of lung cancer

◆ Weight loss may occur

◆ The patient may report bone pain, chest pain or tightness, joint aching, and shoulder and arm pain

◆ Superior vena cava syndrome may cause edema of the face, neck, and upper torso as well as dilated veins in the abdomen and chest

■ Diagnosis and treatment

◆ Chest X-ray, computed tomography (CT) scan, magnetic resonance imaging (MRI), bronchoscopy, sputum cytology, pulmonary function

tests, ABG studies, brain and bone scans, and lymph node biopsy may be prescribed
◆ Specimens may be obtained for culture by way of bronchoscopy, transthoracic needle biopsy, mediastinoscopy, open lung biopsy (thoracotomy), or thoracentesis
◆ Surgical procedures — such as lobectomy, pneumonectomy, and wedge resection — are used to treat lung cancer
◆ Chemotherapy, immunosuppressant therapy, and radiation therapy also may be used (see Nursing implications in oncology care, page 351)
◆ Serial thoracentesis or chest tube placement is used for recurrent pleural effusions
◆ Laser therapy through a bronchoscope is a palliative measure that relieves endobronchial obstructions caused by nonresectable tumors
■ Nursing interventions
　◆ Monitor a patient who has undergone surgery
　　▶ Assess the incision for signs of infection
　　▶ Check the dressing for drainage and the chest tube for proper functioning, air leakage, and amount of drainage
　　▶ Assess lungs for signs of atelectasis
　　▶ Assess the intensity and quality of pain
　　▶ Assess the patient for heart failure caused by fluid overload, hyponatremia, and renal failure
　　▶ Monitor electrolyte levels to detect hyponatremia or hyperkalemia
　　▶ Assess fluid intake and output
　　▶ Assess nutritional status
　◆ Administer oxygen to improve PaO_2, and maintain adequate oxygenation
　◆ Suction the patient's airway as needed to maintain patency and to clear secretions
　◆ Provide pain relief as needed to reduce anxiety, and encourage coughing, deep breathing, and early ambulation
　◆ Position the patient for comfort
　◆ Teach relaxation techniques to alleviate anxiety
　◆ Intervene appropriately for a postoperative patient
　　▶ Ensure adequate hydration to liquefy secretions; thin secretions are easier to expectorate
　　▶ Provide chest physiotherapy; postural drainage uses gravity to clear secretions, and percussion and vibration loosen secretions, making them easier to expectorate
　　▶ Teach effective coughing and deep breathing to promote lung expansion and prevent atelectasis
　　▶ Encourage early ambulation and frequent position changes to prevent complications and promote lung expansion
　　▶ Increase the patient's caloric intake to 2,500 calories daily
　　　● Although patients may have a poor appetite, their metabolic needs are increased
　　　● Administer medications to control diarrhea, nausea, and vomiting
　　　● Encourage the patient to eat frequent, small meals

- Encourage family members and friends to provide nutritious food that the patient likes
- Have a patient who has undergone thoracotomy practice arm exercises to promote lung expansion and maintain arm mobility
- Encourage the patient to express concerns to reduce anxiety, decrease pain, and promote healing
- If the patient is a smoker, discuss the effects of smoking, and help get him into a smoking cessation program
- Teach the patient how to improve his quality of life by conserving energy and reorganizing the home so that frequently used items are within reach, and consider employing a homemaking service

❖ Pleural effusion

Description

- Pleural effusion is an accumulation of fluid in the pleural space (the thin space between the visceral and parietal pleura); although it isn't a disease itself, it occurs secondary to other disease states
- Empyema is the accumulation of pus and necrotic tissue in the pleural space; blood (hemothorax) and chyle (chylothorax) may also collect in this space
- A pleural effusion can be classified either as exudative (caused by inflammation of the pleura) or transudative (caused by excessive hydrostatic pressure or decreased osmotic pressure)
  - Common causes of exudative effusions are bacterial or fungal empyema or pneumonitis, chest trauma, collagen disease, malignancy, myxedema, pancreatitis, pulmonary embolism, subphrenic abscess, and tuberculosis
  - Common causes of transudative effusions are heart failure, hepatic disease with ascites, hypoalbuminemia, and peritoneal dialysis

Signs and symptoms

- The most common symptoms are pleuritic pain and dyspnea
- Physical examination may reveal decreased chest wall movement, decreased breath sounds over the affected area, and dullness on percussion
- Infection from empyema may produce cough, fever, and night sweats

Diagnosis and treatment

- Chest X-ray can diagnose pleural effusion; other tests that may be prescribed include CT scan of the chest, bronchoscopy, pleurocentesis, and ultrasonography
- Treat the underlying cause if it can be identified
- Thoracentesis is performed to remove fluid; chest tubes may be placed for continued drainage
- Thoracotomy may be needed if thoracentesis isn't effective
- An antibiotic is prescribed to treat empyema; the specific antibody used depends on the causative organism

Nursing interventions

- Explain thoracentesis to the patient, and support him during the procedure
- Watch for respiratory distress or pneumothorax after thoracentesis

Pneumocystis jiroveci (carinii) pneumonia

Pneumocystis jiroveci pneumonia commonly results from an infection of *P. jiroveci* in an immunocompromised patient. Its onset is abrupt and may be a flare-up of a latent disease. Its signs and symptoms may include crackles over the affected areas, cyanosis, dyspnea or tachypnea, fever, hypoxemia, irritability or restlessness, and nonproductive cough.

Diagnostic tests may include chest X-ray, arterial blood gas analysis to check for hypoxemia, and needle or open biopsy to obtain lung tissue specimens for culture. The drugs of choice for treating this type of pneumonia are pentamidine isethionate, an inhaled antibiotic, and co-trimoxazole (also known as sulfamethoxazole-trimethoprim).

Care for a patient with *P. jiroveci* pneumonia resembles that of a patient with other types of pneumonia. Key nursing interventions include administering oxygen and an analgesic as needed, practicing good hand-washing techniques throughout care, limiting activity and encouraging rest periods, and teaching techniques to reduce the spread of infection and reduce stress.

◆ Administer oxygen to improve oxygenation

◆ Encourage deep-breathing exercises and incentive spirometry to promote lung expansion

◆ Maintain the integrity of the chest tube drainage system; monitor amount, color, and consistency of drainage; and check for air leaks

❖ Pneumonia
- Description
  - ◆ Pneumonia is an acute lung infection with inflammation accompanied by accumulation of exudate in the alveoli (see Pneumocystis jiroveci [(carinii)] *pneumonia*)
  - ◆ The risk of pneumonia increases with aspiration, central nervous system depression, chronic illness, COPD, dehydration, existence of a tracheostomy opening, immobility, immunosuppression, intubation, pain in the thoracic cavity, and use of general anesthesia
  - ◆ It may result from a bacterial, fungal, or viral infection or from exposure to a chemical irritant, through aspiration or gas inhalation
  - ◆ Pneumonia remains a major cause of morbidity and mortality among elderly and chronically ill people
- Signs and symptoms
  - ◆ Dyspnea or tachypnea, fatigue, and fever commonly occur
  - ◆ Signs of cyanosis or hypoxia may occur in those with advanced disease
  - ◆ Irritability or restlessness may signal cerebral hypoxia
  - ◆ Sputum may vary in amount, color, and consistency, depending on the causative agent
  - ◆ Lung auscultation may reveal crackles, rhonchi, or wheezes over the affected areas; breath sounds may be decreased in those with advanced disease
- Diagnosis and treatment

◆ Chest X-ray, ABG studies, sputum culture (for bacterial infection), and serologic testing (for viral infection) may be prescribed

◆ Needle or open biopsy may obtain lung tissue specimens (for fungal infection), and cold agglutinins may reveal antibodies associated with *Mycoplasma pneumoniae* infection

◆ Pneumonia is treated with antibiotics to eradicate the infecting organism

◆ A bronchodilator is used to open narrowed airways

■ Nursing interventions

◆ Teach effective coughing and deep breathing to improve airway clearance

◆ Provide adequate hydration to liquefy secretions; thin secretions are easier to expectorate

◆ Implement chest physiotherapy; postural drainage uses gravity to clear secretions, and percussion and vibration loosen secretions, making them easier to cough up

◆ Administer oxygen to aid ventilation, improve PaO_2, and preserve oxygenation

◆ Suction the patient's airway as needed to maintain patency and to clear secretions

◆ Advise the patient to limit activity and to rest for long periods to decrease oxygen consumption

◆ Provide pain medication as needed to allow effective coughing and deep breathing

◆ Maintain adequate nutrition to offset the increased use of calories secondary to infection

◆ Teach the patient how to contain secretions to reduce the risk of spreading infection

◆ Practice good hand-washing techniques to reduce the risk of spreading infection

◆ Teach relaxation and stress-reduction techniques; anxiety can compromise the immune system and increase the risk of infection

❖ Pulmonary edema

■ Description

◆ Pulmonary edema is the collection of fluid in the extravascular tissues of the lungs

◆ It can result from ARDS, fluid overload, left-sided heart failure, mitral stenosis, myocardial infarction, or pulmonary emboli

◆ With pulmonary edema, the left ventricle can't effectively pump blood from the heart

❱ Fluid backs up into the lungs

❱ Surface tension increases, the alveoli shrink, and the lungs become stiff, making breathing more difficult

❱ Hypoxemia and an altered ventilation-perfusion ($\dot{V}/\dot{Q}$) ratio develop

❱ Fluid moves into the larger airways, where it's coughed up as pink, frothy sputum

■ Signs and symptoms
  ◆ Tachycardia may be accompanied by narrowed pulse pressures and hypotension; third and fourth heart sounds may be present; skin may be cold and clammy
  ◆ Dyspnea, increased respiratory rate, orthopnea, and pulmonary hypertension may occur
  ◆ Jugular veins may be distended, and PAWP may be elevated
  ◆ Coughing may produce blood-tinged or pink, frothy sputum
  ◆ Lung auscultation may reveal dependent crackles
  ◆ Other signs and symptoms may include confusion, decreased urine output, diaphoresis, drowsiness, lethargy, and restlessness
■ Diagnosis and treatment
  ◆ Chest X-ray, pulse oximetry, and ABG studies typically are prescribed
  ◆ A PA catheter is inserted to measure pressures
  ◆ A diuretic is administered to decrease edema
  ◆ Other drugs that may be administered include an inotropic drug to increase myocardial contractility, nitroglycerin to reduce preload and afterload, I.V. nitroprusside to reduce preload and afterload, and a vasopressor to maintain blood pressure
  ◆ Intubation and mechanical ventilation may be necessary to treat respiratory distress
  ◆ Morphine is administered to decrease preload, respiratory rate, and anxiety
  ◆ Patients who don't respond to drug therapy may be treated with an intra-aortic balloon pump, which temporarily assists the failed left ventricle, or with surgery (such as angioplasty, coronary artery bypass grafting, or valvular repair), depending on the underlying heart condition
■ Nursing interventions
  ◆ Administer oxygen to aid ventilation, improve PaO_2, and reverse hypoxemia
  ◆ Place the patient in semi-Fowler's position to maximize oxygenation and increase comfort
  ◆ Carefully monitor fluid intake and output to assess the effectiveness of diuretic therapy and prevent sudden increases in venous return caused by oral and I.V. intake
  ◆ Medicate for pain as needed to reduce anxiety and increase comfort
  ◆ Frequently change the patient's position to prevent pressure ulcers and encourage lung expansion

❖ Pulmonary embolism
■ Description
  ◆ Pulmonary embolism is a blockage in the pulmonary artery
  ◆ Risk factors include atrial fibrillation; COPD; a family history of pulmonary embolism; oral contraceptive use; prior thromboembolic disease; venous injury caused by abdominal, pelvic, or thoracic surgery or leg or pelvic trauma; and venous stasis caused by age (older than age 55), burns, obesity, pregnancy, or prolonged immobility

◆ Pulmonary embolism is commonly caused by dislodged thrombi from deep veins in the pelvis or legs or from any systemic veins

◆ In this disorder, an embolism lodges in a branch of the pulmonary artery; the embolism may consist of bone, air, fat, amniotic fluid, thrombus, or a foreign object

▶ The area of the lung below the embolism isn't perfused, causing altered $\dot{V}/\dot{Q}$ ratio, which can cause alveolar collapse and lead to atelectasis and hypoxemia

▶ Pulmonary infarction may occur, destroying lung tissue

▶ A massive pulmonary embolism can cause pulmonary hypertension as a result of increased vascular resistance, right-sided heart failure as a result of increased right ventricular workload, or ventricular hypertrophy as a result of increased right ventricular workload

■ Signs and symptoms

◆ Dyspnea may occur suddenly, accompanied by chest pain

◆ Pleuritic chest pain may indicate pulmonary infarction

◆ Cough may produce hemoptysis

◆ Anxiety, increased restlessness, hypotension, and tachycardia may occur

◆ Lung auscultation may reveal crackles, pleural friction rub, and wheezes

◆ Low-grade fever and tachypnea may occur

◆ Signs of cor pulmonale and right-sided heart failure may develop

◆ If the patient has a massive pulmonary embolism, he may experience arrhythmias, cyanosis, or diaphoresis

◆ If the patient has a fat embolism, he may experience confusion, dyspnea, or petechiae on his chest and axillae

◆ The patient's legs may have signs and symptoms of deep vein thrombosis, such as edema, redness, tenderness, and warmth

■ Diagnosis and treatment

◆ Several tests are used to diagnose pulmonary embolism: ABG studies, chest X-ray, electrocardiography, lung scintigraphy, MRI, pulmonary angiography, and $\dot{V}/\dot{Q}$ lung scanning

◆ Several tests are used to diagnose deep vein thrombosis, which can lead to pulmonary embolism: contrast venography, Doppler ultrasonography, impedance plethysmography, and leg scan after injection of fibrinogen

◆ After an initial I.V. bolus of heparin, a therapeutic heparin infusion is given to inhibit clot formation, prevent emboli development, and maintain the partial thromboplastin time (PTT) between 1.5 and 2 times the control (60 to 70 seconds)

◆ If the patient needs long-term therapy, warfarin (Coumadin) is administered to maintain the prothrombin time (PT) between 1.5 and 2 times the control (11 to 12 seconds) or the International Normalized Ratio (INR) between 2 and 3; once the therapeutic dose of warfarin is achieved, the heparin infusion may be discontinued

◆ If the patient has a life-threatening embolism, a thrombolytic is administered, or a surgical embolectomy is performed

◆ If the patient can't tolerate anticoagulant therapy or continues to develop clots despite taking these drugs, surgical insertion of a vena caval filter may be needed

◆ A diuretic may be prescribed for a patient with a fat embolism; an antibiotic, for a patient with a septic embolism

◆ An antiarrhythmic may be used to correct heart rhythm disturbances caused by ischemia

■ Nursing interventions

◆ Administer oxygen to improve PaO_2, reverse hypoxemia, and promote lung expansion

◆ Some patients may require mechanical ventilation

◆ Teach effective coughing and deep breathing to help clear secretions and prevent atelectasis

◆ Provide adequate hydration to liquefy secretions; thin secretions are easier to expectorate

◆ Encourage early ambulation to prevent clot formation in deep veins; encourage range-of-motion (ROM) exercises or perform passive ROM exercises if the patient can't walk

◆ Use antiembolism stockings or compression boots to divert blood flow to the large veins, prevent emboli formation, and promote venous return

◆ Don't raise the patient's knees; this obstructs venous flow and increases the risk of deep vein thrombosis

◆ Elevate the legs to prevent venous stasis

◆ Maintain the heparin infusion, and monitor the PTT

◆ Administer warfarin daily, as prescribed, and monitor the PT or INR

◆ Test all stool for blood caused by anticoagulant-induced GI bleeding

◆ Provide analgesia and comfort measures to reduce anxiety

◆ Teach the patient about anticoagulant therapy to reduce the risk of bleeding, and help the patient maintain therapeutic PT or INR

◆ Have the family or home health nurse check the home for hazards, especially those that may cause falls; a safe environment is necessary because a patient receiving an anticoagulant has an increased tendency to bleed

◆ Instruct the patient not to cross his legs, sit for long periods, or wear restrictive clothing; these activities inhibit venous return and promote clot formation

❖ Severe acute respiratory syndrome

■ Description

◆ Severe acute respiratory syndrome (SARS) is a life-threatening viral infection believed to be coronavirus

◆ A theory suggests that coronavirus may have mutated from pigs, birds, and other animals, allowing transmission to and infection of humans

◆ The incubation period is estimated to range from 2 to 7 days (average is 3 to 5 days)

◆ Risk factors include close contact with an infected person, contact with exhaled droplets and bodily secretions from an infected person, or travel to endemic areas

■ Signs and symptoms
   ◆ In early stages, signs and symptoms include nonproductive cough, rash, high fever, headache, body aches, and pneumonia
   ◆ Shortness of breath and respiratory distress occur in later stages

■ Diagnosis and treatment
   ◆ Serum electrophoresis to detect antibodies to the coronavirus
   ◆ Sputum Gram stain and culture to isolate the coronavirus
   ◆ SARS-specific polymerase chain reaction test to detect SARS-CoV ribonucleic acid
   ◆ Isolation (strict respiratory and mucosal barrier) to prevent spread of disease
   ◆ Antivirals to treat viral infection, and a combination of corticosteroids and antimicrobials to treat inflammation and infection
   ◆ Mechanical ventilation to treat respiratory failure

■ Nursing interventions
   ◆ Maintain isolation for the patient
   ◆ Practice good hygiene to prevent further transmission
   ◆ Maintain a patent airway through suctioning if mechanical ventilation is required
   ◆ Monitor vital signs and nutritional, fluid, and respiratory status

❖ Tuberculosis

■ Description
   ◆ Tuberculosis (TB) is an infectious disease that commonly affects the lungs; it typically occurs only after repeated, close contact with a person infected with *Mycobacterium tuberculosis*
   ◆ Risk factors for tuberculosis include alcoholism, immunosuppression, low economic status, and malnutrition; elderly people, areas of crowded populations (for example, shelters and prisons), and immigrants from areas with high incidence of TB (such as Africa, Southeast Asia, and the Caribbean islands) are also more susceptible
   ◆ The incidence of TB has increased in proportion to the increase in patients who are infected with the human immunodeficiency virus
   ◆ *M. tuberculosis* is spread by way of infected airborne droplets; after infected droplets are inhaled into the terminal bronchioles, localized pneumonia develops, initiating an inflammatory response
      ▶ Bacilli are phagocytized by macrophages but remain viable within the phagocyte
      ▶ Tubercles form and grow in the lungs
      ▶ The lesion center forms a yellow, cheesy mass called caseous necrosis
      ▶ Healing begins, walling off the initial infection, and adenopathy occurs
      ▶ Systemic infection may develop

◆ Within 6 weeks after exposure to the infected droplets, cellular immunity occurs, and skin test results become positive

◆ TB can become active years after exposure, when resistance is lowered

■ Signs and symptoms

◆ Anorexia, fatigue, malaise, and weight loss may be accompanied by dehydration

◆ Cough increases sputum production, which may include hemoptysis (late disease)

◆ Lung auscultation may reveal crackles, pleural effusions, and rhonchi

◆ Low-grade fever and night sweats may occur

■ Diagnosis and treatment

◆ Purified protein derivative (of tuberculin) skin test, sputum analysis (using an early-morning sample), chest X-ray, pulmonary function tests, pleural fluid analysis, and bronchoscopy may be prescribed to detect TB

◆ Preventive treatment with isoniazid for 9 to 12 months is recommended for other members of the patient's household, those with recently converted positive skin tests, and those with positive skin tests (depending on medical history)

◆ If the patient has active TB, an antituberculotic is used for 6 to 9 months; isoniazid with rifampin usually is the first choice; other antituberculotics include ethambutol, pyrazinamide, and streptomycin

■ Nursing interventions

◆ Teach the patient how to contain airborne droplets and secretions to reduce the risk of spreading the infection

◆ Practice good hand-washing techniques to reduce the risk of spreading the infection

◆ Explain disease transmission to the patient and the need for prolonged therapy to help increase his compliance with the treatment plan

◆ Teach the patient about the prescribed drugs, including how to recognize adverse reactions (especially the symptoms of hepatotoxicity)

◆ Encourage the patient to maintain adequate dietary intake to maintain nutritional status, build strength, and improve the body's defense mechanisms

◆ Weigh the patient daily to assess nutritional status

Review questions

1. A patient with pneumonia in the right lower lobe is prescribed percussion and postural drainage. When performing percussion and postural drainage, the nurse should position him:

○ **A.** in semi-Fowler's position with his knees bent.

○ **B.** in a right side-lying position with the foot of his bed elevated.

○ **C.** in a prone or supine position with the foot of his bed elevated higher than his head.

○ **D.** bent at the waist leaning slightly forward.

Correct answer: C The aim of percussion and postural drainage is to mobilize pulmonary secretions, so they can be effectively expectorated. When a patient has pneumonia in the right lower lobe, the nurse should position him with his right side up or lower lobes elevated above the upper lobes so that gravity can help mobilize pulmonary secretions. Options A and D are incorrect because semi-Fowler's position and being bent forward at the waist would hamper mobilization of secretions from the right lower lobe. Option B is incorrect because the patient should be positioned with his right side up.

2. A patient with acquired immunodeficiency syndrome (AIDS) develops *Pneumocystis jiroveci (carinii)* pneumonia. Which nursing diagnosis has the highest priority for this patient?

○ **A.** Impaired gas exchange

○ **B.** Impaired oral mucous membranes

○ **C.** Imbalanced nutrition: Less than body requirements

○ **D.** Activity intolerance

Correct answer: A Although all these nursing diagnoses are appropriate for a patient with AIDS, *Impaired gas exchange* is the priority nursing diagnosis for the patient with *P. jiroveci* pneumonia. Airway, breathing, and circulation take top priority for any patient.

3. A patient has chronic bronchitis. The nurse is teaching him breathing exercises. Which point should the nurse include in her teaching?

○ **A.** Make inhalation longer than exhalation.

○ **B.** Exhale through an open mouth.

○ **C.** Use diaphragmatic breathing.

○ **D.** Use chest breathing.

Correct answer: C In patients with chronic bronchitis, the diaphragm is flat and weak. Diaphragmatic breathing helps to strengthen the diaphragm and maximizes ventilation. Option A is incorrect because exhalation should be no longer than inhalation to prevent collapse of the bronchioles. Because a patient with chronic bronchitis should exhale through pursed lips to prolong expiration, keep the bronchioles from collapsing, and prevent air trapping, option B is incorrect. Option D is incorrect because diaphragmatic breathing, not chest breathing, increases lung expansion.

4. A patient with ARDS is intubated and placed on mechanical ventilation. His Pao_2 is 60 mm Hg on 1.0 Fio_2. To improve his Pao_2 without raising the Fio_2, the patient will most likely be placed on:

○ **A.** time-cycled ventilation.

○ **B.** volume-cycled ventilation.

○ **C.** pressure support.

○ **D.** PEEP.

Correct answer: D   PEEP is widely used during mechanical ventilation of the patient with ARDS to improve gas exchange over the alveolar capillary membrane. Time- or volume-cycled ventilation, options A and B, are less likely to be used for a patient with ARDS than pressure-cycled ventilation. Pressure support, option C, depends on the patient's inspiratory effort and isn't as effective as PEEP in treating ARDS.

CHAPTER 10

Neurologic disorders

❖ Introduction

■ The nervous system is the communications center of the body

■ It coordinates all sensory and motor activities essential to proper physiologic functioning; it also plays a significant role in maintaining homeostasis

■ Nursing history

   ◆ The nurse asks the patient about his *chief complaint*
      ▶ The most common complaints concerning the neurologic system include changes in level of consciousness (LOC), confusion, dizziness, faintness, headache, and impaired mental status
      ▶ The patient may also report a change in balance or gait

   ◆ The nurse then questions the patient about his *present illness*
      ▶ Ask the patient about his symptom, including when it started, associated signs and symptoms, location, radiation, intensity, duration, frequency, and precipitating and alleviating factors
      ▶ Ask the patient about any dizziness, numbness, paralysis, seizures, tingling, tremors, or weakness
      ▶ Question him about problems with any of his senses or with keeping his balance, swallowing, urinating, or walking
      ▶ Ask about headaches and photophobia
      ▶ Ask the patient how he rates his memory and ability to concentrate
      ▶ Question him about trouble speaking or understanding people
      ▶ Ask about difficulties reading or writing

   ◆ The nurse asks about *medical history*
      ▶ Question the patient about other neurologic disorders
      ▶ Ask about chronic diseases, major illnesses, accidents, injuries, surgeries, and allergies

   ◆ The nurse then assesses the *family history*
      ▶ Ask about a family history of neurologic diseases, such as amyotrophic lateral sclerosis, cerebrovascular accident (stroke), migraines, and seizures
      ▶ Question the patient about a family history of diabetes mellitus, coronary artery disease, and hypertension

   ◆ The nurse obtains a *social history*
      ▶ Ask about work, exercise, diet, use of recreational drugs, alcohol, and hobbies
      ▶ Also ask about stress, support systems, and coping mechanisms

■ Physical assessment

◆ The nurse assesses neurologic function in these five areas: mental status and speech, cranial nerve function, sensory function, motor function, and reflexes

◆ The nurse assesses *mental status* and *speech*

❯ Note the patient's appearance, mannerisms, posture, facial expression, grooming, emotions, speech, and tone of voice

❯ Check for orientation to person, place, and time and for memory of recent and past events

❯ To test intellect, ask the patient to count backward from 100 by 7s, to read aloud, or to interpret a common proverb, and see how well he understands and follows commands

❯ Describe the patient's response to verbal, motor, and sensory stimuli; use the Glasgow Coma Scale for a standardized assessment

◆ The nurse assesses *cranial nerve function*

❯ Assess each of the 12 pairs of cranial nerves

❯ Note whether the patient has motor or sensory deficits, or both

◆ The nurse assesses *sensory function*

❯ Assess the patient for sensation to superficial pain, light touch, vibration, position, and discrimination

❯ Compare the patient's response bilaterally

◆ The nurse assesses *motor function*

❯ To test cerebellar function, inspect muscle size, contour, and symmetry, observing the patient for abnormal movements, such as tics, tremors, and fasciculations; note coordination, gait, and balance

❯ Assess the patient's muscle tone and strength

❯ Compare assessment findings bilaterally

◆ The nurse assesses *reflexes*

❯ Test the patient's deep tendon, superficial, and primitive reflexes

❯ Compare the findings bilaterally

❖ Alzheimer's disease

■ Description

◆ Alzheimer's disease is a progressive, degenerative disorder of the cerebral cortex; it's irreversible

◆ It's associated with brain cell atrophy, decreased levels of acetylcholine, enlarged ventricles, neuritic plaques in brain tissue, and neurofibrillar tangles

◆ The exact cause is unknown; it may be caused by abnormal protein in the brain, environmental toxins, genetic factors (for example, a variant of apolipoprotein E), and inadequate cerebral blood flow

■ Signs and symptoms

◆ Altered behavior and memory may include recent memory loss and impaired judgment (see *Stages of Alzheimer's disease,* page 158)

◆ Muscle rigidity, myoclonic jerks, and restlessness may occur

◆ Obsessive behaviors may develop

◆ The patient may develop anomia (inability to remember one's name) and aphasia (impaired ability to communicate verbally or in writing due to brain center dysfunctions)

Stages of Alzheimer's disease

Early stage	Intermediate stage	End stage
• Recent memory loss • Inability to learn and retain new information • Difficulty finding words • Personality changes and mood swings • Progressive difficulty performing activities of daily living	• Inability to learn and recall new information • Reduced ability to remember past events • Increased need for assistance with activities of daily living • Wandering • Agitation, hostility, or physical aggressiveness • Lack of orientation to time and place • Bladder and bowel incontinence	• Inability to walk • Total incontinence • No recent or remote memory • Inability to swallow and eat • No intelligible speech

◆ During the final stages, the patient loses almost all mental abilities, including self-care skills, speech, and voluntary movement

■ Diagnosis and treatment

◆ Alzheimer's disease typically is diagnosed when other dementia-producing conditions have been ruled out

◆ A definitive diagnosis can be made only if neuritic plaques and neurofibrillar tangles are found in the brain during a postmortem examination

◆ Treatment calls for supportive measures, such as relieving specific symptoms, providing for patient safety, and providing emotional support to the patient and family

◆ The anticholinergics donepezil and tacrine may improve memory in the early stages of the disease

■ Nursing interventions

◆ Make sure the patient carries identification, such as an ID card or bracelet so that if he wanders off, he can be brought home

◆ Speak in calm, friendly tones; even if the patient can't understand the content of what's being said, he can perceive emotional undertones

◆ Give simple instructions; the patient may become frustrated trying to follow complicated directions

◆ Plan a full schedule of daily activities, especially music therapy and stretching to music, to facilitate sleep at night and provide diversion from an otherwise monotonous day

◆ Provide a quiet, calm environment. Most Alzheimer's patients can't tolerate overstimulation, including bright colors and noises

◆ Maintain the patient's nutritional status; the patient may not eat unless reminded to do so, may not be able to use utensils, and may need help preparing food and eating

◆ Assist the patient with dressing and toileting

◆ Give the patient and family information about Alzheimer's disease; refer family members to a local support group to enhance their ability to cope

◆ Provide a safe environment for the patient, and discuss with the family the possible need for a home care aide; the patient may lack the judgment to drive safely, use appliances, or manage personal finances

◆ As soon as a diagnosis is made, discuss the possibility of power of attorney with the patient and family

◆ Provide emotional support and affection; the family may be so exhausted and frustrated that they can't display affection toward the patient

❖ Brain tumor

■ Description

◆ Brain tumors, which grow in the cranial cavity, can be malignant or benign, primary or metastatic

◆ Brain tumors may cause serious consequences as they compress or invade adjacent tissue; symptoms are caused by the destruction of neurons, displacement of brain structures, and increased intracranial pressure (ICP)

◆ Common primary sites for metastatic cranial tumors are the lungs, breasts, and colon

◆ The most common primary brain tumors in adults are gliomas and meningiomas

■ Signs and symptoms

◆ Symptoms vary not only by cell type but also by tumor location

◆ Generalized signs and symptoms include dizziness, headache, mental changes, progressive neurologic deficits, and seizures

◆ Signs and symptoms of increased ICP include alteration in LOC, bradycardia, difficulty with temperature regulation, headache, nausea and vomiting, personality changes, pupillary changes, respiratory pattern alterations, visual disturbances, and widened pulse pressure

◆ Frontal tumors can lead to expressive aphasia, memory loss, and personality changes; occipital tumors, to visual changes or blindness; temporal tumors, to seizures that are precipitated by olfactory or visual auras, receptive aphasia, or dysarthria; tumors in the dominant hemisphere, to communication problems; tumors near the optic tract, to visual difficulties; and acoustic tumors, to hearing difficulties

■ Diagnosis and treatment

◆ Diagnosis of brain tumors involves various tests, including computed tomography (CT) scan, EEG, magnetic resonance imaging (MRI), and skull X-ray

◆ Stereotactic surgery is the definitive diagnostic method to acquire tumor tissue and make an exact tissue diagnosis

◆ Specific treatments vary with the tumor's histologic type, radiosensitivity, and location and may include surgery, radiation therapy, chemotherapy, and decompression of increased ICP with drugs or shunting of cerebrospinal fluid (CSF)

■ Nursing interventions
  ◆ Assess neurologic status, including signs of increased ICP to establish a baseline and facilitate early intervention
  ◆ Maintain a patent airway to ensure adequate oxygenation; monitor and report respiratory changes
  ◆ Maintain seizure precautions, and administer an anticonvulsant as ordered
  ◆ Monitor the patient's temperature; fever commonly follows hypothalamic anoxia, but it can also indicate meningitis; use hypothermia blankets before and after surgery to keep the patient's temperature down and minimize cerebral metabolic demands
  ◆ Turn and position the patient every 2 hours to prevent pressure ulcer development and encourage lung expansion
  ◆ After surgery, monitor the patient's neurologic status, and look for signs of increasing ICP, such as changes in LOC; after supratentorial craniotomy, position the patient with the head of the bed elevated about 30 degrees to promote venous drainage; after infratentorial craniotomy, keep the patient flat for 48 hours
  ◆ Consult with occupational and physical therapists to encourage independence in daily activities; assist with self-care as required; if the patient is aphasic, arrange for consultation with a speech pathologist
  ◆ Provide emotional support to the patient and his family to help them cope with the diagnosis, treatment, potential disabilities, and changes in lifestyle

❖ Head trauma
■ Description
  ◆ Head trauma, a term that encompasses several types of injuries, is the leading cause of disability
  ◆ Head trauma is a general term for injuries to the head, ranging from a minor concussion to life-threatening hematoma and herniation
  ◆ Primary injuries are directly caused by the trauma; secondary injuries are indirectly caused by the trauma (see *Types of head injury*)
■ Signs and symptoms
  ◆ Depending on the severity and location of the injury, the patient will have varying neurologic deficits, such as motor and sensory changes, pupillary changes, reduced LOC, and seizures
  ◆ If the patient has increased ICP, he may experience bradycardia, decerebrate or decorticate posturing, focal neurologic signs, headache, increased blood pressure, pupillary changes (including sluggish or absent response to light and unequal size), reduced LOC (including agitation, coma, confusion, lethargy, and restlessness), seizures, vomiting, and widened pulse pressure
  ◆ If CSF leakage occurs, the patient may experience frequent swallowing, otorrhea, and rhinorrhea
■ Diagnosis and treatment
  ◆ Diagnosis may be based on skull X-ray, CT scan of the head and cervical spine, MRI, lumbar puncture, cerebral angiography, and EEG

Types of head injury

Primary and secondary head injuries result from trauma in different ways.

Injury	Description	Mechanisms
Primary injuries		
Concussion	Brief period of cerebral paralysis; full recovery usually occurs in 12 hours, but postconcussion syndrome (characterized by difficulty concentrating, fatigue, headache, and photophobia) sometimes occurs	Sudden blow to the head that causes anterograde and retrograde brain injury
Contusion	Bruising of the brain; may be a *coup* injury (hemorrhage and edema under the injury site) or a *contrecoup* injury (hemorrhage and edema opposite from the injury site)	Sudden impact, commonly resulting from acceleration-deceleration forces, that displaces cerebrospinal fluid and causes the brain to hit the inside of the skull
Laceration	Tearing of the cortical surface	High-velocity acceleration-deceleration injury or a penetrating trauma, such as a stab wound or gunshot wound
Secondary injuries		
Cerebellar herniation	Pushing of the cerebellar tonsils through the foramen magnum	Force that pushes the brain contents into another compartment, compressing the medulla
Epidural hemorrhage or hematoma	Arterial bleeding between the dura and the skull; initially causes loss of consciousness, followed by a brief lucid period and progressive neurologic deterioration	Tearing of the medial meningeal artery by a temporal bone fracture
Intracerebral hemorrhage or hematoma	Bleeding within the cerebrum; may lead to increased intracranial pressure and permanent neurologic damage	Contusion or laceration
Subarachnoid hemorrhage or hematoma	Arterial bleeding in the subarachnoid space; sudden symptoms can include chills, decreased level of consciousness, diaphoresis, dizziness, nausea, severe headache, and vomiting	Force that causes bleeding immediately or long after an injury
Subdural hemorrhage	Venous bleeding between the dura and arachnoid membrane	Acute process (causing symptoms within 48 hours of injury), subacute process (causing symptoms within 2 to 14 days), or chronic process (causing symptoms 2 or more weeks after the injury)
Supratentorial (central) herniation	Pushing of the cerebral ventricles through the incisura of tentorium	Force, such as a supratentorial mass, that pushes the brain contents into another compartment, compressing the diencephalon and midbrain
Uncal (lateral transtentorial) herniation	Shifting of the temporal lobe across the tentorium into the posterior fossa	Force that shifts the brain contents into another compartment, compressing the midbrain and brain stem

◆ Place a cervical collar on the patient's neck until a cervical injury is ruled out

◆ Treatment depends on the severity of the injury

❯ For a concussion, neurologic function is monitored for 24 hours

❯ For a contusion, neurologic function is monitored in a controlled environment for possibly increased ICP

❯ For laceration, diagnostic procedures are implemented for early identification of secondary injuries

◆ Continuous ICP monitoring may be indicated

◆ If present, clots are removed surgically; hematomas may need to be evacuated; in the presence of hydrocephalus, a drain may be placed in the ventricles

◆ Supportive measures—such as drug therapy for increased ICP (see "Increased intracranial pressure," page 163), intubation and mechanical ventilation, invasive hemodynamic monitoring, and invasive ICP monitoring—are initiated

■ Nursing interventions

◆ Monitor vital signs every 15 minutes until the patient's condition is stable to detect increased ICP

◆ Perform neurologic assessments every 15 minutes until the patient's condition is stable to detect increased ICP; assess LOC according to the Glasgow Coma Scale (see *Using the Glasgow Coma Scale*)

◆ Initiate I.V. therapy while strictly monitoring input and output to maintain hydration and prevent cerebral edema

❯ Excessive urine output may indicate diabetes insipidus (antidiuretic hormone deficiency) due to pituitary gland damage; it's treated with vasopressin

❯ Fluid retention may indicate syndrome of inappropriate antidiuretic hormone (SIADH) due to craniocerebral trauma; it's treated with fluid restriction

◆ Provide respiratory care to maintain a patent airway and adequate ventilation; turn and encourage frequent deep breathing in a nonintubated patient, suction an intubated patient, and remember that hypoxemia and hypercapnia increase ICP

◆ Provide a safe, quiet, dimly lit environment

◆ Take seizure precautions and keep emergency equipment nearby; a patient with head trauma is at risk for seizures and respiratory insufficiency

◆ Provide bed rest with positioning appropriate to the injury

❯ Elevate the head of the bed as prescribed to reduce cerebral edema; immediately after cranial surgery, the patient may need to lie in a supine position for 24 hours; early elevation of the head of the bed after infratentorial craniotomy can increase the risk of postoperative herniation

❯ Change the patient's position frequently to prevent complications stemming from immobility, and position him accordingly to prevent deformity

Using the Glasgow Coma Scale

The Glasgow Coma Scale assesses levels of consciousness by testing and scoring three observations: eye opening, motor response, and response to verbal stimuli. Patients are scored on their best responses as shown below, and these scores are totaled. The highest score is 15.

Eye opening	Motor response	Verbal response
4 (spontaneous)	6 (obeys commands)	5 (oriented to person, place, and time)
3 (to sound)	5 (localizes pain)	4 (confused conversation)
2 (to pain)	4 (normal flexion)	3 (inappropriate words)
1 (no response)	3 (abnormal flexion)	2 (incomprehensible sounds)
	2 (extension)	1 (no response)
	1 (no response)	

◆ Watch for signs of acute respiratory distress syndrome and traumatic delirium; if the patient experienced an open head injury, look for signs of infection, which could point to meningitis or brain abscess

◆ Initiate range-of-motion (ROM) exercises (unless contraindicated by increased ICP) to prevent complications of immobility

◆ Provide appropriate nutritional support, including enteral or parenteral feedings if the patient can't eat; nutritional deficits impede healing and lead to muscle wasting; check cough and gag reflex to prevent aspiration

◆ Provide emotional support to the patient and his family; remember that the injury may be fatal or severely alter the patient's lifestyle and that the patient may require extensive rehabilitation

❖ Increased intracranial pressure

■ Description

◆ ICP is a measure of the pressure in the cranial cavity; 0 to 15 mm Hg is normal, 16 to 20 mm Hg is mildly elevated, 21 to 30 mm Hg is moderately elevated, and 31 mm Hg or more is severely elevated

◆ The adult skull has a fixed volume of intracranial components, which consist of 80% brain tissue, 10% blood, and 10% CSF

▶ According to the Monro-Kellie doctrine, an increase in any of the three components must be offset by a decrease in the others

▶ If this balancing out doesn't occur, ICP increases

◆ Autoregulation adjusts cerebral blood flow and CSF production and reabsorption to maintain normal ICP; it can no longer maintain normal pressure when ICP exceeds 33 mm Hg or the mean arterial pressure (MAP) exceeds 160 mm Hg

◆ Cerebral perfusion pressure (CPP) is the pressure at which the brain cells are perfused; CPP = MAP − ICP; CPP is normally 60 mm Hg

◆ Several factors may increase ICP: cerebral edema resulting from infection, intracranial or subarachnoid bleeding, or brain tumor; cytotoxic cerebral edema resulting from a metabolic disorder; interstitial cerebral edema caused by blocked CSF reabsorption; intracranial or subarachnoid bleeding; or vasogenic cerebral edema caused by trauma

■ Signs and symptoms

◆ An altered LOC is usually the earliest sign of increased ICP

▶ The patient may exhibit partial or total loss of motor and sensory function

▶ Pupillary changes may occur, such as unequal size, constriction, dilation, or reduced or absent responses to light

▶ Cushing's triad (bradycardia, bradypnea, and hypertension) is a late sign of increased ICP

◆ Other signs and symptoms include changes in respiratory patterns, headache, seizures, vomiting, and a widening pulse pressure

■ Diagnosis and treatment

◆ Diagnosis is based on CT scan, skull X-rays, and ICP monitoring

◆ The goal of treatment is to normalize ICP and avoid complications

◆ Pressures are carefully monitored by means of epidural monitoring, subarachnoid screw and bolt, or intraventricular monitoring

◆ CSF blockage is corrected by surgical placement of shunts; tumor or hematoma also is removed surgically; craniectomy or burr holes may be required for decompression

◆ Drug therapy may include an antibiotic to treat or prevent infection, an anticonvulsant to prevent seizures, and a diuretic to prevent cerebral edema

◆ Hyperventilation therapy is used to reduce the partial pressure of carbon dioxide in arterial blood level, which decreases cerebral edema and ICP

◆ Metabolic disorders are corrected

◆ Lumbar puncture is contraindicated in a patient with increased ICP because it can cause life-threatening herniation (shifting of brain contents into another compartment)

■ Nursing interventions

◆ Provide bed rest, with the head of the bed elevated 30 to 45 degrees to promote venous drainage from the cranium

◆ Avoid neck extension, flexion, and rotation to promote optimal venous drainage

◆ Avoid hip flexion above 60 degrees, which can lead to increased intra-abdominal pressure that increases ICP

◆ Monitor and document fluid intake and output until the patient's condition is stable to ensure proper hydration

▶ Excessive urine output may indicate diabetes insipidus due to posterior pituitary gland damage; it's treated with vasopressin

▶ Fluid retention may indicate SIADH due to craniocerebral trauma; it's treated with fluid restriction

◆ Slowly infuse I.V. bolus medications; rapid infusion can trigger an abrupt increase in brain fluid volume

◆ Administer an analgesic, an antibiotic, an anticonvulsant, and a diuretic as prescribed

◆ Perform neurologic assessments hourly until the patient's condition is stable, to help prevent complications, and then every 4 hours or as prescribed; watch for changes in LOC and motor responses using the Glasgow Coma Scale (see *Using the Glasgow Coma Scale*, page 163)

◆ Monitor vital signs hourly until the patient's condition is stable

◆ Monitor patient for signs of bleeding and hypovolemia—for example, by checking stools, urine, and vomitus for occult blood; systemic bleeding may signal coagulopathy, which increases the risk of intracranial bleeding

◆ Place pads loosely over the ears or under the nose to absorb leaking CSF (a clear liquid that leaves yellow halos on linen and tests positive for glucose); change pads frequently to prevent pathogens from migrating through the CSF to the brain

◆ Use aseptic technique to prevent systemic or intracranial infection, which increases the risk of further increases in ICP

◆ Closely monitor respiratory status by auscultating breath sounds and checking tissue oxygenation with noninvasive pulse oximeters; encourage deep breathing

  ❭ Hypoxemia and hypercapnia further elevate ICP; coughing and inspired spirometry temporarily increase ICP

  ❭ Bed rest and altered LOC increase the risks of atelectasis and pneumonia

◆ Assist with turning in bed, and teach the patient to breathe while moving to avoid straining, which can increase ICP

◆ Maintain a quiet environment: limit noise, light, visitors, and emotional stress; overstimulation can increase ICP

◆ Provide nutritional support as appropriate to maintain normal fluid and electrolyte balance; tube feedings may be required

◆ Teach the patient to avoid performing Valsalva's maneuver; also, tell him to avoid coughing, holding his breath while lifting, sneezing, straining during defecation, and vomiting; all of these actions increase ICP

◆ Provide emotional support to the patient and his family

❖ Meningitis

■ Description

  ◆ Meningitis is an infection of the subarachnoid space and meninges

  ◆ Exudate formation causes meningeal irritation and increased ICP

  ◆ Meningococcal meningitis is caused by *Neisseria meningitidis,* a highly contagious organism

  ◆ *Haemophilus influenzae* meningitis is the most common bacterial meningitis in infants and children

  ◆ Pneumococcal meningitis is caused by *Streptococcus pneumoniae;* it can be a severe complication of an upper respiratory tract infection, is the most common type of meningitis after neurosurgery, and has a high mortality rate

  ◆ Tuberculous meningitis is a bacterial infection caused by *Mycobacterium tuberculosis;* it's generally self-limiting and benign

◆ Infecting organisms gain entry to the subarachnoid space through basilar skull fractures with dural tears, chronic otitis media or sinusitis, neurosurgical contamination, penetrating head wounds, or septicemia

■ Signs and symptoms

◆ The cardinal signs and symptoms of meningitis are those of infection (including chills, fever, and malaise) and those of increased ICP (including headache and vomiting)

◆ Other signs and symptoms include changes in LOC, irritability, and seizures

◆ Signs and symptoms of brain and spinal cord irritation may include Brudzinski's sign (leg adduction and flexion when the neck is flexed), Kernig's sign (resistance to extension when thigh is flexed up to the abdomen), nuchal rigidity, and severe headache

◆ Irritation of cranial nerve (CN) II may cause blindness and papilledema; of CN III, IV, and VI, diplopia, impaired ocular movement, ptosis, and unequal pupils; of CN V, photophobia; of CN VII, facial paresis; and of CN VIII, tinnitus or deafness and vertigo

■ Diagnosis and treatment

◆ Diagnosis may be based on physical examination findings and the results of lumbar puncture, serologic studies, and cultures of blood, urine, nasal or pharyngeal mucosa, sputum, and skin lesions

◆ Meningitis is treated with organism-specific antibiotic therapy

◆ An anticonvulsant may be administered to decrease the risk of seizures; an analgesic may be given to reduce headache, which is common with meningitis

◆ Prophylactic antibiotic therapy may be prescribed for family members and other people who have had close contact with a patient who has bacterial meningitis

◆ Supportive measures include reducing fever, ensuring adequate hydration and nutrition, providing mechanical ventilation, if necessary, and preventing and treating increased ICP

■ Nursing interventions

◆ Perform neurologic examinations, and check vital signs hourly; early detection of increased ICP, hyperthermia, hydrocephalus, and shock can help prevent complications

◆ Implement isolation techniques if the causative agent is highly contagious; bacterial meningitis is transmitted by direct and sometimes indirect contact with respiratory droplets from infected people and carriers

◆ Report meningococcal meningitis to local health authorities; report other bacterial meningitis in endemic areas only

◆ Monitor fluid intake and output to prevent overhydration, which can lead to cerebral edema and increased ICP

◆ Provide nutritional support to maintain immune response and fluid and electrolyte balance; enteral feedings may be required

◆ Provide proper positioning, skin care, and ROM exercises to prevent complications of immobility, such as contracture deformities, muscle wasting, pneumonia, and pressure ulcers

◆ Provide a comfortable, quiet, dimly lit environment to help prevent seizures and to reduce the discomfort of photophobia
◆ Give emotional support to the patient and family
◆ Provide referrals for rehabilitation if neurologic deficits are permanent

❖ Multiple sclerosis
- ■ Description
  - ◆ Multiple sclerosis is a progressive, neurologic disease caused by destruction, injury, or malformation of the myelin sheaths that cover nerves
  - ◆ Plaques (areas of demyelination) can occur anywhere in the nervous system but are most common on the white matter of the brain and spinal cord and the optic nerves; plaques slow or stop saltatory conduction, the normally rapid conduction of nerve impulses
  - ◆ Although the exact cause is unknown, multiple sclerosis may be triggered by a slow, progressive viral disease; an autoimmune disorder; or an allergic reaction to an infection
  - ◆ Multiple sclerosis is characterized by unpredictable exacerbations and remissions; symptoms worsen with each episode
- ■ Signs and symptoms
  - ◆ Symptoms of multiple sclerosis may be transient, variable, and bizarre
  - ◆ The first symptoms are usually sensory and visual problems, such as burning, electrical sensations, and pins and needles
  - ◆ Ocular disturbances may include blurred vision, diplopia, nystagmus, ophthalmoplegia, and optic neuritis
  - ◆ Muscle dysfunction — including gait ataxia, hyperreflexia, intention tremor, paralysis ranging from monoplegia to quadriplegia, spasticity, and weakness — may also occur
  - ◆ Urinary disturbances may include frequency, incontinence, urgency, and frequent infections
  - ◆ Bowel problems include constipation and involuntary evacuation
  - ◆ Fatigue is usually the most debilitating symptom; speech disturbance may also occur
- ■ Diagnosis and treatment
  - ◆ Diagnostic tests may include lumbar puncture, CT scan, evoked response, and MRI of the brain and spinal cord to detect plaques from multiple sclerosis; optic atrophy typically is present, and evoked potential of the brain stem and rolandic somatosensory responses may be abnormal
  - ◆ Because multiple sclerosis has no cure, treatment aims to decrease the length and severity of exacerbations and diminish or reverse the deficits caused by exacerbations
  - ◆ Drug therapy consists of a corticosteroid and a muscle relaxant; interferon beta-1b may be used to reduce the frequency of exacerbations in patients with relapsing-remitting multiple sclerosis; glatiramer acetate may also be helpful in reducing the frequency of relapses in such patients
  - ◆ Occupational, physical, and speech therapies and nutritional counseling are used to help the patient manage the disorder's effects
  - ◆ The patient may also need home care, or he may need to stay in an extended-care facility

■ Nursing interventions
 ◆ Teach the patient and his family about the disease and strategies for avoiding stress, fatigue, and infections, factors that can exacerbate it
 ◆ Administer carbamazepine, phenytoin, or amitriptyline to control pain from dysesthesias or other pain syndromes such as trigeminal neuralgia; transcutaneous electrical nerve stimulation and alternative measures such as relaxation techniques can also help
 ◆ Encourage the patient to participate in physical therapy to maintain muscle strength and decrease spasms
 ◆ Encourage the patient to eat a balanced diet to maintain proper functioning of the immune system and avoid constipation
 ◆ Initiate bowel and bladder training; loss of muscle and sphincter tone may require self-catheterization and daily suppositories
 ◆ Encourage good respiratory hygiene; tell the patient and family to contact the health care provider if the patient develops dyspnea, shortness of breath, or pulmonary infection
 ◆ Teach the patient and caregivers how to prevent complications of immobility; if bed rest or a wheelchair is required, discuss transfer techniques and proper turning and positioning to prevent deformity
 ◆ Develop alternative forms of communication for use during exacerbations, such as eyelid blinking or using letter or picture boards
 ◆ Teach the patient to alternate rest and activity, avoid temperature extremes, and reduce stress
 ◆ Refer the patient to a support group or a local chapter of the Multiple Sclerosis Society

❖ **Myasthenia gravis**
 ■ Description
 ◆ Myasthenia gravis is a chronic autoimmune disorder of neuromuscular transmission characterized by extreme, abnormal muscle weakness during activity; weakness can be relieved by rest
 ◆ It may be caused by a defect of the postsynaptic receptor sites or acetylcholine deficiency
 ◆ It affects neuromuscular transmission at the myoneural junction, leaving sensation intact and preventing muscle atrophy
 ■ Signs and symptoms
 ◆ The dominant symptoms of myasthenia gravis are skeletal muscle fatigability and weakness; typically, muscles are strongest in the morning but weaken throughout the day, especially after exercise
 ◆ The first indications may include weak eye closure, diplopia, and ptosis
 ◆ The face may be blank and expressionless; the voice, nasal
 ◆ The patient experiences difficulty chewing and swallowing
 ◆ Weakened respiratory muscles may make breathing difficult, leading to respiratory distress
 ■ Diagnosis and treatment
 ◆ Diagnostic tests may include thymus scan (to rule out the presence of thymoma and thymic hyperplasia, both of which are associated with

myasthenia gravis), chest X-ray, thyroid studies, electromyography, and Tensilon test (to evaluate muscle contractility); if the Tensilon test is inconclusive, a neostigmine test is done

   ◆ An anticholinesterase alleviates symptoms but is ineffective during a crisis

   ◆ Corticosteroid and immunosuppressive therapy and thymectomy (if thymomas are present) may alter the course of the disease

   ◆ Plasmapheresis may relieve symptoms; it may be used to prepare the patient for thymectomy and during a respiratory crisis

   ◆ Ventilator support may be needed during a myasthenic crisis

■ Nursing interventions

   ◆ Support respiratory function, encourage coughing and deep breathing, and use nasotracheal or oral tracheal suction when necessary to keep the airway open; use mechanical ventilation or a tracheostomy tube, if prescribed

   ◆ Schedule activity 20 to 30 minutes after medication is given, when strength is greatest, and space activities to avoid fatigue

   ◆ If the patient can't chew and swallow solid food, provide a semisoft diet; make sure he doesn't choke on liquids as a result of cranial nerve weakness

   ◆ Assess the patient for signs and symptoms of myasthenic crisis, such as anxiety, fever, increased weakness, problems with chewing and swallowing, and respiratory distress

   ◆ Assess the patient for signs and symptoms of cholinergic crisis, such as abdominal cramps, bradycardia, diarrhea, dyspnea, general weakness, lacrimation, muscle cramps, myasthenic crisis, nausea, respiratory distress, salivation, sweating, vomiting, and wheezing

   ◆ Teach the patient and his family about the disease, and suggest lifestyle changes such as scheduling activities during energy peaks

   ◆ Teach the patient and his family the signs of anticholinesterase toxicity—such as diaphoresis, dyspnea, increased muscle weakness, nausea, and ptosis—to ensure prompt intervention

   ◆ Teach the patient and his family the signs of respiratory distress and failure

   ◆ Provide emotional support, and refer the patient to the Myasthenia Gravis Foundation of America

❖ Parkinson's disease

■ Description

   ◆ Parkinson's disease is a chronic, degenerative disease of the basal ganglia, substantia nigra, and corpus striatum of the brain; it's associated with a deficiency of the neurotransmitter dopamine

   ◆ Although the exact cause of Parkinson's disease is unknown, possible causes include exposure to a toxic agent such as carbon monoxide and manganese, genetic factors, vascular (arteriosclerotic) changes, and viral infection

◆ Iatrogenic Parkinson's disease can result from the use of major tranquilizers, methyldopa, and reserpine; it's generally reversible within 2 weeks of discontinuing the drug

■ Signs and symptoms

◆ Movement changes may include bradykinesia (extreme slowness of movement), cogwheel tremor or rigidity (jerky limb movement), festination (tendency to speed up each step to compensate for a displaced center of gravity), pill-rolling tremor (repeated rotary movement of the thumb and forefinger), and a slow, shuffling gait

◆ Other symptoms include decreased blinking; dysarthria; dysphagia; excessive drooling; micrographia (handwriting that becomes progressively smaller); oculogyric crisis (involuntary deviation and fixation of the eyeballs); slow, slurred, monotone speech; and wide-eyed, blank facial expression

■ Diagnosis and treatment

◆ Physical examination and health history findings may be confirmed by electromyography

◆ Treatment aims at slowing the progression of symptoms and providing supportive care

◆ Antiparkinsonians are prescribed: Levodopa decreases muscle rigidity and an anticholinergic decreases rigidity and tremors

◆ The antiviral amantadine is used early on to reduce tremors and rigidity

◆ The dopamine receptor agonists bromocriptine (Parlodel), pergolide (Permax), pramipexole dihydrochloride (Mirapex), and ropinirole (Requip) activate dopamine receptors in the basal ganglia

◆ The monoamine oxidase type B inhibitor selegiline allows conservation of dopamine and enhances the therapeutic effect of levodopa

◆ The catechol-O-methyltransferase inhibitors entacapone and tolcapone inhibit the breakdown of dopamine and may be useful as adjuncts to levodopa

◆ Patients may benefit from physical therapy

◆ Referrals may be provided for home health assistants, visiting nurses, adult day care, or nursing home placement

■ Nursing interventions

◆ Administer medications as prescribed

◆ Encourage physical therapy to maintain muscle function as long as possible

◆ Teach the patient and family about the disease and the drugs' adverse effects

◆ Teach the patient and family about home safety; suggest they remove throw rugs and loose carpeting and install grab bars and elevated toilet seats in the bathrooms; recommend the use of a cane or walker for a patient in the later stages of Parkinson's disease

◆ Teach the patient and his family about preventing constipation by encouraging adequate nutrition and hydration; stress the importance of establishing a regular pattern of elimination

◆ Provide emotional support for the patient and family, and refer them to Parkinson's disease support groups

❖ Seizure disorders
- ■ Description
  - ◆ Seizures are sudden paroxysmal discharges of a group of neurons that interfere with normal mental and behavioral activities
  - ◆ Seizures may be triggered by toxic states, electrolyte imbalances, tumors, anoxia, CNS inflammation, increased ICP, or idiopathic causes
- ■ Signs and symptoms
  - ◆ Seizure symptoms vary with the type of seizure (see *Differentiating seizures*, page 172)
  - ◆ Seizures have three phases
    - ▶ The prodromal phase occurs before the seizure and produces auras (sensory signals that warn of an approaching seizure), such as a flash of light, mood or behavior changes, or a sudden sensation of smell or taste; this phase lasts from seconds to days
    - ▶ The ictal phase is the seizure itself
    - ▶ The postictal phase occurs after the seizure and may produce amnesia, confusion, inability to be aroused for minutes or hours, or sleepiness
- ■ Diagnosis and treatment
  - ◆ Diagnosis may be based on CT scan, MRI, EEG, cerebral angiography, medical history, and neurologic examination
  - ◆ Lumbar puncture may be performed to rule out an infectious cause
  - ◆ An anticonvulsant is prescribed to prevent seizures
  - ◆ If the seizures don't respond to drug therapy, the seizure focus may be resected
  - ◆ Brain tumors, if present, are surgically removed
- ■ Nursing interventions
  - ◆ Take seizure precautions during hospitalization to prevent injury
  - ◆ Protect the patient during a seizure
    - ▶ Don't insert a tongue blade into the patient's mouth during an active seizure; forcing one in may break his teeth and lead to aspiration
    - ▶ Safeguard the patient from nearby objects, but don't restrain him; restraining limbs can fracture bones; loosen tight clothing
    - ▶ To maintain a patent airway, turn the patient to his side to prevent aspiration of saliva or stomach contents
  - ◆ After a seizure occurs, document your observations
    - ▶ Note prodromal signs and the time of onset
    - ▶ Write down the specific types of movements and the order in which they occurred, including body parts involved
    - ▶ Note changes in the patient's respiratory pattern
    - ▶ Document eye deviation and pupillary response
    - ▶ Record the time the seizure stopped and any postictal response
  - ◆ Teach the patient and his family about the therapeutic and adverse effects of the prescribed anticonvulsant, the importance of taking medications exactly as prescribed to maintain therapeutic levels, and the need to return for laboratory work to monitor serum drug levels and detect adverse reactions

Differentiating seizures

Seizures can be classified as partial or generalized. Some patients may be affected by more than one type.

Partial seizures

Partial seizures arise from a localized area in the brain and cause specific symptoms. In some patients, partial seizure activity spreads to the entire brain, causing a generalized seizure. Partial seizures include simple partial (Jacksonian motor-type and sensory-type), complex partial (psychomotor or temporal lobe), and secondarily generalized partial seizures.

Simple partial (jacksonian motor-type) seizure
A simple partial seizure begins as a localized motor seizure, which is characterized by a spread of abnormal activity to adjacent areas of the brain. Typically, the patient experiences a stiffening or jerking in one extremity, accompanied by a tingling sensation in the same area. For example, the seizure may start in the thumb and spread to the entire hand and arm. The patient seldom loses consciousness, although the seizure may secondarily progress to a generalized tonic-clonic seizure.

Simple partial (sensory-type) seizure
Perception is distorted in a simple partial seizure. Symptoms can include hallucinations, flashing lights, tingling sensations, a foul odor, vertigo, or déjà vu (the feeling of having experienced something before).

Complex partial (psychomotor or temporal lobe) seizure
Symptoms of a complex partial seizure vary but usually include purposeless behavior. The patient may experience an aura and exhibit overt signs, including a glassy stare, picking at his clothes, aimless wandering, lip-smacking or chewing motions, and unintelligible speech. The seizure may last for a few seconds or as long as 20 minutes. Afterward, mental confusion may last for several minutes; as a result, an observer may mistakenly suspect psychosis or intoxication with alcohol or drugs. The patient has no memory of his actions during the seizure.

Secondarily generalized partial seizure
A secondarily generalized partial seizure can be either simple or complex and can progress to generalized seizures. An aura may precede the progression. Loss of consciousness occurs immediately or within 1 to 2 minutes of the start of the progression.

Generalized seizures

As the term suggests, generalized seizures cause a generalized electrical abnormality in the brain. They include several distinct types, including absence (petit mal), myoclonic, generalized tonic-clonic (grand mal), and akinetic.

Absence (petit mal) seizure
An absence seizure commonly occurs in children but also may affect adults. It usually begins with a brief change in the level of consciousness, indicated by blinking or rolling of the eyes, a blank stare, and slight mouth movements. The patient retains his posture and continues preseizure activity without difficulty. Typically, the seizure lasts from 1 to 10 seconds. The impairment is so brief that the patient is sometimes unaware of it. If not properly treated, these seizures can recur as often as 100 times a day. An absence seizure can progress to a generalized tonic-clonic seizure.

Myoclonic seizure
A myoclonic seizure — also called bilateral massive epileptic myoclonus — is marked by brief, involuntary muscular jerks of the body or extremities, which may occur in a rhythmic manner, and a brief loss of consciousness.

Generalized tonic-clonic (grand mal) seizure
Typically, a generalized tonic-clonic seizure begins with a loud cry, precipitated by air rushing from the lungs through the vocal cords. The patient falls to the ground, losing consciousness. The body stiffens (tonic phase) and then alternates between episodes of muscle spasm and relaxation (clonic phase). Tongue biting, incontinence, labored breathing, apnea, and subsequent cyanosis may also occur. The seizure stops in 2 to 5 minutes, when abnormal electrical conduction of the neurons is completed. The patient then regains consciousness but is somewhat confused and may have difficulty talking. If he can talk, he may complain of drowsiness, fatigue, headache, muscle soreness, and arm or leg weakness. He may fall into a deep sleep after the seizure.

Akinetic seizure
An akinetic seizure is characterized by a general loss of postural tone and a temporary loss of consciousness. This type of seizure occurs in young children. Sometimes it's called a drop attack because it causes the child to fall.

◆ Advise the patient to avoid oral thermometers, which can be swallowed or broken if a seizure occurs

◆ Instruct the patient to avoid alcohol and nicotine; these stimulants can precipitate a seizure

◆ Tell the patient he should always carry identification stating that he has seizures and listing the name and phone number of his practitioner

◆ Refer the patient to the Epilepsy Foundation for additional support and strategies for living with epilepsy

❖ Spinal cord injury

■ Description

◆ Spinal cord injury usually results from traumatic force on the vertebral column, which, in turn, injures the spinal cord

◆ Spinal cord injury includes concussion, contusion, hemorrhage, herniated disk syndrome, laceration, transection, and vertebral fractures (see *Types of spinal cord injury,* page 174)

◆ *Complete spinal cord injury* or lesion causes loss of voluntary motor function, all sensations, and proprioception below the level of the lesion

▶ Paraplegia (paralysis of both legs) results from spinal cord injuries from the level of T1 down

▶ Quadriplegia (paralysis of all arms and legs) results from spinal cord injuries of one or more cervical vertebrae

◆ *Incomplete spinal cord injury* or lesion leaves some motor or sensory function intact

▶ Central cord syndrome is damage to the central fibers of the spinal cord; it commonly results from a forced hyperextension injury, causes arterial disruption to the spinal cord, and leads to motor function deficit in the arms and, possibly, the legs

▶ Anterior cord syndrome is damage to the anterior two-thirds of the spinal cord; it usually results from a flexion injury, disrupts the anterior spinal artery, and leads to paralysis and loss of pain and temperature sensation below the lesion (senses of touch, vibration, position, and motion remain intact)

▶ Posterior cord syndrome is damage to the posterior gray and white matter of the spinal cord; it usually results from an extension injury and impairs vibratory sensation, light touch, and proprioception (motor function, pain, and temperature sensation remain intact)

▶ *Brown-Séquard's syndrome* is damage to one side of the spinal cord; it results from a penetrating injury (such as a gunshot or stab wound)

● Rotation-flexion injury causes unilateral damage

● Ipsilateral damage below the lesion affects motor function, pressure and touch sensations, and the senses of vibration and position

● Contralateral damage causes loss of pain and temperature sensations

▶ *Horner's syndrome* can occur as part of Brown-Séquard's syndrome or result from damage to the midbrain; it occurs ipsilaterally to a cervical lesion and causes anhidrosis (lack of sweat), ptosis, and pupillary contraction on the affected side of the face

Types of spinal cord injury

Different spinal cord injuries produce different effects.

Injury	Description	Possible effects
Concussion	Severe shaking	Temporary loss of function for 24 to 48 hours
Contusion	Bruising of the spinal cord	Spinal cord compression by bleeding and edema, causing varying degrees of damage
Dislocated vertebrae	Rupture of spinal ligaments and disruption of vertebral alignment	Spinal cord disruption
Hemorrhage	Bleeding from an aneurysm or other rupture	Spinal cord irritation by blood and edema, causing neurologic deficits
Herniated disk syndrome	Anterior, lateral, or posterior displacement of intervertebral disk, especially in lumbar and lumbosacral areas	Spinal cord injury caused by displaced tissue that compresses nerve roots and narrows the spinal canal
Laceration	Tear in the spinal cord	Spinal cord compression by bleeding and edema, causing permanent damage
Transection	Severing of the spinal cord	Complete or incomplete loss of spinal cord function
Vertebral fracture • Comminuted (burst)	Shattering of vertebrae	Fragment penetration of spinal cord
• Compressed	Compression or anterior wedging of vertebrae	Spinal cord compression
• Odontoid (hangman's)	Fracture of odontoid process of second cervical vertebra	Typically fatal injury of spinal cord and all organs below the fracture
• Simple	Single break, usually of a transverse or spinous process	Spinal cord unaffected if vertebrae remain aligned
• Stable	Fracture without bone displacement	No permanent damage if properly immobilized
• Unstable	Fracture with bone displacement	Spinal cord injury, instant quadriplegia, and loss of respiratory function

◆ Spinal cord injury may result from trauma (see *Mechanisms of spinal cord injury*); it also can result from organic causes, such as arteriovenous malformation, emboli, hematoma, infection, and tumor
■ Motor loss caused by spinal cord injury
 ◆ Paralysis is a temporary or permanent loss of function
  ❱ Spastic paralysis is the loss of voluntary movement caused by damage to upper motor neurons; the lower motor neurons may be intact, in which case, the reflex arc remains intact

---

Mechanisms of spinal cord injury

Spinal cord injury may result from various types of trauma.

Mechanism	Possible effects
Compression injury Caused by vertical fall, such as diving into shallow water	● Vertebral and spinal cord damage
Flexion Caused by violent impact to back of head	● Anterior dislocation of vertebrae ● Rupture of posterior ligaments
Hyperextension (whiplash) Caused by violent impact to the chin	● Rupture of anterior ligaments ● Rupture of intervertebral disks and vertebrae
Penetrating injury Caused by a gunshot wound or stab injury	● Spinal cord damage that disrupts tissue function
Rotation injury Caused by violent rotation in opposite directions of top and bottom of body	● Rupture of ligaments, vertebrae, and disks

---

▮ Flaccid paralysis is the loss of voluntary movement caused by damage to the lower motor neurons; reflexes, including deep tendon reflexes, are lost

◆ Deep tendon reflexes include the biceps reflex, triceps reflex, brachioradialis reflex, patellar reflex, and Achilles tendon reflex; they're graded as 0 (absent), 1+ (diminished), 2+ (normal), 3+ (increased), or 4+ (hyperactive)

◆ Superficial reflexes comprise the abdominal reflex, cremasteric reflex, plantar reflex, and gluteal reflex; they're graded as 0 (absent), +/− (diminished or inconsistent), or + (normal)

■ Level of spinal cord injury and associated motor loss

◆ Injury to the cord at the C1 to C4 level causes quadriplegia and loss of respiratory function

◆ Injury to the cord at the C4 to C5 level causes quadriplegia and may affect respiratory function if edema damages the phrenic nerve

◆ Injury to the cord at the C5 to C6 level causes quadriplegia; gross motor movement of the arms remains intact with use of the scapular elevators; diaphragmatic breathing remains intact but may not be able to support ventilation because of the loss of intercostal muscle innervation

◆ Injury to the cord at the C6 to C7 level causes quadriplegia; diaphragmatic breathing remains intact but may not be able to support ventilation; arm muscles remain innervated and capable of elbow flexion, wrist extension, and weak thumb grasp

◆ Injury to the cord at the C7 to C8 level causes quadriplegia; diaphragmatic breathing remains intact, but ventilation and airway secretion removal may be compromised because of loss of intercostal muscle innervation; biceps and triceps muscles respond to voluntary control, and wrist flexion may be possible

◆ Injury to the cord between the T1 and L1 to L2 levels causes paraplegia; voluntary motor function of the arms remains intact; loss of some intercostal muscle innervation may impede ventilation and secretion removal

◆ Injury to the cauda equina causes mixed loss of motor, sensory, bowel, bladder, and sexual function and depends on which roots are damaged

◆ Injury to the sacral spinal nerves causes loss of bowel, bladder, and sexual function

■ Spinal shock

◆ Spinal shock is caused by sudden, severe spinal cord damage and initially produces flaccid paralysis; areflexia below the level of the lesion and loss of cutaneous and proprioceptive sensations occur in the first few hours and may last for weeks

◆ Recovery occurs over time; reflex activity returns in 3 to 6 weeks; flexion spasms affect paralyzed limbs 6 to 16 weeks after injury; alternating flexion and extension spasms affect paralyzed limbs about 6 months after injury; extension spasms predominate after 6 months

■ Autonomic dysreflexia

◆ Autonomic dysreflexia is a complication of complete spinal cord injury

◆ Injuries at or above T6 present the greatest risk, but autonomic dysreflexia has been observed in injuries occurring at the T8 level

◆ Autonomic dysreflexia is a clinical emergency and is caused by stimulation of the autonomic reflexes below the level of the lesion

◆ Autonomic dysreflexia causes decreased heart rate, pallor, pilomotor spasm (goose bumps and hair erection), and severe, persistent hypertension

◆ Other findings include blotchy skin, diaphoresis, flushing, nasal congestion, pounding headache, and vasodilation above the lesion

◆ Autonomic dysreflexia can be precipitated by various sensory stimuli, including a full bladder or rectum, painful stimuli (such as pressure on the skin, pressure ulcers, and surgical incisions), other skin stimulation (such as pressure on the glans penis or perianal or periurethral area), and visceral contractions (such as bladder spasms and uterine contractions of pregnancy)

◆ Treatment aims to control blood pressure while locating and removing the sensory stimulus

■ Diagnosis and treatment

◆ Diagnosis is based on anterior and lateral X-rays of the spine, CT scan, and MRI

◆ Emergency life support is required to maintain vital function and avoid further injury; priorities include maintaining a patent airway; ensuring adequate ventilation (spontaneous or mechanical); maintaining adequate circulation; and performing neurologic assessments

◆ To prevent further injury, the spine is immobilized with a cervical collar, cervical traction or cervical tongs (such as Gardner-Wells, Crutchfield, Barton, Cone, and Vinke), kinetic bed with cervical tongs for skeletal traction, halo brace with vest (for long-term use), or surgery (by means of Harrington rods, Weiss springs, laminectomy, or spinal fusion)

◆ Clots, fragments, and tumors are surgically decompressed

◆ A steroid is administered for the first 24 hours after the injury to reduce edema and inflammatory response

◆ An analgesic and an opioid may be administered to control pain

◆ A muscle relaxant is given to reduce muscle spasm

◆ An antacid and an antihistamine are given to prevent gastric ulcers (traumatic events, such as spinal cord injury, can precipitate gastric ulcer formation)

◆ Anticoagulant therapy is initiated to prevent deep vein thrombosis; therapy may include low doses of heparin, thigh-high antiembolism stockings (which compress superficial veins and prevent peripheral blood pooling), and sequential pneumatic compression devices (which massage the veins, mimic muscle action, and prevent peripheral blood pooling and thrombus formation)

◆ Rehabilitative management includes surgical release of tendons for persistent muscle spasm of paralyzed muscles and surgical correction for cervical support (laminectomy and spinal fusions)

◆ Rehabilitation referrals include those for occupational and physical therapies, nutritional counseling, social services, and psychiatric evaluation and assistance

■ Nursing interventions

◆ Provide respiratory support for a patient with a spinal cord injury above L1 to L2; support ranges from deep-breathing exercises to diaphragmatic coughing (exertion of abdominal pressure during coughing) to mechanical ventilation

◆ Continuously monitor and assess neurologic function to detect early signs of deterioration

◆ Modify the patient's environment to decrease dependence on others and increase his feelings of self-worth; discuss modifications with the patient and his family before discharge; modifications may include manual or electric wheelchairs, ramps, widened doorways, structural changes to bathroom facilities, and home care aides

◆ Provide frequent and proper positioning, skin care, and proper hydration and nutrition to prevent complications of immobility

◆ Teach the patient and his family about the recovery process, therapeutic and adverse effects of prescribed drugs, possible drug interactions, nutritional needs, exercise, bowel and bladder training, ways to prevent constipation and urinary tract infection, self-catheterization techniques, skin care, proper positioning, ways to avoid infection (especially respiratory infection), symptoms to report to the practitioner, and local support groups

◆ Provide emotional support to the patient and family; permanent physical disabilities can be devastating to self-concept, relationships, and lifestyle; emotional support, particularly from others with similar experiences, can facilitate healing

❖ **Stroke**
- ■ Description
  - ◆ Stroke is a disruption in cerebral circulation, causing permanent neurologic deficits
  - ◆ An occlusive stroke may result from atherosclerotic plaque, an embolism, or vasospasm
  - ◆ A thrombotic ischemic stroke occurs when the occlusion evolves from partial to complete and may be heralded by a transient ischemic attack
  - ◆ A hemorrhagic stroke may result from a ruptured or leaking aneurysm, an arteriovenous malformation, a bleeding disorder, trauma, or an arterial rupture (as caused by hypertension)
- ■ Signs and symptoms
  - ◆ Symptoms of stroke vary with the affected artery (see *Signs and symptoms of stroke*)
  - ◆ Symptoms also vary according to the severity of the damage and the extent of collateral circulation
- ■ Diagnosis and treatment
  - ◆ CT scan, MRI, cerebral arteriography, lumbar puncture, Doppler flow studies, and EEG may be used to diagnose stroke
  - ◆ Carotid endarterectomy removes plaque to improve cerebral blood flow
  - ◆ Surgical evacuation of the clot or hematoma relieves increased ICP
  - ◆ Although anticoagulants are contraindicated in a patient with a hemorrhagic stroke, they may be useful in a patient with a nonhemorrhagic thrombolytic event
  - ◆ An anticonvulsant is used to prevent or treat seizures
  - ◆ Tissue plasminogen activator can improve neurologic function when given within 3 hours of the onset of symptoms in a patient with a thrombotic stroke
  - ◆ An analgesic is used to relieve discomfort such as headache
  - ◆ An antihypertensive is used to lower blood pressure and, thus, prevent additional bleeding
  - ◆ A diuretic is used to lower blood pressure and reduce cerebral edema
  - ◆ Physical therapy and occupational therapy help maintain muscle and joint function while teaching the patient needed home management techniques
- ■ Nursing interventions
  - ◆ Provide emergency care; the patient may require lifesaving measures because of cardiopulmonary arrest triggered by the injury; administer oxygen, if needed, to promote oxygenation within the cerebral tissue
  - ◆ Maintain a patent airway; the patient may be unable to protect his airway because of impaired cough and gag reflexes and inability to support his head; suction the patient as necessary

Signs and symptoms of stroke

Signs and symptoms of stroke vary with the artery affected, the severity of the damage, and the extent of collateral circulation. Typical arteries affected and their associated signs and symptoms are described below.

Middle cerebral artery

When a stroke occurs in the middle cerebral artery, the patient may experience:
- altered level of consciousness (LOC)
- aphasia
- contralateral hemiparesis (more severe in the face and arm than in the leg)
- contralateral sensory deficit
- dysgraphia
- dysphagia
- dyslexia
- visual field cuts

Carotid artery

When a stroke occurs in the carotid artery, the patient may experience:
- altered LOC
- aphasia
- bruits over the carotid artery
- headaches
- numbness, paralysis, sensory changes, visual disturbances, and weakness on the affected side
- ptosis

Vertebrobasilar artery

When a stroke occurs in the vertebrobasilar artery, the patient may experience:
- amnesia
- ataxia

- diplopia
- dizziness
- dysphagia
- numbness around the lips and mouth
- poor coordination
- slurred speech
- visual field cuts
- weakness on the affected side

Anterior cerebral artery

When a stroke occurs in the anterior cerebral artery, the patient may experience:
- confusion
- impaired motor and sensory function
- incontinence
- loss of coordination
- numbness and weakness on the affected side
- personality changes

Posterior cerebral arteries

When a stroke occurs in the posterior cerebral arteries, paralysis is usually absent; however, the patient may experience:
- coma
- cortical blindness
- dyslexia
- sensory impairment
- visual field cuts

◆ Make sure the patient maintains bed rest until the cause of the stroke is known because activity can cause bleeding to recur

◆ Position the patient to prevent deformity; loss of muscle tone leads to flexion contractures; turn and position him every 2 hours to prevent pressure ulcers

◆ Implement physical therapy to maintain strength and prevent contractures; provide passive range of motion to prevent venous thrombosis and contractures

◆ Speak slowly and simply; the patient may not be able to understand rapid speech and may become confused

◆ Monitor vital signs at least hourly until the patient's condition is stable; alterations can indicate further injury

◆ Assess neurologic status hourly until the patient's condition is stable; early identification and treatment of increased ICP (signs include abnormal posturing, bradycardia, decreased LOC, decreased motor response, increased systolic blood pressure, and widened pulse pressure) may prevent further injury

◆ Monitor fluid input and output hourly to ensure hydration until the patient's condition is stable

◆ Ensure nutritional status by helping the patient to eat or by providing enteral or parenteral feedings when necessary

◆ Provide for toileting needs; use aseptic technique with indwelling urinary catheters to prevent infections, and begin a bowel retraining program to reestablish continence

◆ Modify nursing care for left- and right-hemisphere stroke

> ◗ Left-hemisphere stroke causes expressive, global, or receptive aphasia (in most people, the left side is dominant for speech); right-sided hemiparesis or hemiplegia; right visual field deficit; and slow, cautious behavior

> ◗ Right-hemisphere stroke causes apparent unawareness of the deficits of the affected side, leading to accidents; distractibility, impulsive behavior, and poor judgment; left-sided hemiparesis or hemiplegia; left visual field deficit; and spatial-perceptual deficits

◆ Teach the patient and his family how to use assistive devices, such as walkers and braces

◆ Refer the patient and his family to the American Stroke Association for support groups

Review questions

1. The nurse is caring for a patient with a C7 spinal cord injury who develops bradycardia, hypertension, and sweating. Which intervention should the nurse perform first?

○ **A.** Palpating the patient's bladder

○ **B.** Lying the patient flat in bed

○ **C.** Covering the patient with a blanket

○ **D.** Performing a rectal examination

Correct answer: A   Bradycardia, hypertension, and sweating are signs of autonomic dysreflexia, a complication that may occur with a spinal cord injury at or above T6. Because a distended bladder is one of the most common causes of autonomic dysreflexia, the nurse should palpate the patient's bladder for fullness. If the patient has an indwelling urinary catheter, the nurse should check it for patency and kinks. Option B is incorrect because appropriate interventions for autonomic dysreflexia include elevating the head of the bed to promote cerebral venous return; dangling the patient's feet over the side of the bed, if possible, to promote an orthostatic reduction in blood pressure; and keeping the patient from lying flat. Option C is incorrect because anything that may stimulate the skin, such as a blanket or shoes, should be removed. Although a distended rectum is another common cause of autonomic dysreflexia, option D is incorrect because the nurse shouldn't check for fecal impaction until an anesthetic has been applied to reduce stimulation.

2. The nurse is caring for a comatose patient who has suffered a closed head injury. Which intervention should the nurse implement to prevent increases in ICP?

○ **A.** Suctioning the airway every hour and as needed

○ **B.** Elevating the head of the bed 30 to 45 degrees

○ **C.** Turning the patient and changing his position every 2 hours

○ **D.** Maintaining a well-lit room

Correct answer: B   To facilitate venous drainage and avoid jugular compression, the nurse should elevate the head of the bed 30 to 45 degrees. Option A is incorrect because patients with increased ICP poorly tolerate suctioning and shouldn't be suctioned on a regular basis. Option C is incorrect because turning from side to side increases the risk of jugular compression and rises in ICP. Option D is incorrect because the room should be kept quiet and dimly lit.

3. The nurse is teaching the patient with multiple sclerosis. When teaching the patient how to reduce fatigue, the nurse should tell the patient to:

○ **A.** take a hot bath.

○ **B.** rest in an air-conditioned room.

○ **C.** increase the dose of his muscle relaxant.

○ **D.** avoid naps during the day.

Correct answer: B   Fatigue is a common symptom in patients with multiple sclerosis. Lowering the body temperature by resting in an air-conditioned room may relieve fatigue; however, extreme cold should be avoided. Option A is incorrect because a hot bath or shower can increase body temperature and produce fatigue. Option C is incorrect because muscle relaxants are prescribed to reduce spasticity and can cause drowsiness and fatigue. Option D is incorrect because taking frequent rest periods and naps can relieve fatigue. Other measures to reduce fatigue in the patient with multiple sclerosis include treating depression, using occupational therapy to learn energy conservation techniques, and reducing spasticity.

4. To encourage adequate nutritional intake for a patient with Alzheimer's disease, the nurse should:

○ **A.** stay with the patient, and encourage him to eat.

○ **B.** help the patient fill out his menu.

○ **C.** give the patient privacy during meals.

○ **D.** fill out the menu for the patient.

Correct answer: A   Staying with the patient and encouraging him to feed himself will ensure adequate food intake. A patient with Alzheimer's disease can forget to eat. Filling out the patient's menu (option B), allowing privacy during meals (option C), or filling out the menu for the patient (option D) don't ensure adequate nutritional intake.

5. The nurse is teaching a patient and his family about dietary practices related to Parkinson's disease. A priority for the nurse to address is risk of:

○ **A.** fluid overload and drooling.

○ **B.** aspiration and anorexia.

○ **C.** choking and diarrhea.

○ **D.** dysphagia and constipation.

Correct answer: D   Eating problems associated with Parkinson's disease include aspiration, choking, constipation, and dysphagia. Option A is incorrect since fluid overload isn't specifically related to Parkinson's disease and, although drooling occurs with Parkinson's disease, it doesn't take priority. Anorexia (option B) and diarrhea (option C) aren't specifically associated with Parkinson's disease.

Musculoskeletal disorders

❖ Introduction
- ■ The musculoskeletal system provides the structure and leverage that permits mobility
  - ◆ Bones of the skeletal system serve as a reservoir for calcium and a manufacturing facility for red blood cells, white blood cells (WBCs), and platelets
  - ◆ Alterations in the musculoskeletal system can result from soft-tissue injury, bone fractures, infections, and tumors
- ■ Various tests are used to assess musculoskeletal integrity

❖ Nursing history
- ■ The nurse asks the patient about his *chief complaint*
  - ◆ The patient with a joint injury may report a joint deformity, pain, stiffness, swelling, or sensory alteration
  - ◆ A patient with a fracture may report deformity or pain
  - ◆ A patient with a muscular injury may report pain, swelling, weakness, or sensory alteration
- ■ The nurse then questions the patient about his *present illness*
  - ◆ Ask the patient about his symptom, including when it started, associated symptoms, location, radiation, intensity, duration, frequency, and precipitating and alleviating factors
  - ◆ Ask the patient if activities of daily living are affected; question him about the use of assistive devices, such as a cane, walker, or crutches
  - ◆ Ask about the use of prescription and over-the-counter drugs, herbal remedies, and vitamin and nutritional supplements
- ■ The nurse asks about *medical history*
  - ◆ Question the patient about other musculoskeletal disorders, such as arthritis, gout, osteoporosis, and trauma
  - ◆ Ask the female patient whether she uses an oral contraceptive or is undergoing hormone therapy and whether she's premenopausal or postmenopausal
- ■ The nurse then assesses the *family history*
  - ◆ Ask about a family history of musculoskeletal problems
  - ◆ Also ask about a family history of chronic and genetic disorders
- ■ The nurse obtains a *social history*
  - ◆ Ask about work, exercise, diet, use of recreational drugs and alcohol, and hobbies
  - ◆ Also ask about stress, support systems, and coping mechanisms

◆ Assess how the patient functions at home; determine his ability to get around, climb stairs, and drive
■ Physical assessment
  ◆ The nurse begins with *inspection*
    ❱ Note the size and shape of joints, limbs, and body regions; note body symmetry
    ❱ Inspect the skin and tissues around joint, limb, or body region for color, swelling, masses, and deformities
    ❱ Observe how the patient stands and moves; watch him walk, noting his gait, posture arm movements, and coordination
    ❱ Inspect the curvature of his spine
    ❱ To check range of motion (ROM), ask the patient to abduct, adduct, and flex or extend affected muscles
    ❱ Inspect major muscle groups for tone, strength, symmetry, and abnormalities; note contractures and abnormal movements, such as spasms, tics, tremors, fasciculations
  ◆ Next, the nurse uses *palpation*
    ❱ Palpate the patient's bones, noting any deformities, masses, or tenderness
    ❱ Evaluate the patient's muscle tone, mass, and strength
    ❱ Palpate joints for tenderness, nodes, crepitus, and temperature at rest and during passive ROM
    ❱ Palpate arterial pulses, and check capillary refill time
    ❱ Check neurovascular status, including movement and sensation

❖ **Dislocations**
  ■ Description
    ◆ A dislocation occurs when the articulating surfaces of a joint come out of position
    ◆ Dislocations may result from trauma, diseases that affect the joint, or congenital weaknesses
    ◆ Dislocations may cause injury to blood vessels and nerves, change in contour of joint, length of the extremity, and change in the axis of the dislocated bones
  ■ Signs and symptoms
    ◆ The patient experiences pain at the affected joint
    ◆ Neurovascular compromise may occur, including loss of movement, paresthesia, and pulselessness
  ■ Diagnosis and treatment
    ◆ Diagnosis is based on patient history, physical examination, and X-rays
    ◆ Treatment consists of open or closed reduction, immobilization, and pain relief
  ■ Nursing interventions
    ◆ Immobilize and elevate the affected joint; apply ice as indicated
    ◆ Assess neurovascular status before and after reduction, including strength of pulse, capillary refill time, sensation, movement, pain, and color of skin

Types and causes of fractures

Type of fracture	Description	Force causing the fracture
Avulsion	Fracture that pulls bone and other tissues from their usual attachments	Direct force with resisted extension of the bone and joint
Closed	Skin is closed but bone is fractured	Minor force
Compression	Fracture in which the bone is squeezed or wedged together at one side	Compressive, axial force applied directly above the fracture site
Greenstick	Break in only one cortex of the bone	Minor direct or indirect force
Impacted	Fracture with one end wedged into the opposite end or into the fractured fragment	Compressive, axial force applied directly to the distal fragment
Linear	Fracture line runs parallel to bone's axis	Minor or moderate direct force applied to the bone
Oblique	Fracture at an oblique angle across both cortices	Direct or indirect force with angulation and some compression
Open	Skin is open, bone is fractured, and soft tissue trauma may occur	Moderate to severe force that is continuous and exceeds tissue tolerances
Pathologic	Transverse, oblique, or spiral fracture of a bone weakened by tumor	Minor direct or indirect force
Spiral	Fracture curves around both cortices	Direct or indirect twisting force, with the distal part of the bone held or unable to move
Stress	Crack in one cortex of a bone	Repetitive direct force, as from jogging, running, or osteoporosis
Transverse	Horizontal break through the bone	Direct or indirect force toward the bone

❖ **Femoral fractures**
- Description
  - ◆ A femoral fracture is a break in the femur anywhere along its shaft
  - ◆ Transverse, oblique, and comminuted fractures are the most common types of femoral fractures and may be open or closed (see *Types and causes of fractures*)
  - ◆ A femoral fracture can occur at any age, as a result of a fall, an accident, a gunshot wound, or other injury
- Signs and symptoms
  - ◆ Pain occurs at the fracture site
  - ◆ Discoloration and deformity may also be present

◆ The fractured limb can't bear weight and may be shortened and externally rotated

◆ Other findings may include an open wound, edema, and bruising

◆ Leg fractures may produce any or all of the five Ps: pain, pallor, paralysis, paresthesia, and pulse loss

■ Diagnosis and treatment

◆ Diagnosis is based on patient history, physical examination, and X-rays that show the type and severity of the fracture

◆ Ice bags are applied to the fracture site

◆ An opioid analgesic and a muscle relaxant are given to relieve pain

◆ If the patient has an open fracture or has undergone surgery to correct the fracture, an antibiotic is administered; tetanus prophylaxis may also be required

◆ Reduction of the fracture restores the displaced bone segments to their normal position

▶ With closed reduction, the bones are aligned by manual manipulation or traction; immobilization is by splint, cast, or traction

▶ With open reduction, the fracture is surgically reduced and immobilized with rods, plates, or screws, and a cast is usually applied

◆ When a splint or cast fails to maintain the reduction, immobilization requires skin or skeletal traction, using a series of weights and pulleys (see *Skeletal and skin tractions*)

▶ With skin traction, elastic bandages and moleskin coverings are used to attach the traction devices to the patient's skin

▶ With skeletal traction, a pin or wire is inserted through the bone distal to the fracture and attached to a weight, allowing more prolonged traction

■ Nursing interventions

◆ Perform neurovascular checks, which will provide data needed to formulate a care plan (see *Neurovascular checks,* page 189)

◆ Assess vital signs, and monitor patient for signs of shock because significant blood loss may occur with a femur fracture

◆ Assess patient for signs of fat embolism — including confusion, dyspnea, hypotension, petechiae on trunk, tachycardia, and tachypnea — can occur following the fracture of a long bone

◆ Apply ice bags to the fracture site; ice causes vasoconstriction, which decreases bleeding and edema and lessens pain

◆ Check and maintain the traction setup, if used (see *Nursing considerations for patients in skeletal or skin traction,* page 190)

◆ Provide good cast care to prevent skin breakdown and other complications

◆ Provide appropriate postoperative care

▶ Keep the fractured leg elevated on a pillow to reduce edema by increasing venous return

▶ Apply ice bags to reduce bleeding and edema

▶ Help the patient sit in a chair with his leg elevated; upright positions increase peripheral circulation, which decreases edema

Skeletal and skin tractions

Type and description	Purpose	Nursing considerations
Skeletal traction **Balanced suspension to femur** Used in patients age 3 and older on the upper tibia and thigh with 20 to 35 lb (9 to 16 kg) of weight	● Realignment of fractures of the femur ● Relief of muscle spasms associated with femoral fractures	● Steinmann pin or Kirschner wire is inserted through the upper tibia. The thigh and leg are suspended in a splint and leg attachment. ● Thigh and leg suspension is counterbalanced by traction to the top of the thigh splint. ● The patient should be recumbent, but he can turn about 30 degrees to either side briefly for back care or lift himself up using the trapeze and the uninjured leg and foot. ● Neurovascular checks are vital to assess circulatory status and prevent compartmental syndrome. ● Tissue pressure monitoring is performed.
Cervical traction via skull tongs Used in patients of any age, but especially in young adults, bilaterally on skull bones with 20 to 30 lb (9 to 14.5 kg) of weight	● Realignment of fractures of cervical vertebrae ● Relief of pressure on cervical nerves	● Patients may be severely injured and may have quadriplegia.
Halo-pelvic traction Used in adolescents and young adults on the skull and pelvis with no weight (bars extending between the skull and pelvic portions hold the body in the desired position)	● Preoperative straightening of scoliosis curvature	● Pins are inserted into the skull in four areas to hold the halo. Pins are inserted through the iliac pelvic bones to hold the pelvis. ● Straightening is accomplished by tightening the bars, which overcomes muscle contractions. ● Traction is "comfortable" after the patient has recovered from the insertional trauma. ● Dressing is complicated because the vertical bars interfere with clothing. ● Traction may remain in place postoperatively to be replaced by a brace or cast. ● Halo-pelvic traction is a variant of halo-femoral traction, in which the pins are inserted through the distal femurs instead of the pelvic bones, and the skull pins pull away from the femoral pins.
Skin traction **Buck's extension** Most commonly used in adults on one or both legs with 5 to 8 lb (2.5 to 3.5 kg) of weight per leg	● Preoperative traction for hip fractures ● "Pulling" contracted muscles ● Relief of leg or back muscle spasms	● Patient generally lies recumbent. ● Patient may be turned to either side if no fracture is present or turned to the unaffected side if fracture is present. ● An older patient's skin is more friable and subject to loosening because of less subcutaneous fat. ● Patient may complain of burning under tape, moleskin, or traction boot. ● Traction may be removed for skin care even if fracture is present.

(continued)

Skeletal and skin tractions *(continued)*

Type and description	Purpose	Nursing considerations
Skin traction (continued) **Cervical head halter** Used in adults under the chin and around the face and back of the head with 5 to 15 lb (2.5 to 7 kg) of weight	● Relief of muscle spasms caused by degenerative or arthritic conditions of the cervical vertebrae or by muscle strain	● Halter should be applied so that the pull comes from the occipital area, not through the chin portion. ● Patients may be in low- or high-Fowler's position, depending on the purpose of the traction. ● If the patient complains of pain in the chin, teeth, or temporomandibular joint, the halter may be incorrectly positioned. Side straps should be adjusted to relieve these complaints. ● Patients should be removed from traction for sleeping. ● Patients can use this type of traction at home for cervical arthritic conditions.
Cotrel's traction Used in adolescents and young adults with a head halter (5 to 7 lb [2.5 to 3 kg]) and a pelvic belt (10 to 20 lb [4.5 to 9 kg])	● Preoperative muscle stretching in patients with scoliosis	● Pulling in opposite directions may cause pain or discomfort. ● Traction can be removed briefly for massage and skin care.
Dunlop's traction Used in adolescents and young adults on the lower humerus (5 to 7 lb) and forearm (3 to 5 lb [1.5 to 2.5 kg])	● Realignment of fractures of the humerus	● Body is used for countertraction by slightly elevating side of bed of arm in traction. ● Forearm is held at a right angle to the humerus for comfort, by using Buck's extension on the forearm. ● Dunlop's traction can be used for skin traction (using Buck's extension to the humerus) or skeletal traction (using a Steinmann pin inserted through the distal humerus); use of skin or skeletal traction depends on the patient's injury. ● Traction to the forearm should be removed daily for skin care.
Pelvic belt or girdle Used in older adolescents and adults on the abdomen or pelvis with 20 to 35 lb of weight	● Relief of muscle spasms and pain associated with disk conditions	● Pull comes from iliac crests to relieve spasm. ● Patient may be placed in the William's position, which permits 45-degree knee and hip flexion to relax the lumbosacral muscles. ● Orders typically are "in traction 2 hours, out 2 hours" and out of traction at night. ● Traction straps shouldn't put pressure on sciatic nerves.
Pelvic sling Used in adults under the pelvis and buttocks like a hammock with 20 to 35 lb of weight	● Holding of fractured pelvic bones	● Buttocks must be slightly off the bed. ● Patients are comfortable in the sling even with extensive pelvic bruising. ● They may become dependent on the sling and may require gradual weaning. ● The sling should be kept clean and dry. ● Patients can be removed from the sling for care and toileting if facility policy permits.
Russell traction Used in patients age 5 and older on one or both legs with 2 to 5 lb (1 to 2.5 kg) of weight per leg	● Preoperative traction for hip fractures ● "Pulling" contracted muscles ● Treatment of Legg-Calvé-Perthes disease	● Pulley placement and amount of weight used are based on the principle that "for every force in one direction, there is an equal force in the opposite direction." ● Patient is positioned on back for most effective pull. ● Knee sling can be loosened for skin care and checking pulses in popliteal area.

Neurovascular checks

Fractures may cause nerve or arterial damage, producing any or all of the five Ps: pain, pallor, paralysis, paresthesia, and pulselessness. When performing a neurovascular check, compare findings bilaterally and above and below the fracture.

Pain

Ask the patient if he's having pain. Assess the location, severity, and quality of the pain as well as anything that seems to relieve or worsen it. Pain that is unrelieved by an opioid or that worsens with elevating the limb (elevation reduces circulation and worsens ischemia) may indicate compartment syndrome.

Pallor

Paleness, discoloration, and coolness of the injured site may indicate neurovascular compromise from decreased blood supply to the area. Check capillary refill time. Tissues should return to normal color within 3 seconds. Palpate skin temperature with the back of your hand.

Paralysis

Note any deficits in movement or strength. If the patient can't move the affected area or if movement causes severe pain and muscle spasms, he might have nerve or tendon damage. For a femoral fracture, assess peroneal nerve injury by checking for sensation over the top of the foot between the first and second toes.

Paresthesia

Ask the patient about changes in sensation, such as numbness or tingling. Check for loss of sensation by touching the injured area with the tip of an open safety pin or the point of a paper clip. Abnormal sensation or loss of sensation indicates neurovascular involvement.

Pulselessness

Palpate peripheral pulses distal to the injury, noting rate and quality. If a pulse is decreased or absent, blood supply to the area is reduced.

❯ Help the patient use an ambulatory aid when prescribed; weight bearing is restricted until some bone union occurs
❯ Administer an opioid analgesic, or monitor the use of patient-controlled analgesia
❯ Encourage the patient to perform leg and foot exercises to maintain muscle and joint strength and decrease venous stasis
❯ Change dressings as needed, using strict aseptic technique, and administer an antibiotic, if prescribed; the patient is susceptible to wound infection and, possibly, osteomyelitis
❯ Provide good pin care by covering the ends with cork or tape to prevent injury, and assess pin site for signs of inflammation or infection
❯ Assess patient for signs of compartment syndrome (for example, pallor; paresthesia; paralysis; and pain that is throbbing, intensifies with elevation, is unrelenting, and uncontrolled with analgesics)
❯ Monitor fluid intake and output to ensure fluid balance
◆ Help with discharge planning by anticipating the patient's discharge needs

Nursing considerations for patients in skeletal or skin traction

Nursing action	Rationale
Check ropes, knots, pulleys, freedom of movement, and intactness.	These actions help ensure that the traction is functioning properly.
Check the entire traction setup, pin site, and all suspension apparatus for tightness or signs of loosening.	These actions help ensure that the traction is functioning properly.
Check weights to ensure that they're hanging freely.	This action helps ensure that there is a proper amount of traction.
Make sure the weights aren't "lifted" during care.	This action helps to avoid pain caused by sudden muscle contraction and disrupted fragments of the injured or fractured bone. (Patients in skeletal traction should be moved for position changes without lifting or releasing the weights.)
Take care not to bump the weights or weight holders.	This action helps to avoid pain caused by rope movements that affect the traction bow and pin.
Check all skin surfaces for signs of tolerance or pressure areas (especially on the occipital area of the head, shoulder blades, elbows, coccyx, and heels).	These actions may uncover signs of pressure, which include redness, tenderness or pain, soreness caused by excoriation, and numbness.
Provide physical and psychological comfort. Answer questions honestly, answer the call light promptly, provide prompt and thorough care, encourage patient participation in care, provide diversionary activities, and prepare the patient and family for discharge.	These actions help ensure that the patient participates in and is prepared for self-care.

❖ **Hip fracture**
- Description
  - ◆ Hip fracture is a fracture of the head, neck, trochanteric, or subtrochanteric regions of the femur
    - ▶ *Intracapsular* fractures are those of the femoral head and neck, which are inside the hip capsule; the hip capsule is made up of ligaments surrounding the hip joint
    - ▶ *Extracapsular* fractures are those of the femoral trochanteric and subtrochanteric regions, which lie outside the ligaments of the hip capsule
  - ◆ Hip fractures are most common in older people, particularly elderly women; many are associated with osteoporosis and falls
- Signs and symptoms
  - ◆ The fractured limb is shortened and rotated externally; it can't bear weight
  - ◆ Other findings include hip discoloration, pain, and tenderness
- Diagnosis and treatment
  - ◆ Diagnosis is based on patient history, physical examination, and X-rays

◆ Buck's extension or Russell traction to the affected limb is used before surgery to increase comfort and reduce muscle spasms

◆ Intracapsular fracture requires open reduction with prosthetic replacement because of the high risk of loss of blood supply to the head of the femur, which leads to avascular necrosis

◆ Extracapsular fracture requires insertion of a sliding compression hip nail, hip nail with side plate, or multiple pins

■ Preoperative nursing interventions

◆ Monitor traction setup and functioning; skin traction is used as a temporary measure to reduce muscle spasms and increase patient comfort and safety

◆ Monitor neurovascular status; trauma disrupts arterial and venous vessels, leading to bruising, edema, pain, and color changes

◆ Monitor vital signs; fluctuating vital signs may be caused by shock (up to 1,000 ml of blood may be lost into the hip joint), trauma, or a preexisting vascular condition; temperature typically is below normal unless a urinary or respiratory tract infection exists

◆ Perform other preoperative care, such as giving the patient nothing by mouth, having him empty his bladder, and checking his vital signs

◆ Send an abduction pillow to the operating room if the patient is receiving a prosthesis; the pillow helps keep the prosthesis in the hip joint until muscles and ligaments heal

■ Postoperative nursing interventions

◆ Monitor vital signs and neurovascular status; surgical repair of hip fracture is traumatic because of bone and tissue injuries and can lead to complications, such as thrombophlebitis and fat or pulmonary embolism

◆ Monitor the amount and type of wound drainage; drainage should be serosanguineous and should total no more than 200 ml over 3 days

◆ Position the affected limb properly to prevent dislocation; use abduction if a prosthesis was inserted, but use a neutral position if another internal fixation device was inserted

◆ Turn the patient on the nonoperative side as prescribed to facilitate circulation and recovery while easing tired muscles and relieving pressure; prop the operative limb with an abduction pillow if the patient has a prosthesis or with pillows if the patient has another internal fixation device

◆ Encourage deep breathing and coughing every 2 hours, and use an incentive spirometer every 1 to 2 hours to prevent pulmonary complications

◆ Auscultate all lung lobes for breath sounds, which should be clear

◆ Check the color and amount of sputum, which should be clear

◆ Monitor fluid intake and output and I.V. infusions; intake should be 3,000 ml daily; output should include 2,300 ml of urine and 300 to 700 ml of insensible water loss and perspiration

◆ Provide a regular diet as prescribed, and monitor bowel sounds; a patient with good bowel sounds who is passing flatus can receive regular foods; nerve involvement from the hip may cause mild abdominal distention

◆ Assess skin, and provide skin care to pressure areas (for example, heels, back, sacrum, shoulders, and elbows)

◆ Help the patient sit on the bed or in a chair on the first postoperative day; initially, weight-bearing activity is prohibited because it can cause excessive pressure on internal fixation devices; therefore, the patient must use a walker, which provides stability and allows ambulation with little or no weight bearing

◆ Make sure the hip isn't flexed more than 90 degrees for up to 2 months after surgery; during the first 10 postoperative days, even less flexion may be allowed

◆ Administer an opioid analgesic, or monitor the use of patient-controlled analgesia

◆ To prevent thrombophlebitis, administer an anticoagulant as ordered, and use external pneumatic compression devices and thigh-high antiembolism stockings

◆ Perform dressing changes as needed using aseptic technique; the wound may be left uncovered after draining ceases

◆ Encourage the patient to perform foot and ankle exercises, including dorsiflexion and plantar flexion, to increase venous return and prevent thrombophlebitis

◆ Teach the patient about proper use of a walker and use of the prescribed amount of weight bearing

❖ Lower back pain

- ■ Description
  - ◆ Lower back pain is pain that occurs in the lumbar region of the back
  - ◆ Lower back pain affects most of the population at some time
  - ◆ Most lower back pain is musculoskeletal; other common causes are degeneration and disk disease
  - ◆ Risk factors for lower back pain include obesity, poor body mechanics, lifting of heavy objects, and lack of exercise or physical activity
- ■ Signs and symptoms
  - ◆ The patient reports lower back pain, which may radiate to one or both legs
  - ◆ Associated symptoms include impaired bladder and bowel function, paresthesia, and reduced motor function
- ■ Diagnosis and treatment
  - ◆ Diagnosis is based on patient history, physical examination, and radiographic procedures, including X-rays, computed tomography (CT) scan, magnetic resonance imaging (MRI), myelogram, electromyogram, diskogram, and somatosensory evoked potentials
  - ◆ A nonsteroidal anti-inflammatory drug (NSAID) and an analgesic are administered for pain, and muscle relaxants may be used to relieve muscle spasms
  - ◆ Bed rest may be indicated initially
  - ◆ Physical therapy, intermittent pelvic traction, ultrasound, heat or ice, and whirlpool may be helpful

◆ Surgical intervention may include discectomy, discotomy, laminectomy, and spinal fusion
■ Nursing interventions
◆ Help the patient achieve a comfortable position; elevate the head of the bed 30 degrees, and have the patient flex his hips and knees slightly
◆ Alternate the application of cold and heat, and administer an analgesic as indicated
◆ Teach the patient the proper use of assistive devices
◆ Demonstrate proper body mechanics to the patient

❖ Osteoarthritis

■ Description
◆ Osteoarthritis is a noninflammatory joint disease characterized by degenerative changes in the articular cartilage; it primarily affects weight-bearing joints in the hips, knees, and vertebrae but may also affect the ankles, shoulders, wrists, fingers, and toes
◆ Osteoarthritis affects more than 50 million American men and women, primarily those older than age 45
◆ Osteoarthritis has been associated with aging, obesity, and wear and tear on the joints; however, a defective gene may account for many cases of idiopathic osteoarthritis
◆ Osteoarthritis may be *idiopathic* (occurring without a previous injury or known cause) or *secondary* (resulting from another injury or disease)
◆ Both types of osteoarthritis begin with the breakdown of the hyaline cartilage covering the ends of the bones on either side of the joint; the underlying bones become roughened, and bone cysts, fissures, or spurs develop on the bone surface; eventually, the joint space is lost as cartilage loss increases, and the joint ROM is progressively restricted
■ Signs and symptoms
◆ Joint stiffness and soreness may be accompanied by dull, aching pain that worsens with joint use and weight bearing; rest may relieve the pain
◆ ROM is decreased, and crepitus may be felt with joint movement
◆ Joints exhibit deformities, such as Heberden's nodes (bony outgrowths on the distal interphalangeal joints) and Bouchard's nodes (bony outgrowths on the proximal interphalangeal joints); the joints may also appear enlarged and edematous
◆ Muscle weakness and joint changes may lead to ulnar drift or wrist deviation, valgus deviation of the great and other toes, and increased or decreased lordosis in the lumbar spine
◆ Bone spurs may press on peripheral nerves, causing numbness or paralysis and hypoesthesia of the arms, forearms, hands, legs, and feet
◆ Carpal tunnel syndrome and tarsal tunnel syndrome may result from pressure of bony growths on nerves
◆ Gait analysis may show a discrepancy in leg length and joint alignments
◆ The patient may have a positive Trendelenburg's test (the buttock and pelvis rise when the opposite leg is raised, indicating hip dysplasia)

■ Diagnosis and treatment
  ◆ Patient history, physical examination, X-rays, CT scan, MRI, arthro-centesis, arthrogram, and bone scan may be ordered; serologic studies, including complete blood count, erythrocyte sedimentation rate (ESR), creatinine level, mineral assays, and humoral tests for immunoglobulins, also may be performed
  ◆ Support and stabilize the joint, if necessary, with a cane, crutches, a walker, braces, a cervical collar, or traction
  ◆ Weight reduction is encouraged in an obese patient
  ◆ Moist heat and paraffin dips are applied as needed
  ◆ The joints are massaged to increase circulation
  ◆ ROM exercises are performed for all joints
  ◆ Properly fitted shoes are used to help maintain correct posture, decrease pressure on affected tissues, and increase ambulation
  ◆ Medications such as salicylates, NSAIDs, muscle relaxants, and intra-articular steroids may be prescribed to relieve soreness (systemic steroids aren't used to treat osteoarthritis because it isn't an inflammatory disease)
  ◆ Studies indicate that glucosamine and chondroitin may be useful in controlling symptoms and reducing functional impairment
  ◆ Surgery is considered when other treatments have failed; total or partial joint replacement, joint fusion (arthrodesis), or osteotomy may be performed
■ Nursing interventions
  ◆ Explain the proposed treatment regimen to the patient
  ◆ Apply warm compresses, paraffin dips, or other ordered treatments to the joint
  ◆ Administer medications as prescribed
  ◆ Consult a physical therapist about exercise and other treatments
  ◆ Help the patient achieve a comfortable position, using pillows as needed, to promote rest
  ◆ Teach the patient how to use an ambulatory aid; walkers, canes, and other aids decrease weight on the affected joints and help to minimize cartilage erosion; teach proper body mechanics to prevent injury
  ◆ Encourage the patient to perform activities of daily living when possible to maintain muscle strength and joint ROM
  ◆ Provide skin care to maintain skin integrity

❖ Osteomyelitis
■ Description
  ◆ Osteomyelitis is an acute or a chronic infection of the bone or bone marrow
    ❯ The acute form may result from an infection in other tissues (hematogenic osteomyelitis) or from an open fracture with bacterial contamination
    ❯ The chronic form may result from inadequate initial therapy or lack of response to treatment (relapse occurs when the patient's resistance is lowered)

◆ The metaphyseal area in long bones is usually affected; the longer and larger the bone, the more susceptible it is to osteomyelitis; such bones include the femur, tibia, humerus, and vertebrae

◆ Common pathogenic organisms are *Staphylococcus aureus* (which causes 90% of osteomyelitis), *Streptococcus pyogenes, Pseudomonas aeruginosa, Escherichia coli, Neisseria gonorrhoeae, Haemophilus influenzae,* and *Salmonella typhi*

◆ Once the pathogens locate in the metaphysis, they grow and reproduce until they have formed a mass; leukocytes help wall off and localize the infection; bone cells in the area die, and purulent matter spreads along the bone, eventually penetrating through the tissues to the skin surface

■ Signs and symptoms

◆ The patient may complain of site pain and pressure; heat, edema, and tenderness may also be present

◆ Associated systemic signs and symptoms include chills, fever, malaise, nausea, and tachycardia

◆ The affected limb may be sore with use

◆ An open, draining area may appear

■ Diagnosis and treatment

◆ Diagnosis may be based on patient history, bone scan, MRI, physical examination, X-rays of the involved bone, culture of the drainage, WBC count, and ESR

◆ An antibiotic is administered I.V. in large doses after blood cultures are taken

◆ Aspirin or acetaminophen is given to control fever and pain

◆ Tetanus toxoid or antitoxin is given if the patient has an open wound

◆ Hyperbaric oxygen treatments at twice the atmospheric pressure for 2 hours per day up to six times per week may be prescribed

◆ After antibiotic therapy is completed, the bone is surgically scraped to clear away the dead bone and residue of infection

▶ Bone grafts may be used to aid bone healing and prevent fracture

▶ Tubes or catheters may be inserted to flush the site with an antibiotic to clear any residual organisms

▶ An external fixator may be placed above and below the osteomyelitic site to decrease the possibility of bone fracture

◆ Surgery to drain infection may be necessary

◆ Immobilization of the infected bone may be necessary using a cast, traction, or bed rest

■ Nursing interventions

◆ Monitor the type and amount of pain to determine the disease's status

◆ Administer an antibiotic, an analgesic, or tetanus toxoid or antitoxin as prescribed

◆ Administer I.V. fluids to maintain hydration

◆ Perform neurovascular checks, and monitor vital signs

◆ Use strict aseptic technique when required; the patient is more susceptible to additional infection or nosocomial infection

◆ Help the patient achieve a comfortable position to relieve pressure on the affected tissues

◆ Encourage the patient to perform ROM exercises for all unaffected tissues and joints to maintain strength

◆ Teach the patient how to use an ambulatory aid (or arm sling)

◆ Discuss concerns about the length and types of treatment

◆ Provide and encourage diversionary activities to help the patient maintain a positive outlook

❖ Osteoporosis

■ Description

◆ Osteoporosis is a systemic disease in which bone density and bone mass decrease because of a disturbance in the balance between bone resorption and bone deposition

◆ Osteoporosis begins to develop after age 30 but progresses rapidly in postmenopausal women; 70% of women older than age 45 have osteoporosis

◆ Causes of osteoporosis include menopausal decreases in estrogen, family history, immobility, insufficient intake of calcium and vitamin D, alcohol use, smoking, corticosteroid use, and caffeine intake

◆ Patients with osteoporosis are susceptible to fractures (particularly of the femur, radius, and ulna) and compression or crush injuries of the vertebrae

■ Signs and symptoms

◆ Pain may affect the lower back or thoracic spinal area

◆ Kyphosis, or dowager's hump, may be present

◆ A minor twist or turn can cause a sudden fracture

◆ Numbness or tingling in arms or legs may occur

■ Diagnosis and treatment

◆ Diagnosis may be based on patient history, physical examination, dual photon absorptiometry, and CT scans

◆ Calcium intake is increased to 1,500 mg daily

◆ Estrogen and progesterone are prescribed to restore hormonal balance

◆ Calcitonin and bisphosphonates (etidronate and panidronate) are prescribed to prevent bone resorption; alendronate, ibandronate, raloxifene, and risedronate are also used to treat osteoporosis

◆ Back or neck supports are used to prevent stress fractures

◆ Active exercises are encouraged to help retain calcium in the bones

■ Nursing interventions

◆ Monitor amount and type of pain to determine its extent

◆ Give an analgesic as prescribed to relieve pain and promote mobility

◆ Teach the patient how to use an ambulatory aid to maintain mobility, and apply a neck or back support, if ordered

◆ Teach the patient about dietary sources of calcium and calcium supplements; increased calcium intake decreases the risk of fractures

◆ Refer the patient to a practitioner for possible estrogen replacement therapy (controversial)

◆ Discuss methods of dressing to camouflage kyphosis

◆ Discuss how to ensure a safe home environment to decrease the risk of falls, for example, by removing loose rugs and avoiding long, uncovered electrical cords

◆ Encourage the patient to participate in active, weight-bearing exercises, such as walking and swimming, to maintain calcium in bones and preserve muscle strength

◆ Encourage the patient to modify lifestyle choices by avoiding smoking, alcohol, caffeine, and carbonated beverages, and increasing protein intake

❖ Rhabdomyolysis

■ Description

◆ Rhabdomyolysis is the breakdown of muscle tissue and may cause myoglobinuria

◆ Muscle tissue breakdown usually follows muscle trauma, especially a crush injury

◆ May lead to renal failure if not treated

◆ Causes of rhabdomyolysis, besides trauma, are excessive muscle activity (such as status epilepticus or severe dystonia), familial tendency, infection, medications (such as antihistamines, salcylates, fibric acid derivatives, HMG-CoA reductase inhibitors, neuroleptics, anesthetics, paralytic agents, corticosteroids, tricyclic antidepressants, and selective serotonin reuptake inhibitors), and sporadic strenuous exertion (for example, running in a marathon)

■ Signs and symptoms

◆ Tenderness, swelling, and muscle weakness resulting from muscle trauma and pressure

◆ Dark, reddish brown urine caused by myoglobin release

■ Diagnosis and treatment

◆ Diagnosis is based on patient history that reveals myalgias or muscle pain; physical examination; elevated levels of creatinine kinase, serum potassium, phosphate, and creatinine; and CT scan, MRI, and bone scintigraphy, which detects muscle necrosis

◆ Treatment should focus on the underlying cause

◆ I.V. crystalloids may be given to increase intravascular volume and glomerular filtration rate

◆ Analgesics may be given for pain

◆ If compartment syndrome develops, and venous pressure is greater than 25 mm Hg, immediate fasciotomy and debridement may be needed to relieve pressure and prevent tissue death

◆ Urine alkalinization and osmotic or loop diuretics may be implemented to prevent renal failure

■ Nursing interventions

◆ Administer I.V. fluids and diuretics to reduce nephrotoxicity

◆ Monitor intake and output

◆ Recommend exercise modification to prevent recurrence of rhadomyolysis

Review questions

1. A patient in balanced suspension traction for a fractured femur needs to be repositioned toward the head of the bed. During repositioning, the nurse should:

○ **A.** place slight additional tension on the traction cords.

○ **B.** release the weights, and replace them immediately after positioning.

○ **C.** lift the traction and the patient during repositioning.

○ **D.** maintain the same degree of traction tension.

Correct answer: D Traction is used to reduce the fracture and must be maintained at all times, including during repositioning. Options A, B, and C are incorrect because it isn't appropriate to increase traction tension or release or lift the traction during repositioning.

2. A patient undergoes cast placement for a fractured left radius. The nurse should suspect compartment syndrome if the patient experiences pain that:

○ **A.** intensifies with the elevation of the left arm.

○ **B.** disappears with the flexion of the left arm.

○ **C.** increases with the arm in a dependent position.

○ **D.** radiates up the arm to the left scapula.

Correct answer: A Pain is the most common symptom of compartment syndrome. Because the pain is the result of ischemia, elevating the limb reduces circulation, worsens the ischemia, and intensifies the pain. Options B and C are incorrect because these positions don't alter the pain of compartment syndrome. Option D is incorrect because the pain of compartment syndrome doesn't radiate up the arm to the scapula.

3. A patient received a right hip prosthesis after a fall. In the immediate postoperative period, the nurse should:

○ **A.** maintain the leg in an adducted position.

○ **B.** maintain the leg in an abducted position.

○ **C.** maintain the leg in a neutral position.

○ **D.** maintain the leg with the hip flexed greater than 90 degrees.

Correct answer: B After receiving a hip prosthesis, the affected leg should be kept abducted. Adduction (option A) may dislocate the hip. Option C would be correct if an internal fixation device was used. Option D is incorrect because the hip must not be flexed more than 90 degrees for the first 2 months and even less than that for the first 10 days.

4. A 78-year-old patient has a history of osteoarthritis. Which signs and symptoms would the nurse expect to find on physical assessment?

○ **A.** Joint pain, crepitus, Heberden's nodes

○ **B.** Hot, inflamed joints; crepitus; joint pain

○ **C.** Tophi, enlarged joints, Bouchard's nodes

○ **D.** Swelling, joint pain, tenderness on palpation

Correct answer: A Signs and symptoms of osteoarthritis include joint pain, crepitus, Heberden's nodes, Bouchard's nodes, and enlarged joints. Joint pain occurs with movement and is relieved by rest. As the disease progresses, pain may also occur at rest. Heberden's nodes are bony growths that occur at the distal interphalangeal joints. Bouchard's nodes involve the proximal interphalangeal joints. Hot, inflamed joints (option B) rarely occur with osteoarthritis. Tophi (option C) are deposits of sodium urate crystals that occur with chronic gout, not osteoarthritis. Swelling, joint pain, and tenderness on palpation (option D) occur with a sprain injury.

5. The nurse is caring for an elderly female patient who has osteoporosis. When teaching her, the nurse should include information about which major complication?

○ **A.** Bone fracture

○ **B.** Loss of estrogen

○ **C.** Negative calcium balance

○ **D.** Dowager's hump

Correct answer: A Bone fracture is a major complication of osteoporosis that results when loss of calcium and phosphate increases the fragility of bones. Option B is incorrect because estrogen deficiencies result from menopause, not osteoporosis. Option C is wrong because calcium and vitamin D supplements may be used to support normal bone metabolism, but a negative calcium balance isn't a complication of osteoporosis. Option D is incorrect because dowager's hump results from bone fractures. It develops when repeated vertebral fractures increase spinal curvature.

Gastrointestinal disorders

❖ Introduction
- The GI, or digestive, system breaks down food and prepares it for absorption by the body's cells; nonabsorbable ingested substances pass through the system and are eliminated as solid waste
- Although not part of the alimentary canal, the liver, gallbladder, and pancreas are essential accessory components of the GI system

❖ Nursing history
- The nurse asks the patient about his *chief complaint*
  - ◆ The patient with a GI problem may report a change in appetite, heartburn, nausea, pain, or vomiting
  - ◆ The patient may also report a change in bowel habits, such as constipation, diarrhea, or stool characteristics
- The nurse then questions the patient about his *present illness*
  - ◆ Ask the patient about his symptom, including when it started, associated symptoms, location, radiation, intensity, duration, frequency, and precipitating and alleviating factors
  - ◆ Ask about the use of prescription and over-the-counter drugs, herbal remedies, and vitamin and nutritional supplements; ask about the use of laxatives
  - ◆ If the patient's chief complaint is diarrhea, find out if he recently traveled abroad
  - ◆ Ask the patient about changes in appetite and in bowel habits (for example, a change in the amount, appearance, or color of his stool or the appearance of blood in it) and difficulty eating or chewing
- The nurse asks about *medical history*
  - ◆ Question the patient about other GI disorders, such as gallbladder disease, GI bleeding, inflammatory bowel disease, or ulcers
  - ◆ Also, ask about previous abdominal surgery or trauma
- The nurse then assesses the *family history*
  - ◆ Ask about a family history of diseases with a hereditary link, such as alcoholism, colon cancer, Crohn's disease, stomach ulcers, and ulcerative colitis
  - ◆ Also, question the patient about a family history of chronic diseases
- The nurse obtains a *social history*
  - ◆ Ask about work, exercise, diet, use of recreational drugs and alcohol, caffeine intake, and hobbies
  - ◆ Also ask about stress, support systems, and coping mechanisms

■ Physical assessment
  ◆ When assessing the abdomen, use this sequence: inspection, auscultation, percussion, and palpation; palpating or percussing the abdomen before you auscultate can change the character of the patient's bowel sounds and lead to an inaccurate assessment
  ◆ The nurse begins with *inspection*
    ❯ Observe the patient's general appearance, and note his behavior
    ❯ Inspect the skin for turgor, color, and texture; note abnormalities such as bruising, decreased axillary or pubic hair, edema, petechiae, scars, spider angiomas, and stretch marks
    ❯ Observe the patient's head for color of the sclerae, sunken eyes, dentures, caries, lesions, breath odor, and tongue color, swelling, or dryness
    ❯ Check the size and shape of the abdomen, noting distention, peristalsis, pulsations, contour, visible masses, and protrusions
    ❯ Observe the rectal area for abnormalities
  ◆ The nurse continues by using *auscultation*
    ❯ Note the character and quality of bowel sounds in each quadrant
    ❯ Auscultate the abdomen for vascular sounds
  ◆ Then the nurse *percusses* the abdomen
    ❯ Percuss the abdomen to detect the size and location of the abdominal organs
    ❯ Note the presence of air or fluid
  ◆ Next, the nurse uses *palpation*
    ❯ Palpate the abdomen to determine the size, shape, position, and tenderness of major abdominal organs and to detect masses and fluid accumulation
    ❯ Note abdominal muscle tone and tenderness
    ❯ Palpate the rectum, noting any abnormalities

❖ Cholecystitis
  ■ Description
    ◆ Cholecystitis is an acute or a chronic inflammation of the gallbladder; commonly associated with cholelithiasis (presence of gallstones)
    ◆ Cholecystitis is caused by a bacterial infection or gallstones
  ■ Signs and symptoms
    ◆ Sharp abdominal pain may affect the right upper quadrant of the abdomen, especially after ingestion of fatty foods, and may be referred to the right shoulder area
    ◆ Other GI effects include abdominal tenderness and muscle rigidity on palpation, eructation, flatulence, nausea, and vomiting
    ◆ Fever may result from acute infection
    ◆ Positive Murphy's sign (painful inspiration due to severe tenderness) may be present
    ◆ Jaundice may occur if gallstones obstruct the common bile duct
  ■ Diagnosis and treatment
    ◆ Diagnosis is based on ultrasonography of the upper abdomen and oral cholecystography that shows enlarged gallbladder and gallstones

◆ Percutaneous transhepatic cholangiography supports the diagnosis of obstructive jaundice and reveals calculi in the ducts

◆ Levels of serum alkaline phosphate, lactate dehydrogenase, aspartate aminotransferase, and total bilirubin are elevated

◆ The patient is placed on a low-fat diet

◆ An anticholinergic, such as propantheline or dicyclomine, is given to decrease spasms of the common bile duct

◆ An analgesic is prescribed for pain

◆ An antibiotic may be given to prevent or treat infection

◆ Chenodeoxycholic acid or ursodeoxycholic acid may be administered to dissolve gallstones; it must be taken for up to 2 years to be effective

◆ If pain persists, the gallbladder and gallstones are surgically removed by means of laparoscopic microsurgery or abdominal laparotomy; lithotripsy may also be performed to break up gallstones using ultrasonic waves

■ Preoperative nursing interventions

◆ Monitor the patient for abdominal pain in the right upper quadrant that may radiate to the right shoulder

◆ Check the skin and conjunctivae for jaundice

■ Postoperative nursing interventions

◆ Monitor vital signs every 1 to 2 hours for 4 to 8 hours and then every 4 hours to detect fluid imbalances, hemorrhage, or shock

◆ Monitor bowel sounds every 4 hours and bowel output to determine return of GI functions

◆ Check the wound area for signs of bleeding and inflammation

◆ Change the wound dressing as needed; the wound may be left uncovered if no drainage is present

◆ Monitor drainage from the T tube, if present; a T tube is used if gallstones were in the common bile duct because it lets bile pass into the small intestine and decreases duct inflammation

◆ Administer an opioid analgesic every 4 hours as needed and I.V. antibiotics every 6 to 8 hours as prescribed to maintain comfort and prevent infection

◆ Make sure the patient maintains nothing-by-mouth status as prescribed; administer I.V. fluids (up to 3,000 ml daily) to maintain fluid balance, also monitor fluid intake and output every 8 hours

◆ Start giving the patient clear liquids, then progress to a regular diet as prescribed; fat restrictions may be lifted because gallbladder removal increases the patient's tolerance to fatty foods

◆ Help the patient sit on the bed or in a chair and ambulate as prescribed to promote recovery from the surgery

◆ Record pertinent data in the patient's chart for continuity of care

❖ **Cirrhosis of the liver**

■ Description

◆ Cirrhosis is a chronic, progressive disease that causes extensive degeneration and destruction of parenchymal liver cells; it's twice as common in men as in women, and it's the fourth leading cause of death among middle-aged people

◆ Common types of cirrhosis include *micronodular* (Laënnec's), which is caused by excessive alcohol intake; *macronodular* (postnecrotic, toxin-induced), which is caused by chemicals, bacteria, and viruses; *biliary,* which is caused by irritating biliary products; *pigment,* which is caused by hemochromatosis; and *cardiac,* which is caused by right-sided heart failure and chronic liver disease

■ Signs and symptoms

◆ GI effects include anorexia, constipation or diarrhea, dull abdominal pain and heaviness, marked flatulence, nausea, vomiting, and weight loss

◆ The liver may be enlarged and have nodules; jaundice and hepatic encephalopathy may occur

◆ Hematologic effects may include anemia and thrombocytopenia

◆ Fever and malaise may be present

◆ Ascites, esophageal varices, and peripheral edema may occur

◆ Skin lesions may include petechiae, purpura, and spider angiomas; dry skin and pruritus also may occur

◆ Asterixis (liver flap, a hand-flapping tremor commonly seen in patients with hepatic coma), lethargy, mental changes, slurred speech, and peripheral neuropathies may occur

◆ Endocrine effects may include gynecomastia and impotence in men and amenorrhea in women

■ Diagnosis and treatment

◆ Diagnosis is based on patient history (especially excessive alcohol intake or hepatitis), physical examination, liver biopsy and liver function studies, ultrasonography, computed tomography (CT) scan, magnetic resonance imaging (MRI), and serologic studies, including complete blood count (CBC), serum electrolyte levels, and prothrombin time (PT)

◆ Paracentesis may be used to remove ascitic fluid

◆ For intractable chronic ascites, peritoneovenous shunt may be inserted to transfer ascitic fluid into the venous system for eventual excretion in the urine

◆ A potassium-sparing diuretic is used to decrease ascites and peripheral edema

◆ An antiemetic is used to reduce nausea and vomiting

◆ Vitamin K is used to reduce bleeding tendencies stemming from hypothrombinemia

◆ Lactulose is used to treat hepatic encephalopathy; lactulose decreases ammonia levels by trapping ammonia ions in the bowel

◆ Bleeding esophageal varices are treated by administering vasopressin and a beta-adrenergic blocker; performing endoscopic sclerosis; and inserting a Sengstaken-Blakemore tube or various surgical shunts (such as a portacaval shunt)

◆ Blood transfusions may be required for massive hemorrhage; I.V. therapy using colloid volume expanders or crystalloids may be given for volume expansion

◆ The recommended diet is typically high in calories and has moderate to high protein, moderate to low fat, and low sodium content; fluids are restricted

■ Nursing interventions

◆ Make sure the patient maintains bed rest; reposition him every 2 hours to help keep the skin intact and prevent pressure ulcers

◆ Encourage active range-of-motion exercises, and use special mattresses to relieve pressure

◆ Encourage deep breathing, and listen for breath sounds in all lung lobes

◆ Observe closely for changes in behavior or personality, such as stupor, lethargy, hallucinations, or neuromuscular dysfunction

◆ Administer an antiemetic as prescribed to control nausea and vomiting

◆ Administer a diuretic as prescribed; weigh the patient daily, and measure fluid intake and output; note signs of hypokalemia

◆ Measure abdominal girth, and note changes

◆ Check the patient's level of consciousness, neurologic status, and vital signs to detect encephalopathy or developing infection

◆ Monitor the patient for bleeding by checking vomitus and stool for blood; apply pressure to injection sites to prevent bleeding

◆ Monitor the results of laboratory tests and other studies; report abnormal findings to the practitioner

◆ Consult the dietitian regarding a low-sodium, fluid-restricted diet; provide four to six small meals daily, including foods that the patient likes, when possible

◆ Perform oral hygiene before meals and as needed to prevent stomatitis and remove characteristic fetid or ammonia-like mouth odor; have the patient use a soft toothbrush

◆ Provide meticulous skin care to prevent excoriation; check for edema, jaundice, petechiae, pruritus, purpura, spider angiomas, and ulcerations

◆ Tell the patient to avoid straining when turning, moving in bed, or defecating to lessen pressure on varices or hemorrhoids

◆ Explain upcoming diagnostic tests or treatments as needed

◆ Instruct the patient to avoid spicy or irritating foods, nonsteroidal anti-inflammatory drugs (NSAIDs), and aspirin

◆ Discuss patient concerns about the disease and lifestyle or body image change; provide a psychological referral, if needed

◆ Encourage the use of community agencies or services to help the patient control alcohol intake; stress the importance of abstaining from alcohol

◆ Record all data in the patient's chart for continuity of care

❖ **Diverticular disease**

■ Description

◆ Diverticular disease is characterized by diverticula (bulging pouches) in the GI wall that push the mucosal lining through the surrounding muscle

◆ There are two clinical forms: diverticulosis (diverticula are present but may cause only mild or no symptoms) and diverticulitis (diverticula are inflamed and may cause potentially fatal obstruction, infection, or hemorrhage)

◆ Results from high intraluminal pressure on an area of weakness in the GI wall, where blood vessels enter

◆ Retained undigested food and bacteria accumulate in diverticular sac, cutting off blood supply, and leading to inflamation, perforation, abscess, peritonitis, obstruction, or hemorrhage

◆ Causes are defects in the wall strength of the colon, diminished colonic motility and increased intraluminal pressure, and a low-fiber diet

■ Signs and symptoms

◆ In mild diverticulitis, moderate left lower abdominal pain, low-grade fever, and leukocytosis may occur

◆ In severe diverticulitis, abdominal rigidity from rupture of the diverticula, abscesses and peritonitis, left lower quadrant pain, high fever, chills, and hypotension from sepsis may occur

◆ In chronic diverticulitis, constipation, ribbonlike stools, intermittent diarrhea, abdominal distention resulting from intestinal obstruction, abdominal rigidity and pain, diminishing or absent bowel sounds, and nausea and vomiting secondary to intestinal obstruction may occur

■ Diagnosis and treatment

◆ Diagnosis may rely on patient history, barium enema, or colonscopy, which reveals diverticula

◆ A high-residue diet may be recommended for the treatment of diverticulosis after pain has subsided

◆ Antibiotics may be given to treat infection of the diverticula

◆ Analgesics may be prescribed to control pain and to relax smooth muscle

◆ Colon resection with removal of involved segment may be done to correct refractory cases; a temporary colostomy may be placed to drain abscess and to rest the colon

■ Nursing interventions

◆ Make sure the patient understands the importance of fiber in the diet

◆ Advise the patient to relieve constipation with stool softeners or bulk-forming cathartics

◆ Observe stools for frequency, color, and consistency

◆ If bleeding of the diverticulum occurs, the patient may need angiography and placement of a catheter for infusing vasopressin

◆ After surgery, watch for signs of infection and bleeding; encourage the patient to cough and breathe deeply

◆ Teach the patient how to care for his ostomy

❖ Gastroesophageal reflux disease

■ Description

◆ Gastroesophageal reflux disease (GERD) is the backflow of gastric contents or duodenal contents, or both, past the lower esophageal sphincter (LES) into the esophagus without associated belching or vomiting

---

Factors affecting LES pressure

Various dietary and lifestyle factors can increase or decrease lower esophageal sphincter (LES) pressure. Take these factors into account when you plan the patient's treatment program.

Factors that increase LES pressure	Factors that decrease LES pressure
• Protein	• Fat
• Carbohydrates	• Whole milk
• Nonfat milk	• Orange juice
• Low-dose ethanol	• Tomatoes
	• Antiflatulent (simethicone)
	• Chocolate
	• High-dose ethanol
	• Cigarette smoking
	• Lying on the right or left side
	• Sitting

◆ Occurs when the LES pressure is deficient or pressure in the stomach exceeds LES pressure

◆ Degree of mucosal injury is based on the amount and concentration of refluxed gastric acid, proteolytic enzymes, and bile acids

◆ Causes include anything that lowers LES pressure, such as alcohol, smoking, hiatal hernia, increased abdominal pressure with obesity or pregnancy, medications (such as morphine, diazepam, calcium channel blockers, meperidine, or anticholenergic), nasogastric (NG) intubation for more than 4 days, and weakened esophageal sphincter

■ Signs and symptoms

◆ Burning pain in the epigastric area, possibly radiating to the arms and chest, resulting from reflux of gastric contents into the esophagus

◆ Pain, usually after a meal or when lying down, secondary to increased abdominal pressure causing reflux

◆ Feeling of fluid accumulation in the throat without a sour or bitter taste because of hypersecretion of saliva

■ Diagnosis and treatment

◆ Diagnosis is based on patient history that reveals heartburn, physical examinaion, esophagoscopy, barium swallow, upper GI series, esophageal acidity test, and an acid perfusion test

◆ Abdominal pressure may be reduced by eating small, frequent meals and not eating before bedtime (see *Factors affecting LES pressure*)

◆ Patient positioning may be helpful in reducing abdominal pressure and preventing reflux (for example, sitting up during and after meal times or sleeping with the head of the bed elevated)

◆ Antacids may help to neutralize the acidic content of the stomach

◆ Histamine-2 receptor antagonists may be given to inhibit gastric acid secretion

◆ Proton pump inhibitors may be prescribed to reduce gastric acidity

◆ Cholinergic agents may be given to increase LES pressure

◆ Smoking cessation is recommended

■ Nursing interventions

◆ Teach the patient about the causes and symptoms of GERD

◆ Tell the patient how to avoid reflux with an antireflux regimen that includes diet, positioning, and taking antacids

❖ Gastrointestinal bleeding

■ Description

◆ Acute GI bleeding can range from minor to severe

◆ About 85% of GI bleeding involves the upper GI tract

◆ Bleeding may be caused by a disrupted mucosal-epithelial barrier or by a ruptured artery or vein

◆ Common conditions leading to GI bleeding include peptic ulcer disease, esophageal varices, diverticular disease, tumors, or ulcerative colitis

■ Signs and symptoms

◆ The patient may vomit blood or have coffee-ground vomitus

◆ Stools may appear bloody, maroon-colored, or black and tarry

◆ Abdominal cramping may occur

◆ The patient with chronic bleeding may have symptoms of anemia

◆ Signs of hypovolemic shock include cold, clammy skin; hypotension; reduced urine output; and tachycardia

■ Diagnosis and treatment

◆ Diagnosis is based on physical examination and patient history, including previous bleeding abnormalities, current medications, recent illnesses, and alcohol use

◆ Colonoscopy and esophagogastroduodenoscopy can detect the source of the bleeding

◆ Blood tests, such as CBC, coagulation studies, and liver function tests, are also helpful

◆ Treatment depends on the location and cause of GI bleeding

◆ Blood or blood component replacement may be indicated

◆ An NG tube may be inserted and the stomach lavaged with room-temperature fluid to remove blood and clots from the stomach

◆ A Sengstaken-Blakemore tube may be indicated for the treatment of esophageal varices

◆ Bleeding blood vessels may be treated with cauterization or endoscopic injection sclerotherapy

◆ A transjugular intrahepatic portosystemic shunt may be indicated to connect the portal vein and hepatic vein

◆ Commonly administered drugs include antacids, histamine blockers, sucralfate, proton pump inhibitors, and antibiotics for the treatment of *Helicobacter pylori*; vasopressin may be administered to produce vasoconstriction

■ Nursing interventions

◆ Monitor vital signs and other hemodynamic parameters for early detection of bleeding and hypovolemic shock; monitor hourly intake and output; maintain nothing-by-mouth status until bleeding is controlled

◆ Initiate two large-bore I.V. lines for fluid, drug, and blood administration

◆ Ensure patency and proper placement of the NG tube

◆ If the patient has a Sengstaken-Blakemore tube, make sure it's properly positioned and secured; the balloon shouldn't be inflated for more than 72 hours because of the high risk of tissue damage; keep scissors at the bedside to cut the airway lumens for immediate tube removal should airway obstruction occur

◆ During vasopressin administration, continuously monitor electrocardiogram results and blood pressure

◆ Teach patient how to prevent recurrence of GI bleeding by avoiding aspirin and aspirin-containing products

❖ Hepatitis

■ Description

◆ Hepatitis is an acute or a chronic inflammation of the liver

◆ It's caused by viruses, bacteria, trauma, immune disorders, or exposure to chemicals such as vinyl chloride and hydrocarbons

◆ Five major types of viral hepatitis exist: hepatitis A, B, C, D, and E (see *Characteristics of viral hepatitis*); of the 60,000 annual cases of viral hepatitis in the United States, about one-half are hepatitis B; hepatitis G is a newly identified virus thought to be blood-borne, with transmission similar to that of hepatitis C

■ Signs and symptoms

◆ The *prodromal* or *preicteric phase,* which lasts 1 to 2 days, can cause arthralgia, anorexia, aversion to cigarettes (among smokers), constipation or diarrhea, decreased senses of taste and smell, dislike of dietary protein, elevated serologic test results, headache, hepatomegaly, low-grade fever, lymphadenopathy, malaise, nausea, right upper quadrant pain or discomfort, splenomegaly, urticaria with or without rash, vomiting, and weight loss

◆ The *clinical phase,* which lasts 1 to 2 weeks, may produce bilirubinuria, dark urine, fatigue, hepatomegaly, jaundice, light-colored stools, lymphadenopathy, pruritus, right upper quadrant tenderness, and weight loss

◆ The *posticteric* or *recovery phase,* which averages 2 to 12 weeks, may result in easy fatigability, hepatomegaly, malaise, resolving jaundice (early in this phase), and resolving liver tenderness and enlargement

■ Diagnosis and treatment

◆ Diagnosis may rely on patient history, physical examination that reveals hepatomegaly, serologic liver function tests (such as bilirubin and protein levels and PT), and antibody tests for surface or cellular antigens in serum (Serologic assays for hepatitis G are being developed.)

◆ Rest is prescribed, including bed rest if hepatomegaly is severe

◆ Supplements of vitamins B, C, and K are administered

◆ The recommended diet is high in calories and carbohydrates and has moderate to high protein and moderate fat

◆ If the patient has hepatitis B, C, or D, an interferon may be used

Characteristics of viral hepatitis

Characteristic	Hepatitis A	Hepatitis B	Hepatitis C	Hepatitis D	Hepatitis E
Incubation period	15 to 45 days	28 to 180 days	15 to 160 days	28 to 180 days	14 to 63 days
Mode of transmission	Fecal-oral route	Parenteral (serum of infected persons); saliva, semen, and vaginal secretions	Parenteral (serum of infected persons)	Parenteral (serum of infected persons); saliva, semen, and vaginal secretions	Fecal-oral route
Sources of infection	Poor sanitation and personal hygiene; contaminated foods, milk, water, raw or steamed shellfish; persons with subclinical infections	Contaminated needles, syringes, blood products, and other instruments; sexual intercourse; kissing; asymptomatic carriers	Needles, syringes, blood and blood products	Contaminated needles, syringes, blood products, and other instruments; sexual intercourse; kissing; asymptomatic carriers	Poor sanitation, contaminated water
Virus in feces	3 to 4 weeks before jaundice	Degraded by enzymes, if present	Not identified in feces	Not applicable	Probably present in feces
Virus in serum	Briefly	Hepatitis B surface antigen (HBsAg) in serum through course of illness	Yes	Yes	Not applicable
Carrier state	No	Yes	Yes	Yes	Unknown
Prophylaxis	Immune serum globulin (ISG) within 2 weeks of exposure	Hepatitis B immune globulin (HBIG) or ISG within 2 weeks of exposure	Possible (some trials with immunoglobulin)	Avoidance of infection with hepatitis B (must be present for hepatitis D to develop)	Questionable protection with previous inoculation with immunoglobulin
Specific antigen in serum	Hepatitis A antigen	HBsAg, hepatitis B e antigen (HBeAg)	Hepatitis C virus	Hepatitis D virus	Not applicable
Specific antibody in serum	Anti-hepatitis A virus	HBsAg, antibody hepatitis B core antigen (HBcAg), anti-hepatitis E	Anti-hepatitis C virus	Anti-hepatitis D virus	Not applicable
Vaccine	Newly available	Made from serum containing HBsAg	None	None specifically for hepatitis D; vaccine for hepatitis B should be given	None

(continued)

Characteristics of viral hepatitis *(continued)*					
Characteristic	**Hepatitis A**	**Hepatitis B**	**Hepatitis C**	**Hepatitis D**	**Hepatitis E**
Prognosis	Complete recovery common; infection doesn't recur	Persistence in chronic or fulminant form is possible; possible precursor to a malignant liver tumor	Mild or severe and fulminant; many will have chronic infection	Increased mortality	Unknown

- Nursing interventions
  - Use standard precautions to avoid spreading the disease and to protect the patient from other diseases
  - Balance rest and activity to reduce metabolic demands on the liver
  - Monitor patient for changes in signs and symptoms—especially dark-colored urine, fatigue, fever, jaundice, and liver function—to assess the disease's status
  - Monitor fluid intake and output; correct fluid and electrolyte imbalances as prescribed
  - Administer immune serum globulin (ISG) as prescribed to modify the effects of hepatitis A and B
  - Consult a dietitian about the prescribed diet; discuss the patient's food preferences, and intervene to increase the patient's appetite and food retention to ensure adequate calorie and protein intake
  - Discuss the dangers of self-medication, and encourage the patient to use only prescribed medications; an inflamed liver can't metabolize drugs well, and some drugs—especially acetaminophen—may exacerbate inflammation
  - Follow preventive measures for hepatitis A: careful hand washing, good personal hygiene, environmental sanitation, screening and control of food handlers, enteric precautions, and ISG administration
  - Follow preventive measures for hepatitis B: careful hand washing, screening of blood donors for hepatitis B surface antigen, use of disposable needles and syringes, registration of carriers, passive immunization with ISG and hepatitis B immune globulin for exposure to mucous secretions or needle-stick exposure, and active immunization with hepatitis B vaccine for high-risk populations such as health care providers
  - Follow the same preventive measures for hepatitis C as for hepatitis B
  - Follow standard precautions for hepatitis A: Use gloves and a gown if touching soiled or infective material (feces) is likely; place the patient who has poor personal hygiene in a private room, and follow precautions for 7 days after jaundice appears
  - Follow standard precautions for hepatitis B: Use gloves and a gown if touching soiled or infective materials (blood, body fluids, or feces if patient has GI bleeding) is likely

◆ Follow standard precautions for hepatitis C: Use gloves and a gown if touching soiled or infective materials (blood or body fluids) is likely

◆ Provide a referral to a community nurse for continuity of care as needed

❖ Large- and small-bowel obstruction

■ Description

◆ Large-bowel obstruction can occur in the ascending, transverse, or descending colon; the rectum; or several areas simultaneously

◆ Small-bowel obstruction can occur in any area of the duodenum, jejunum, or ileum or in several areas simultaneously

◆ Small- and large-bowel obstructions may result from infection, tumor, or intestinal ulcerations with scar formation that lead to obstruction, volvulus, intussusception, adhesions, or paralytic ileus

◆ Complications of small- and large-bowel obstruction include hypovolemic shock, peritonitis, rupture, septicemia, and death

■ Signs and symptoms

◆ Abdominal pain and distention may be mild to severe

◆ Anorexia and nausea may be accompanied by severe vomiting with a fecal odor

◆ Bowel sounds may be high-pitched or absent

◆ Constipation or obstipation may be present, or diarrhea may occur as liquid intestinal secretions and feces move around the obstruction; blood, mucus, or undigested food may appear in stool

◆ Abdominal girth may increase due to distention

◆ Vital sign changes may include fever and signs of shock, such as hypotension, tachycardia, and tachypnea

◆ Other effects may include anxiety, dehydration, dry skin, fatigue, malaise, and weight loss

■ Diagnosis and treatment

◆ Diagnosis may require patient history, physical examination, abdominal X-rays (such as flat plate of the abdomen, barium enema, and GI series), serologic studies, endoscopy, gastric analysis, stool examination, colonoscopy, and proctoscopy

◆ Maintain nothing-by-mouth status, and administer I.V. therapy to restore fluid balance

◆ An NG or intestinal tube is inserted to relieve abdominal distention and vomiting

◆ An opioid analgesic is used to relieve pain

◆ An antibiotic is administered to treat possible infection

◆ Abdominal girth is measured every 2 to 4 hours

◆ Bowel output is monitored, and stools are checked for occult blood

◆ Surgery may be used to correct the obstruction; exploratory laparotomy can determine the cause, small- or large-bowel resection can remove diseased portions, ileostomy or colostomy may be done to permit waste discharge, total ablation (removal) of the large and most of small intestine may be used if the obstruction is caused by mesenteric artery thrombosis

- Nursing interventions
  - Monitor vital signs, particularly noting signs of shock (increased pulse and respiratory rates and decreased blood pressure) and peritonitis or other infection (increased temperature)
  - Administer prescribed medications promptly to maintain therapeutic blood levels
  - Maintain I.V. therapy to ensure proper hydration because the patient must maintain nothing-by-mouth status
  - Monitor fluid intake and output (including vomitus and diarrhea) carefully; excessive fluid loss can lead to shock and dehydration
  - Monitor, measure, and record drainage from the NG or intestinal tube; check drainage for blood and odor, irrigate the tube as prescribed to maintain patency, and turn the patient as prescribed to facilitate tube passage to the obstruction site
  - Measure abdominal girth every 2 to 4 hours to assess distention
  - Auscultate and characterize bowel sounds; high-pitched sounds indicate anoxia resulting from marked distention or obstruction, whereas absent sounds indicate ileus or obstruction
  - Monitor eructation (a sign of continuing obstruction) or flatus passage (a sign of resolving obstruction)
  - Monitor patient for abdominal pain or tenderness, noting its location; pain may be related to distention or inflammation
  - Encourage the patient to perform deep-breathing exercises every 2 hours; abdominal distention may elevate the diaphragm and decrease deep breathing
  - Prepare the patient for surgery, if indicated
  - Keep the patient and family apprised of the situation

❖ Pancreatitis

- Description
  - Pancreatitis is an inflammation of the pancreas accompanied by the release of digestive enzymes into the gland, resulting in autodigestion of the organ
  - Causes of pancreatitis include alcohol abuse, trauma, infection, drug toxicity, and obstruction of the biliary tract
- Signs and symptoms
  - Pancreatitis is characterized by severe epigastric pain that worsens after meals and may radiate to the shoulder, substernal area, back, and flank
  - Fever and malaise may be present
  - The patient may experience abdominal tenderness and distention, nausea, and vomiting; he may lie in a knee-chest or fetal position or lean forward for comfort
  - Bulky, fatty, foul-smelling stool may occur
  - Signs of hypovolemic shock may be present
- Diagnosis and treatment
  - Diagnosis is based on patient history including alcohol intake and use of prescription and nonprescription drugs

◆ Laboratory tests include increased serum amylase, aspartate amino-transferase, bilirubin, glucose, and lipase levels; increased white blood cell count; and decreased serum calcium levels

◆ Other diagnostic tools include abdominal and chest X-rays, ultrasound, CT scan, MRI, and endoscopic retrograde cholangiopancreatography

◆ Cullen's and Grey Turner's signs are positive

◆ The patient maintains nothing-by-mouth status, and an NG tube is inserted; total parenteral nutrition may be indicated

◆ I.V. fluids are administered, and electrolytes are replaced as indicated

◆ An analgesic and an antibiotic may be prescribed; elevated glucose levels are controlled

◆ Surgical intervention is used to treat the underlying cause, if appropriate

■ Nursing interventions

◆ Make sure the patient maintains nothing-by-mouth status during the acute phase; then begin to introduce bland, low-fat, high-protein diet of small, frequent meals with restricted intake of alcohol, caffeine, and gas-forming foods

◆ Monitor for symptoms of calcium deficiency (such as tetany, cramps, carpopedal spasm, and seizures)

◆ Provide mouth, nares, and skin care

◆ Check the NG tube for patency, and correct placement each shift

◆ Monitor intake and output and vital signs, and obtain daily weights

◆ Administer an analgesic (usually meperidine) as needed

◆ Advise patient to avoid alcohol, caffeine, and spices

◆ Explain the importance of a quiet, restful environment to conserve energy and decrease metabolic demands

❖ Peptic ulcer disease

■ Description

◆ Peptic ulcer disease is characterized by ulcerations in the stomach (gastric) or small intestine (duodenal); 20% of peptic ulcers are gastric, and 80% are duodenal

◆ Peptic ulcer disease is caused by erosion of the lining cells of the stomach or duodenum; factors such as *H. pylori* and NSAIDs disrupt the normal mucosal defense making the mucosa more susceptible to the effects of gastric acid

■ Signs and symptoms

◆ Gastric and peptic ulcers have different signs and symptoms (see *Common symptoms of peptic ulcer disease*, page 214)

◆ Other effects may include anorexia, dizziness, eructation, and lightheadedness or syncope

◆ The patient may have a family history of peptic ulcer disease; medication history of aspirin or other anti-inflammatory drug use; or a personal history of cigarette, alcohol, or caffeine use or of stressful conditions at home or on the job

Common symptoms of peptic ulcer disease

Symptom	Gastric ulcer	Duodenal ulcer
Pain Type	Gnawing, burning, aching, heartburn	Gnawing, burning, cramping, heartburn at times
Duration	Constant unless relieved by food or drugs	Intermittent and relieved by food or drugs (steady pain may be related to a perforated ulcer of the posterior wall of the duodenum)
Site	Upper epigastrium with localization to left of umbilicus	Right epigastric area to right of umbilicus; radiation of pain to right upper quadrant may be due to a perforated ulcer of the posterior wall of the duodenum
Time of day	At night and when stomach is empty	At night and when duodenum is empty
Cause	Presence of hydrochloric acid in stomach	High acid content of chyme moving into duodenum
Periodicity	Recurs daily for a period of time, then disappears for months, only to recur	Recurs daily for a period of time, then disappears for months, only to recur
Nausea	Intermittent	Intermittent
Vomiting	Occasional (more often than with duodenal ulcers)	Occasional
Feeling of fullness	Present at times; eructation common	Present at times
Bleeding	Detected in vomitus, unless hemorrhage occurs	Detected in stools through stool guaiac tests, unless hemorrhage occurs

■ Diagnosis and treatment
   ◆ Diagnosis may be based on patient history, physical examination, gastric endoscopy, barium test, upper-GI series, gastric analysis, gastric cytology, serologic studies, testing for *H. pylori,* and stool tests for occult blood
   ◆ A histamine blocker — such as cimetidine, famotidine, nizatidine, or ranitidine — is used to decrease gastric acid production; an antacid is also prescribed to neutralize hydrochloric acid
   ◆ A proton pump inhibitor, such as omeprazole or lansoprazole, may be used to suppress acid production by halting the mechanism that pumps acid into the stomach
   ◆ Sucralfate, a cytoprotective drug, may be prescribed; it works by forming a protective barrier over the ulcer's surface
   ◆ Misoprostol, a synthetic prostaglandin analogue, may be prescribed to prevent ulcers from forming in patients who take high doses of an

NSAID by protecting the gastric mucous; an antibiotic may be prescribed to treat *H. pylori* infections; bismuth is also used as adjunct therapy against *H. pylori*
◆ Stress-reduction techniques are recommended to prevent development of a stress ulcer or worsening of peptic ulcers
◆ Smoking cessation is recommended
◆ If drug therapy is ineffective, surgical repair may include laser cauterization of a bleeding site, partial gastrectomy with gastroduodenostomy (Billroth I), partial gastrectomy with gastrojejunostomy (Billroth II), or vagotomy with pyloroplasty (rare)
■ Nursing interventions
◆ Administer prescribed medications
◆ Help the patient identify and eliminate foods that cause distress
◆ Teach the patient about the disease, its treatment, and stress-reduction techniques, if needed
◆ Encourage the patient to stop smoking to eliminate the effects of nicotine on ulcers
◆ Provide postoperative care as needed
  ❯ Verify placement and maintain patency of the NG tube
  ❯ Make sure the patient maintains nothing-by-mouth status as prescribed; administer I.V. fluids to maintain fluid and electrolyte balance
  ❯ To help control pain, encourage the patient to use patient-controlled analgesia, or administer an opioid analgesic every 3 to 4 hours
  ❯ Measure abdominal girth to assess abdominal distention or ileus
  ❯ Auscultate bowel sounds to detect the return of peristalsis
  ❯ Help the patient perform deep-breathing exercises every 2 hours and use an incentive spirometer every 2 hours to prevent pulmonary complications
  ❯ Help the patient ambulate as prescribed
  ❯ Take steps to avoid dumping syndrome (a rapid gastric emptying produced by a bolus of food, causing distention of the dodenum or jejunum)
  ❯ Start giving the patient clear liquids when prescribed; observe him for nausea or vomiting, and assess his tolerance of intake, and increase to small, frequent meals
  ❯ Monitor for flatus or bowel movements to determine bowel functions
  ❯ Before discharge, teach the patient about rest, activity restrictions, diet, medications, smoking cessation, and stress control

❖ **Regional ileitis and ulcerative colitis**
■ Description
◆ *Regional ileitis*, also known as Crohn's disease, is an inflammatory disease of the small bowel that also may affect the large intestine; it typically begins in the ileum but can affect all areas of the small intestine and even the esophagus
◆ *Ulcerative colitis* is a chronic inflammatory disease of the large intestine, commonly in the sigmoid and rectal areas

Comparing regional ileitis and ulcerative colitis

The following chart compares some key characteristics of regional ileitis and ulcerative colitis.

Characteristic	Regional ileitis	Ulcerative colitis
Areas affected	All layers of the bowel in various areas of the bowel at the same time	Only the mucosal and submucosal layers
Lesion	"Skip" or discontinuous lesions; edematous, reddish-purple areas with granulomas (scarring)	Continuous, diffuse lesions that don't skip segments; ulcerations with erosion and bleeding
Incidence	Slightly more common in women than men, primarily between ages 20 and 50; more common in Jews and non-Whites	More common in women than men, primarily those between ages 20 and 40; more common in Jews and non-Whites
Cause	Unknown, but may be genetic or immunologic; may be exacerbated by stress	Unknown, but may be genetic, immunologic, or infectious
Signs and symptoms	• Abdominal distention • Anemia • Arthralgia • Cramping abdominal pain and tenderness • Dehydration and fluid and electrolyte imbalances • Flatulence • Low-grade fever • Nausea and vomiting • Three to four semisoft stools daily with no blood, except in patients with advanced disease; some fat is present, and stools may be foul-smelling • Weight loss	• Abdomen distention • Abdominal rigidity at times • Anemia • Bowel distention • Cramping abdominal pain, typically in lower left quadrant • Dehydration and fluid and electrolyte imbalances • Diarrhea (pronounced, 5 to 25 stools daily) with blood, mucus, and pus but no fat • Fever • Nausea and vomiting • Rectal bleeding • Weight loss
Diagnostic tests	• Barium enema • Proctosigmoidoscopy • Stool analysis for occult blood and culture • X-ray of small bowel	• Barium enema • Biopsy of rectal cells • Fiberoptic colonoscopy • Sigmoidoscopy • Stool analysis

■ Signs and symptoms
  ◆ Regional ileitis and ulcerative colitis produce different signs and symptoms (see *Comparing regional ileitis and ulcerative colitis*)
  ◆ The stool of a patient with ulcerative colitis may appear liquid, with blood, pus, and mucus; the patient with regional ileitis typically has diarrhea without visible blood
■ Diagnosis and treatment
  ◆ Regional ileitis and ulcerative colitis are diagnosed differently but managed similarly; regional ileitis is diagnosed by small bowel X-ray, barium enema, and sigmoidoscopy, whereas ulcerative colitis is diagnosed by biopsy with colonoscopy

◆ Tailored to the patient's specific needs, the diet typically restricts raw fruits and vegetables as well as fatty and spicy foods; debilitated patients may require total parenteral nutrition

◆ An anticholinergic is used to manage intestinal spasms; an antidiarrheal to control diarrhea; an anti-inflammatory such as sulfasalazine to reduce inflammation; an antimicrobial to prevent infection; a corticosteroid to decrease inflammation; and an immunosuppressant to decrease antigen-antibody reactions

◆ Surgery is indicated for fistula formation, intestinal obstruction, bowel perforation, hemorrhage, and intractable disease (if ulcerative colitis persists for more than 10 years, cancer may develop)

  ❯ Intestinal resections may need to be performed repeatedly
  ❯ Ileostomy is curative; ileorectal anastomosis may be performed

■ Nursing interventions

◆ Make sure the patient understands the purpose, therapeutic effects, and adverse effects of prescribed medications

◆ Provide postoperative care for a patient undergoing surgery

◆ Maintain patency of the NG tube, if present, by irrigating with normal saline solution every 2 hours as needed

  ❯ Encourage the patient to use patient-controlled analgesia, or administer an opioid analgesic to relieve pain; administer a steroid to prevent adrenal insufficiency and an antibiotic to prevent infection
  ❯ Monitor vital signs every 1 to 2 hours for 4 to 8 hours and then every 4 hours
  ❯ Make sure the patient maintains nothing-by-mouth status as prescribed; monitor I.V. fluids every 1 to 2 hours; up to 3,000 ml of fluid daily is needed
  ❯ Check wound sites for drainage and signs of inflammation, infection, and healing; use aseptic technique to prevent infection
  ❯ Monitor bowel sounds every 2 to 4 hours to detect the return of peristalsis or, possibly, ileus
  ❯ Monitor bowel output to determine return of bowel function
  ❯ Help the patient ambulate as prescribed
  ❯ Encourage the patient to perform deep-breathing exercises and use an incentive spirometer every 2 hours to prevent pulmonary complications
  ❯ Start giving the patient clear liquids when prescribed; the diet initially may be a low-residue one, gradually increasing to a regular diet as tolerated
  ❯ Provide care for a patient with an ileostomy or a colostomy (see *Comparing colostomy and ileostomy,* page 218)
    • Change bags if they start leaking to prevent skin excoriation; the patient may change bags on a regular schedule to prevent leaking
    • Make sure the opening of the bag around the stoma is no larger than ⅛" (3 mm) to prevent skin excoriation
    • Refer the patient to an enterostomal nurse therapist for care of the stoma and colostomy and psychosocial adjustment

Comparing colostomy and ileostomy

Procedure	Type of stool	Appliance and bowel regulation	Nursing considerations
Single-barrel, or end, colostomy	Formed	Requires appliance until discharge becomes regulated; regulates bowel	Bowel is regulated through diet and irrigation (every 2 to 3 days).
Double-barrel and loop colostomy	Semiliquid, semiformed, proteolytic discharge	Requires appliance; doesn't regulate bowel	Stool is discharged from the proximal loop of the colostomy. Mucus may be discharged from a distal stoma. Loop colostomy has a plastic rod under the bowel to hold it to the outer abdominal wall; rubber tubing attached to the ends of the rod prevent it from being dislodged.
Conventional ileostomy	Semiliquid to liquid, frequent discharge of stool, proteolytic discharge	Requires appliance; doesn't regulate bowel	Ileostomy discharge may contain undigested food. Patient may become dehydrated from frequent discharges of semiliquid stool.
Continent ileostomy (Kock pouch)	Semiliquid to liquid, constant, proteolytic discharge	Doesn't require appliance or regulate bowel (ileostomy has one-way valve or nipple to prevent leakage)	Stoma is catheterized every 4 hours to empty Kock pouch.

▶ Provide opportunities for the patient to discuss feelings about the disease and its treatment

▶ Teach the patient how to care for the incision or the colostomy or ileostomy

▶ Refer the patient for continued nursing monitoring or assistance after discharge for continuity of care and support with new self-care procedures

Review questions

1. A patient with peptic ulcer disease secondary to chronic NSAID use is prescribed misoprostol (Cytotec). The nurse would be most accurate in informing the patient that the drug:

○ **A.** reduces the stomach's volume of hydrochloric acid.

○ **B.** increases the speed of gastric emptying.

○ **C.** protects the stomach's lining.

○ **D.** increases LES pressure.

Correct answer: C Misoprostol is a synthetic prostaglandin that, like prostaglandin, protects the gastric mucosa. NSAIDs decrease prostaglandin production and predispose the patient to peptic ulceration. Misoprostol doesn't reduce gastric acidity (option A), improve emptying of the stomach (option B), or increase LES pressure (option D).

2. The nurse is caring for a patient with active upper-GI bleeding. What's the appropriate diet for this patient during the first 24 hours after admission?

○ **A.** Regular diet

○ **B.** Skim milk

○ **C.** Nothing by mouth

○ **D.** Clear liquids

Correct answer: C Shock and bleeding must be controlled before oral intake begins, so the patient should receive nothing by mouth. A regular diet (option A) is incorrect. When the bleeding is controlled, intake is gradually increased, starting with ice chips and then clear liquids. Skim milk (option B) is incorrect because it increases gastric acid production that could prolong the bleeding. A liquid diet (option D) is the first diet offered after bleeding and shock are controlled.

3. A patient is scheduled to have a descending colostomy. He's anxious and has many questions concerning the surgery, the care of a stoma, and lifestyle changes. It would be most appropriate for the nurse to refer the patient to which member of the health care team?

○ **A.** Social worker

○ **B.** Registered dietitian

○ **C.** Occupational therapist

○ **D.** Enterostomal nurse therapist

Correct answer: D An enterostomal nurse therapist is a registered nurse who has received advanced education in an accredited program to care for patients with stomas. The enterostomal nurse therapist can assist with the selection of an appropriate stoma site, teach about stoma care, and provide emotional support. Social workers (option A) provide counseling and emotional support, but they can't provide pre- and postoperative teaching. A registered dietitian (option B) can review any dietary changes and help the patient with meal planning. The occupational therapist (option C) can assist a patient with regaining independence with activities of daily living.

4. The nurse is planning care for a female patient with acute hepatitis A. What's the primary mode of transmission for hepatitis A?

○ **A.** Fecal contamination and oral ingestion

○ **B.** Exposure to contaminated blood

○ **C.** Sexual activity with an infected partner

○ **D.** Sharing a contaminated needle or syringe

Correct answer: A Hepatitis A is predominantly transmitted by the ingestion of fecally contaminated food. Transmission is more likely to occur with poor hygiene, crowded conditions, and poor sanitation. Hepatitis B and C may be transmitted through exposure to contaminated blood and blood products (option B). Sexual activity with an infected partner (option C) and sharing contaminated needles or syringes (option D) may transmit hepatitis B.

5. A patient experiences an exacerbation of ulcerative colitis. Test results reveal elevated serum osmolality and urine specific gravity. What's the most likely explanation for these test results?

○ **A.** Renal insufficiency

○ **B.** Hypoaldosteronism

○ **C.** Diabetes insipidus

○ **D.** Deficient fluid volume

Correct answer: D Ulcerative colitis causes watery diarrhea. The patient loses large volumes of fluid causing hemoconcentration and an elevated serum osmolality and urine specific gravity. Renal insufficiency (option A), hypoaldosteronism (option B), and diabetes insipidus (option C) aren't associated with ulcerative colitis.

CHAPTER 13

Skin disorders

❖ Introduction
- The skin is the largest organ in the body
- It provides a barrier against pathogens, radiation, and trauma; regulates body temperature; and is the site of vitamin D production
- Pressure receptors in the skin provide the sense of touch
- Nursing history
  - ◆ The nurse asks the patient about his *chief complaint*
    - ▶ The most common complaints concerning the integumentary system are itching, lesions, pigmentation abnormalities, and rashes
    - ▶ The patient may also have problems with changes in nail growth or color, hair loss, or increased growth or distribution of hair
  - ◆ The nurse then questions the patient about his *present illness*
    - ▶ Ask the patient about his symptom, including when it started, associated symptoms, location, radiation, intensity, duration, frequency, and precipitating and alleviating factors
    - ▶ Ask how and when skin changes occurred; ask if he has experienced any bleeding, drainage, or itching
    - ▶ Question the patient about any recent insect bites
    - ▶ Ask about the use of prescription and over-the-counter drugs (especially ointments, creams, or lotions), herbal remedies, and vitamin and nutritional supplements
  - ◆ The nurse asks about *medical history*
    - ▶ Question the patient about a history of skin, nail, or hair problems
    - ▶ Ask about previous diseases or conditions
  - ◆ The nurse then assesses the *family history*
    - ▶ Ask about a family history of chronic skin infections, cancer, or other diseases
    - ▶ Question the patient about a family history of disorders of the hair or nails
    - ▶ Ask about a family history of other chronic diseases
  - ◆ The nurse obtains a *social history*
    - ▶ Ask about support systems, work, exercise, diet, use of recreational drugs, alcohol use, stress, hobbies, and coping mechanisms
    - ▶ Ask how much time the patient spends in the sun and whether protective clothing and sunscreen are worn
- Physical assessment
  - ◆ Nurse begins with *inspection*

▶ Examine the patient's mucous membranes, hair, scalp, axillae, groin, palms, soles, and nails; note changes in pigmentation; note the color, size, shape, configuration, pattern of distribution, depth or height, texture, and location of any lesions (see *Differentiating among skin lesions*)

▶ Note the patient's level of hygiene, including any odors

◆ Next, the nurse uses *palpation*

▶ Palpate the skin and note texture, consistency, temperature, moisture, edema, and turgor

▶ Note any areas of tenderness

❖ Basal cell carcinoma

■ Description

◆ Basal cell carcinoma is an epidermal tumor predominantly found on exposed surfaces of the skin

◆ Basal cell carcinoma is a slow-growing, destructive skin tumor that usually occurs in people older than age 40; it's most prevalent in blond, fair-skinned men and is the most common malignant tumor that affects whites; chronic sun exposure is the most common cause

◆ There are four types of basal cell carcinoma: nodular, superficial, morpheaform, and pigmented

■ Signs and symptoms

◆ A pearly papule typically with telangiectasis, raised borders, and superficial ulceration are characteristic of the nodular form

◆ Superficial basal cell carcinoma appears as a well-demarcated erythematous scaly patch without ulceration, commonly on the trunk

◆ A pale, yellow, or white flat or depressed scarlike plaque with indistinct borders suggests morpheaform basal cell carcinoma

◆ Pigmented basal cell carcinoma appears as a pearly papule that contains melanin appearing blue, black, or brown in color

■ Diagnosis and treatment

◆ All types of basal cell carcinomas are diagnosed by their appearance; incisional or excisional biopsy and histologic study may help to determine the tumor type and histologic subtype

◆ Treatment options include surgical excision, electrodesiccation and curettage, cryosurgery, radiation therapy, and Mohs' surgery

◆ Interferon therapy and fluorouracil or imiquimod may also be used

■ Nursing interventions

◆ Monitor the skin after biopsy for bleeding

◆ Assess the patient's skin while you're helping him bathe or perform range-of-motion (ROM) exercises

◆ Explain to the patient which treatments he's receiving

◆ Encourage the patient to express feelings about changes in body image and a fear of dying; offer emotional support and encouragement

◆ Provide postchemotherapy and postradiation nursing care to promote healing

◆ Teach the patient and family members about wound care, protection from the sun, lifestyle modifications, skin examination, and the importance of follow-up examinations

Differentiating among skin lesions

These illustrations depict the most common primary skin lesions.

Primary lesions

Bulla
Fluid-filled lesion more than 2 cm in diameter (also called a blister); occurs in patients with severe poison oak or ivy dermatitis, bullous pemphigoid, or second-degree burns

Patch
Flat, pigmented, circumscribed area more than 1 cm in diameter — for example, herald patch (pityriasis rosea)

Comedo
Plugged, exfoliative pilosebaceous duct formed from sebum and keratin — for example, blackhead (open comedo) and whitehead (closed comedo)

Plaque
Circumscribed, solid, elevated lesion more than 1 cm in diameter that is elevated above skin surface and that occupies larger surface area in comparison with height, as occurs in psoriasis

Cyst
Semisolid or fluid-filled encapsulated mass extending deep into dermis — for example, acne

Pustule
Raised, circumscribed lesion, usually less than 1 cm in diameter, that contains purulent material, making it a yellow-white color — for example, acne or impetiginous pustule and furuncle

Macule
Flat, pigmented, circumscribed area less than 1 cm in diameter — for example, freckle or rash that occurs in patients with rubella

Tumor
Elevated, solid lesion larger than 2 cm in diameter that extends into dermal and subcutaneous layers — for example, dermatofibroma

Nodule
Firm, raised lesion, 0.6 to 2 cm in diameter that is deeper than a papule and extends into dermal layer — for example, intradermal nevus

Vesicle
Raised, circumscribed, fluid-filled lesion less than 1 cm in diameter, as occurs in chickenpox or herpes simplex infection

Papule
Firm, inflammatory, raised lesion up to 0.6 cm in diameter that may be the same color as skin or pigmented — for example, acne papule and lichen planus

Wheal
Raised, firm lesion with intense localized skin edema that varies in size, shape, and color (from pale pink to red) and that disappears in hours — for example, hives and insect bites

❖ Burns
- Description
  - ◆ A burn is a lesion caused by fire, friction or abrasion, heat, caustic substances, electricity, or radiation
  - ◆ Burns are classified by their depth and the amount of tissue damage (see *Burn classification,* page 224)

Burn classification

Characteristic	First-degree burn	Second-degree burn	Third-degree burn
Thickness	Superficial, partial-thickness	Deep, partial-thickness	Full-thickness
Appearance	Dry with no blisters	Weeping, edematous blisters	Dry, leathery, and possibly edematous
Color	Pink	White to pink or red	White to charred
Comfort	Painful	Very painful	Little or no pain
Depth	Epidermis only	Epidermis, dermis, and possibly some subcutaneous tissue	Subcutaneous tissue and possibly fascia, muscle, and bone

■ Treatment in stage 1 (immediate or emergent stage)
  ◆ Stage 1 begins when the patient is burned and continues until the patient's condition is stabilized and fluids have been replaced
  ◆ The burn team implements lifesaving measures
    ▶ A patent airway is established
    ▶ Oxygen is supplied by nasal cannula or endotracheal tube
    ▶ A patent large-bore I.V. line is established for fluid resuscitation, which is titrated to urine output (not burn size)
    ▶ The extent and depth of burn area are determined
    ▶ The patient is assessed for other injuries, including smoke inhalation
  ◆ The severity of the burn is determined
    ▶ The amount of body surface involved is determined by the Rule of Nines: head and neck (9%), arms (9% each), anterior trunk (18%), posterior trunk (18%), legs (18% each), and perineum (1%)
    ▶ The specific body parts involved, such as the face and neck, are identified
    ▶ The burn depth (partial- or full-thickness) is noted
    ▶ The causative agent is identified as thermal, chemical, or electrical
    ▶ The patient's age is documented because it alters body surface area estimates based on body proportions; the Lund-Browder classification is used to estimate body surface area burned in a pediatric patient
  ◆ Fluid and electrolyte balance is the chief concern for up to 48 hours after a major burn; the greatest fluid loss occurs in the first 12 hours; the larger the burned area, the greater the fluid loss
  ◆ Burns initially cause capillaries in the damaged area to dilate
    ▶ Increased hyperpermeability causes fluid to move out of cells into surrounding tissues; this fluid movement causes edema and vesiculation (blistering)

◗ Proteins, plasma, and electrolytes shift to the interstitial compartment; red blood cells remain in the vascular system, causing increased blood viscosity and false hematocrit elevation

◆ Burns also cause acute dehydration and poor renal perfusion

◆ Burn shock is a serious complication caused by decreased fluid volume

◗ Most burn-related deaths result from burn shock

◗ Signs and symptoms of burn shock include decreased urine output, tachycardia, hypotension, tachypnea with shallow respirations, and restlessness

■ Treatment in stage 2 (intermediate or acute stage)

◆ Stage 2 begins 48 to 72 hours after the burn injury

◆ Circulatory overload is the chief concern as fluid shifts back into the cells from the interstitial areas, and the kidneys begin to excrete large volumes of urine (diuresis)

◆ Vital signs, urine output, and level of consciousness must be monitored during this stage

◆ Smoke inhalation damages the respiratory cilia and mucosa, decreases the amount of alveolar surfactant, and can cause atelectasis

◗ Breathing difficulties — especially in patients with burns in the upper chest, neck, and face — may occur immediately or may not occur for several hours

◗ Symptoms of smoke inhalation include hoarseness, productive cough, singed nasal hairs, agitation, tachypnea, flaring nostrils, retractions, and sooty septum

■ Treatment in stage 3 (rehabilitation stage)

◆ Stage 3 begins after the burn area is treated; prevention of infection is the chief concern, and the goal is to return the patient to a productive life

◆ The patient may need to wear elastic garments to decrease scarring and may need cosmetic surgery and psychological and vocational counseling

■ Burn care

◆ Burned areas may be left exposed (open to air) if the burn doesn't encircle the arm, trunk, or leg

◆ An occlusive dressing may be applied (covered with a nonadhesive, water-permeable mesh gauze)

◆ The burn may require primary excision, or debridement (removal of necrotic or damaged tissue)

◆ Skin grafting may be necessary

◗ Autograft is obtained from undamaged parts of the patient's body

◗ Homograft is obtained from a person other than the patient

◗ Xenograft is obtained from a different species such as a pig

◗ Isograft is obtained from an identical twin

■ Nursing interventions

◆ Maintain a patent airway

◆ Monitor vital signs every 15 minutes to evaluate effectiveness of fluid resuscitation and to detect secondary infections

◆ Encourage coughing and deep breathing to promote lung expansion and adequate gas exchange

◆ Establish an I.V. line to initiate fluid replacement with a colloid and crystalloid solution (lactated Ringer's solution) during the first 24 hours

◆ Insert an indwelling urinary catheter to measure urine output and identify potential renal shutdown

◆ If possible, weigh the patient on admission to obtain baseline data

◆ Provide hyperalimentation (concentrated glucose and amino acids) if needed; insert a nasogastric tube as ordered to decompress the stomach and prevent aspiration of stomach contents

◆ If the patient hasn't had a booster shot within the past 5 years, administer tetanus toxoid; the patient may have an injury prone to tetanus

◆ Administer an I.V. analgesic, such as morphine, to reduce discomfort

◆ Administer an antibiotic as prescribed; the patient is more susceptible to infection because the skin's protective function is compromised

◆ Long-term treatment with an antacid and a histamine-2 receptor antagonist may be needed to maintain pH and reduce the risk of Curling's ulcer

◆ Keep the patient warm; he may lose body heat through the burn area and may become hypothermic

◆ Use aseptic technique when assisting the patient in the whirlpool bath (for debridement) and when changing the dressing

◆ Apply the prescribed topical agent to prevent bacterial infections; be aware that silver nitrate produces stains, mafenide acetate (Sulfamylon) can cause temporary stinging and burning (analgesia may be needed before application), and silver sulfadiazine (Silvadene) maintains adequate hydration in a patient receiving sulfonamides

◆ Perform ROM exercises for affected areas, if possible, to maintain function

◆ Encourage the patient and family to discuss feelings and concerns

❖ Lyme disease

■ Description

◆ Lyme disease is an inflammatory, multisystemic disorder caused by a spirochete, which is transmitted by a deer tick bite; the disease is most common in the summer

◆ Lyme disease causes many complications, such as arrhythmias, arthritis, cranial or peripheral neuropathies, encephalitis, meningitis, myocarditis, and pericarditis

■ Signs and symptoms

◆ Lyme disease may cause distinctive, expanding skin lesions that are warm to touch and have an intense red border (bull's-eye rash)

 ❿ The lesions appear 3 days to 4 weeks after the tick bite

 ❿ Common lesion sites are the groin, buttocks, axillae, trunk, upper arms, and legs

◆ Lyme disease occurs in three stages

 ❿ Stage 1 begins with a tick bite and produces chills, fatigue, fever, sore throat, and stiff neck — that is, signs and symptoms that may be mistaken for meningitis; it typically begins with the classic skin lesion called erythema chronicum migrans, beginning as a small papule at the site of the bite, and gradually enlarges into a round or oval ring with central clearing

▶ Stage II is characterized by neurologic effects, such as Bell's palsy, and cardiac effects, such as arrhythmias or heart block

▶ Stage III is characterized by arthritis, usually of the knees; the patient may have recurrent attacks up to 3 years after the rash appears

■ Diagnosis and treatment

◆ Blood tests, including antibody titers to identify *Borrelia burgdorferi,* are the most practical diagnostic tests; enzyme-linked immunosorbent assay has greater sensitivity and specificity

◆ Serologic tests don't always confirm the diagnosis—especially in the early stages before the body produces antibodies—or seropositivity for *B. burgdorferi*

◆ Mild anemia along with elevated aspartate aminotransferase levels, erythrocyte sedimentation rate, serum immunoglobulin M levels, and white blood cell count support the diagnosis

◆ A lumbar puncture may be ordered if Lyme disease involves the central nervous system

◆ As soon as the diagnosis is made, the patient is treated with oral doxycycline, amoxicillin, or erythromycin for 10 to 21 days

◆ Patients in stages II and III are treated with I.V. or I.M. penicillin or ceftriaxone

◆ A salicylate or another nonsteroidal anti-inflammatory drug may be prescribed to reduce inflammation

■ Nursing interventions

◆ Plan care to provide adequate rest

◆ Monitor vital signs to evaluate the patient's response to treatment

◆ Use a cardiac monitor or electrocardiogram to determine cardiac involvement

◆ Check for neurologic signs to assess neurologic involvement

◆ Promote the patient's comfort with position changes and skin care

◆ Educate the patient about the disease, including measures to prevent and avoid exposure to ticks; also explain that if he finds a tick on his body, he should grasp it with tweezers and pull it straight out

◆ Encourage the patient to discuss feelings about the disease

◆ Report infections to the Centers for Disease Control and Prevention

❖ Malignant melanoma

■ Description

◆ Malignant melanoma is a neoplasm derived from dermal or epidermal cells; it's the leading cause of death from skin cancer

◆ Prognosis is related to the thickness of the tumor at the time of diagnosis

◆ Exposure to sunlight increases the risk of malignant melanoma; fair-skinned, blond- or red-haired people are at greater relative risk than persons with darker pigmentation

◆ Melanoma originates in normal skin or an existing mole and metastasizes to other areas of the body; common sites are the back, legs, between the toes, scalp, back of the hands, face, and neck

■ Signs and symptoms

◆ A change in borders, color, size, or shape of a preexisting skin lesion

◆ An irregular, circular bordered lesion with hues of tan, black, or blue

◆ The lesion may produce local soreness and may be accompanied by pruritus, oozing, bleeding, or crusting

■ Diagnosis and treatment

◆ A skin biopsy shows cytology positive for malignant melanoma

◆ Diagnostic studies may include chest X-ray, a gallium scan, bone scan, magnetic resonance imaging, and computed tomography scans of the head, chest, and abdomen to evaluate possible metastases

◆ Treatment depends on lesion thickness; initial treatment includes a wide excision of the lesion and involved lymph nodes in the vicinity of the tumor

◆ A chemotherapeutic agent may be directly infused into the lesion, or a combination of direct infusion and systemic chemotherapeutic treatment may be used

◆ Administration of interferon and interleukin-2 may achieve temporary remission

◆ Radiation therapy may be used for palliative effects

◆ Although still investigational, gene therapy is another treatment being used

■ Nursing interventions

◆ Perform assessments while bathing the patient or performing ROM exercises; this approach is less obvious, and the patient may be more relaxed

◆ Medicate for discomfort, especially if a wide excision is necessary

◆ Teach the patient about the disease, including prevention measures, such as decreasing exposure to ultraviolet rays, using sunscreen, avoiding tanning booths, and performing a monthly self-examination, during which time he should check all skin lesions for changes

◆ Answer the patient's questions to decrease anxiety

◆ Identify resources and support systems to help the patient cope

◆ Encourage the patient to express feelings about the disease

❖ **Squamous cell carcinoma**

■ Description

◆ Squamous cell carcinoma is an invasive tumor arising from keratinizing epidermal cells; it has the potential for metastasis

◆ This type of cancer is most common among men who are fair skinned and older than age 60

■ Signs and symptoms

◆ Basal cell carcinoma lesions appear scaly and keratotic with raised, irregular borders

◆ As the disease progresses, lesions grow outward, are friable, and tend toward chronic crusting
■ Diagnosis and treatment
  ◆ An excisional biopsy provides a definitive diagnosis
  ◆ Local disease treatment may include cryosurgery, electrosurgery, Mohs' surgery, and radiation therapy
  ◆ Regional control includes radiation of lymph nodes, surgical excision, chemotherapy, or combination therapy
■ Nursing interventions
  ◆ Assess the patient's skin while you're helping him bathe or perform ROM exercises
  ◆ Explain the treatment recommendations and the need for follow-up
  ◆ Teach the patient about wound care, protection from the sun, lifestyle modifications, and skin examination

Review questions

1. The nurse is teaching a patient diagnosed with basal cell carcinoma. The most common cause of basal cell carcinoma is:

○ **A.** immunosuppression.

○ **B.** radiation exposure.

○ **C.** sun exposure.

○ **D.** burns.

Correct answer: C Sun exposure is the best known and most common cause of basal cell carcinoma. Immunosuppression (option A), radiation (option B), and burns (option D) are less common causes.

2. A patient received burns to his entire back and left arm. Using the Rule of Nines, the nurse can calculate that he has sustained burns on what percentage of his body?

○ **A.** 9%

○ **B.** 18%

○ **C.** 27%

○ **D.** 36%

Correct answer: C According to the Rule of Nines, each of the posterior and anterior trunks and legs makes up 18% of the total body surface, each of the arms makes up 9%, the head and neck make up 9%, and the perineum makes up 1%. In this case, the patient received burns to his back (18%) and one arm (9%), totaling 27% of his body.

3. A patient is admitted to a burn intensive care unit with extensive full-thickness burns. The nurse is most concerned about the patient's:

○ **A.** fluid and electrolyte status.

○ **B.** risk of infection.

○ **C.** body image.

○ **D.** level of pain.

Correct answer: A   During the early phase of burn care, the nurse is most concerned with fluid resuscitation and electrolyte balance, to correct large-volume fluid loss through the damaged skin. Infection (option B), body image (option C), and pain (option D) are significant areas of concern, but are less urgent than fluid status.

4. A patient undergoes a biopsy to confirm a diagnosis of skin cancer. Immediately following the procedure, the nurse should observe the site for:

○ **A.** infection.

○ **B.** dehiscence.

○ **C.** hemorrhage.

○ **D.** swelling.

Correct answer: C   The nurse's main concern following a skin biopsy procedure is bleeding. Infection (option A) is a later possible consequence of a biopsy. Dehiscence (option B) is more likely in larger wounds such as surgical wounds of the abdomen or thorax. Swelling (option D) is a normal reaction associated with any event that traumatizes the skin.

5. The nurse is caring for a patient with malignant melanoma. The nurse explains that the first and most important treatment for malignant melanoma is:

○ **A.** chemotherapy.

○ **B.** immunotherapy.

○ **C.** radiation therapy.

○ **D.** wide excision.

Correct answer: D   Wide excision is the primary treatment for malignant melanoma and removes the entire lesion and determines the level and staging. Chemotherapy (option A) may be used after the melanoma is excised. Immunotherapy (option B) is experimental. Radiation therapy (option C) is palliative.

CHAPTER

14

Endocrine disorders

❖ Introduction

- The endocrine system plays a significant role in human growth, metabolism, and environmental adaptation
- Along with the nervous system, the endocrine system provides a communication system for the body
- By releasing hormones from various ductless glands, the endocrine system carefully regulates many physiologic functions
- Nursing history
  - ◆ The nurse asks the patient about his *chief complaint*
    - ❯ A patient with an endocrine disorder may report abnormalities of fatigue, mental status changes, polydipsia, polyuria, weakness, and weight change
    - ❯ The patient with an endocrine disorder may also report problems of sexual maturity and function
  - ◆ The nurse then questions the patient about his *present illness*
    - ❯ Ask the patient about his symptom, including when it started, associated symptoms, location, radiation, intensity, duration, frequency, and precipitating and alleviating factors
    - ❯ Ask about the use of prescription and over-the-counter drugs, herbal remedies, and vitamin and nutritional supplements
  - ◆ The nurse asks about *medical history*
    - ❯ Question the patient about other endocrine disorders, such as diabetes mellitus, height and weight problems, sexual problems, and thyroid disease
    - ❯ Ask the female patient about past reproductive problems and use of oral contraceptives and hormones; also ask whether she's premenopausal or postmenopausal
  - ◆ The nurse then assesses the *family history*
    - ❯ Ask about a family history of endocrine disorders, such as diabetes mellitus and thyroid disorders
    - ❯ Question the patient about his cultural background and heredity
  - ◆ The nurse obtains a *social history*
    - ❯ Ask about work, exercise, diet, use of recreational drugs, alcohol use, and hobbies
    - ❯ Also ask about stress, support systems, and coping mechanisms
- Physical assessment
  - ◆ The nurse begins with *inspection*

▶ Observe the patient's general appearance and development, height, weight, posture, body build, proportionality of body parts, and distribution of body fat and hair

▶ Note affect, speech, level of consciousness, orientation, appropriateness of behavior, grooming and dress, and activity level

▶ Assess overall skin color and, for areas of abnormal pigmentation, note any bruising, lesions, petechiae, or striae

▶ Assess the face for erythematous areas, note facial expression, shape, and symmetry of the eyes; also note abnormal lid closure, eyeball protrusion, and periorbital edema, if present

▶ Inspect the tongue for color, size, lesions, tremor, and positioning

▶ Inspect the neck area for symmetry

▶ Evaluate the overall size, shape, and symmetry of the chest, noting any deformities, especially around the nipples

▶ Check for truncal obesity, supraclavicular fat pads, and buffalo hump

▶ Inspect the external genitalia for normal development

▶ Inspect the arms and legs for tremors, muscle development and strength, symmetry, color, and hair distribution

▶ Examine the feet, noting size, deformities, lesions, marks from shoes and socks, maceration, dryness, or fissures

◆ Next, the nurse uses *palpation*

▶ Palpate the thyroid gland for size, symmetry, and shape; note any nodules or irregularities

▶ Palpate the testes for size, symmetry, and shape; note any nodules or deformities

◆ Then the nurse uses *auscultation*

▶ Auscultate the thyroid gland to identify systolic bruits

▶ Auscultate the heart, noting heart rhythm disturbances that may occur in endocrine disorders

❖ Addison's disease

■ Description

◆ Addison's disease is a chronic adrenocortical insufficiency most commonly caused by autoimmune destruction of the adrenal cortex

◆ Other causes of adrenal insufficiency include fungal infection and infectious disease such as tuberculosis; hemorrhage; metastatic disease (rarely); therapy with drugs, such as ketoconazole, phenytoin, and rifampin; after sudden withdrawal of steroid therapy; and surgical removal of both adrenal glands

◆ Addison's disease leads to impaired metabolism, inability to maintain a normal glucose level, and fluid and electrolyte imbalances

◆ Primary insufficiency results from low levels of glucocorticoids and mineralocorticoids; secondary insufficiency results from inadequate pituitary secretion of corticotropin

◆ Lack of cortisol (a glucocorticoid), aldosterone (a mineralocorticoid), and androgens diminish gluconeogenesis, decrease liver glycogen, and increase the sensitivity of peripheral tissues to insulin

◆ Because cortisol is required for a normal stress response, patients with cortisol insufficiency can't withstand surgical stress, trauma, or infection

■ Signs and symptoms

◆ The patient may have a history of fatigue, muscle weakness, and weight loss

◆ The skin and mucous membranes may appear bronze due to increased levels of melanocyte-stimulating hormone

◆ GI effects may include anorexia, nausea, vomiting, and diarrhea

◆ Other effects may include dehydration, hyperkalemia, hypoglycemia, hyponatremia, hypotension, and loss of axillary, extremity, and pubic hair

■ Diagnosis and treatment

◆ Laboratory tests may show low levels of plasma and urine cortisol and elevated levels of plasma corticotropin as well as hyperkalemia, hyponatremia, leukocytosis, and metabolic acidosis

◆ In a corticotropin stimulation test, plasma corticotropin levels may not increase in response to I.V. corticotropin

◆ Treatment consists of replacing glucocorticoids and mineralocorticoids; cortisone is given in two daily doses (usually on arising and at 6 p.m.) to mimic the body's diurnal variations; doses are increased during periods of stress

◆ Treatment also includes prevention of adrenal crisis, which may develop after trauma, infection, or GI upset; prevention requires consistent replacement therapy (without abrupt withdrawal); treatment of crisis requires immediate replacement of sodium, water, and cortisone

◆ Adrenal hemorrhage after septicemia is a rare complication of Addison's disease; it's treated with aggressive antibiotic therapy, an I.V. vasopressor, and massive doses of a steroid

■ Nursing interventions

◆ Monitor the patient for signs and symptoms of adrenal crisis, such as fever, changes in GI function (which may alter drug absorption), decreased sodium and cortisol levels with increased potassium levels (which may signal an impending crisis), dehydration, headache, hypotension, nausea, severe fatigue, tachycardia, and confusion

◆ Ensure strict adherence to the medication schedule to prevent crisis

◆ Decrease environmental stressors as much as possible

◆ Teach the patient and his family how to prevent complications of Addison's disease by never omitting a dose of medication, notifying the practitioner if the patient can't take the medication, avoiding undue stress, and wearing a medical identification bracelet

◆ Instruct the patient and his family to report any symptoms of adrenal crisis to a practitioner

❖ Cushing's syndrome

■ Description

◆ Cushing's syndrome is hyperfunction of the adrenal cortex caused by an overabundance of cortisol

◆ It's classified as corticotropin-dependent or corticotropin-independent

> With corticotropin-dependent Cushing's syndrome, cortical hyperfunction results from excessive corticotropin secretion by the pituitary gland; in 80% of cases, excessive corticotropin secretion is related to a pituitary adenoma

> With corticotropin-independent Cushing's syndrome, cortical hyperfunction is independent of corticotropin regulation; high levels of cortisol are caused by a neoplasm in the adrenal cortex, or islet cell tumor

◆ Cushing's syndrome may be caused by abnormal cortisol production or excessive corticotropin stimulation (spontaneous disorder) or long-term glucocorticoid (such as prednisone) administration (iatrogenic disorder)

◆ For patients with this disorder, excessive cortisol leads to excessive glucose production and interferes with the cells' ability to use insulin; sodium retention, potassium excretion, and protein breakdown occur; body fat is redistributed from the arms and legs to the face, shoulders, trunk, and abdomen; and the immune system becomes less effective at preventing infection

■ Signs and symptoms

◆ Muscle weakness and atrophy may be accompanied by fat deposits on the trunk, abdomen, over the upper back ("buffalo hump"), and face ("moon face")

◆ Skin changes may include acne, bruising, facial flushing, hyperpigmentation, and striae

◆ Gynecomastia may occur in men; clitoral enlargement and menstrual irregularities, in women

◆ Other effects may include arrhythmias, edema, emotional lability, GI disturbances, headaches, hirsutism (fine, downy hair on face and upper body), infection, vertebral fractures, and weight changes

■ Diagnosis and treatment

◆ The dexamethasone suppression test and urine-free cortisol test are standard screening tests for Cushing's syndrome

◆ Laboratory tests may show coagulopathies, hyperglycemia, hypokalemia, hypernatremia, increased aldosterone and cortisol levels, and suppressed plasma corticotropin levels; computed tomography or magnetic resonance imaging may show a tumor

◆ The goal of treatment is normal cortisol activity

◆ Surgery is used if a tumor is causing corticotropin release

> For a confirmed pituitary tumor, transsphenoidal resection is recommended; for a suspected pituitary tumor, cobalt irradiation of the pituitary gland

> For a confirmed adrenal cortex tumor, bilateral adrenalectomy may be done; after surgery, the patient requires lifelong corticosteroid and mineralocorticoid replacement

◆ Drug therapy is used if something else is causing corticotropin release; aminoglutethimide, mitotane, and trilostane interfere with adrenal hormone synthesis or corticotropin production; bromocriptine and cyproheptadine interfere with corticotropin secretion; and glucocorticoids

(such as cortisone, dexamethasone, and prednisone) treat congenital adrenal hyperplasia
■ Nursing interventions
◆ Encourage the patient to express concerns about altered body image
◆ Protect the patient from injury related to loss of bone matrix and abnormal fat distribution by maintaining a safe environment, teaching him how to use a walker or cane, encouraging the use of well-fitting shoes or slippers, and attending to complaints of lower back pain or joint pain
◆ Protect the patient from injury related to easy bruising and protein wasting by avoiding unnecessary venipunctures, using paper tape for dressing changes, avoiding overinflation of the blood pressure cuff, keeping the skin clean and dry, and using a convoluted foam mattress, a water mattress, or an air bed for a patient with skin breakdown
◆ Provide care related to limited mobility and muscle weakness resulting from protein catabolism by planning rest periods, encouraging range-of-motion exercises or daily muscle-strengthening exercises, and referring the patient for physical therapy, if needed
◆ Protect the patient from infection related to decreased immune function by using strict aseptic technique (when appropriate) and discouraging ill family members from visiting the patient
◆ Provide postoperative care after adrenalectomy, including monitoring vital signs frequently, ensuring adequate pain relief and fluid intake and output, and monitoring for complications of hypoglycemia and signs of adrenal crisis
◆ Administer replacement medication as prescribed, and be familiar with its adverse effects
◆ Suggest that the patient wear a medical identification bracelet
◆ Teach the patient and his family about the disease and its treatment

❖ **Diabetes insipidus**
■ Description
◆ Diabetes insipidus is a deficiency of antidiuretic hormone (ADH), resulting in water imbalance; vasopressin is a natural ADH
◆ *Central diabetes insipidus* results from the destruction of vasopressin-producing cells; *nephrogenic diabetes insipidus* results when the renal tubules don't respond to vasopressin
◆ *Syndrome of inappropriate antidiuretic hormone (SIADH)* causes the release of excessive ADH, resulting in water retention (see *Comparing diabetes insipidus and SIADH*, pages 236 and 237)
■ Nursing interventions
◆ Support the patient during the water deprivation test
◆ *For diabetes insipidus:* Treat altered fluid volume related to excessive urine output by maintaining fluid and electrolyte balance, administering replacement therapy as prescribed, and monitoring the patient for signs of therapy-related water intoxication, notifying the practitioner of significant changes in urine output and specific gravity, and observing patient for vital sign changes related to dehydration, such as increased heart rate and decreased blood pressure

Comparing diabetes insipidus and SIADH

This chart summarizes the major characteristics of central and nephrogenic diabetes insipidus and syndrome of inappropriate antidiuretic hormone (SIADH).

Characteristic	Central diabetes insipidus	Nephrogenic diabetes insipidus	SIADH
Cause	• Head trauma or surgery • Pituitary or hypothalamic tumor • Intracerebral occlusion or infection	• Systemic diseases involving the kidney, such as multiple myeloma and sickle cell anemia • Polycystic kidney disease • Pyelonephritis • Medications such as lithium and demeclocycline	• Central nervous system disorders, such as head trauma, infection, intercerebral hemorrhage, or tumor • Pharmacologic agents, including chemotherapeutic agents, phenothiazines, and tricyclic antidepressants • Respiratory disorders and treatment, such as pneumonia, pneumothorax, bronchiogenic tumors, and positive-pressure ventilation
Pathophysiology	• Loss of vasopressin-producing cells, causing deficiency in antidiuretic hormone (ADH) synthesis or release; deficiency in ADH, resulting in an inability to conserve water, leading to extreme polyuria and polydipsia	• Depression of aldosterone release or inability of the nephrons to respond to ADH, causing extreme polyuria and polydipsia	• Inappropriate release of ADH, causing dilutional hyponatremia, leading to cellular swelling and water retention
Signs and symptoms	• Polyuria with urine output of 5 to 15 L daily • Polydipsia, especially a desire for cold fluids • Marked dehydration, as evidenced by dry mucous membranes, dry skin, and weight loss • Anorexia and epigastric fullness • Nocturia and related fatigue from interrupted sleep	• Same as for central diabetes insipidus	• Excessive or inappropriate water retention • Initially, anorexia, headaches, nausea, and vomiting • Later, confusion, irritability, seizures, and coma from severe hyponatremia

Comparing diabetes insipidus and SIADH *(continued)*

Characteristic	Central diabetes insipidus	Nephrogenic diabetes insipidus	SIADH
Diagnostic test results	• High serum osmolality, usually above 300 mOsm/kg of water • Low urine osmolarity, usually 50 to 200 mOsm/kg of water; low urine-specific gravity less than 1.005 • Increased creatinine and blood urea nitrogen (BUN) levels resulting from dehydration • Positive response to water deprivation test: Urine output decreases and specific gravity increases	• Same as for central diabetes insipidus, except that plasma vasopressin levels are elevated in relation to plasma osmolality, and there is no response to exogenous vasopressin administration (decreased urine output and increased specific gravity)	• Low serum osmolality • High urine osmolality • Low serum sodium level • High urine sodium level, usually over 20 mEq/L • Decreased creatinine and BUN levels • Negative response to water deprivation test: Urine output increases and specific gravity decreases
Treatments	• Replacement vasopressin therapy with intranasal or I.V. DDAVP (desmopressin acetate) • Correction of dehydration and electrolyte imbalances	• A thiazide diuretic to deplete sodium and increase renal water reabsorption • Restriction of salt and protein intake	• Restriction of water intake to 1 qt (0.9 L) daily • Infusions of 3% to 5% sodium chloride to replace sodium • A diuretic to decrease volume overload • Demeclocycline to reverse hyperosmolarity

◆ *For SIADH:* Treat altered fluid volume status related to water retention by weighing the patient at the same time daily, reporting weight gains or losses to the practitioner, so treatment with vasopressin or desmopressin can begin, and monitoring patient for signs of water retention, such as dyspnea, edema, hypertension, and tachycardia

◆ Provide oral and skin care, and reposition the patient frequently to prevent skin breakdown

◆ Conserve energy for a patient who is up often during the night to void or drink; encourage short naps to prevent sleep deprivation

◆ Protect the patient from injury related to fatigue, weakness, dehydration, or confusion by providing a safe environment, encouraging a weak patient to request assistance in walking to and from the bathroom, teaching a patient to sit up gradually to prevent dizziness resulting from orthostatic hypotension, and taking seizure precautions for a patient with a low serum sodium level

◆ Teach the patient and family to recognize the signs of diabetes insipidus and SIADH

◆ Teach the patient how to administer intranasal medications

❖ Diabetes mellitus

■ Description

◆ Diabetes mellitus is a chronic systemic disease that alters carbohydrate, fat, and protein metabolism; it's the most common endocrine disorder and the third leading cause of death in the United States. Four general classifications are recognized:

◆ Prediabetes can occur when the fasting blood glucose is > 100 mg/dl and < 126 mg/dl or postprandial blood glucose > 140 mg/dl and < 200 mg/dl

◆ *Type 1 diabetes mellitus* is an absolute deficiency of insulin secretion and may be hereditary; it's associated with histocompatibility antigens, some viruses, abnormal antibodies that attack the islet of Langerhans cells, and toxic chemicals; it causes symptoms when 90% of the pancreatic beta cells have been destroyed

◆ *Type 2 diabetes mellitus* may be hereditary, is associated with obesity, and results from different causes than type 1 diabetes; it's caused by defects in insulin secretion and decreased insulin effectiveness; it accounts for 90% of diabetic patients

◆ *Gestational diabetes mellitus* causes glucose intolerance during pregnancy; it usually disappears after delivery but may develop into type 1 or type 2 diabetes

◆ Other types of diabetes mellitus can be linked to either a disorder (such as an endocrinopathy, a genetic syndrome, an insulin receptor disorder, or a pancreatic disease) or to the use of a drug or a chemical (such as a corticosteroid, epinephrine, furosemide, glucagon, lithium, or phenytoin)

◆ *Impaired glucose tolerance* occurs when glucose levels are outside the normal range following a glucose tolerance test but the patient doesn't meet the criteria for diabetes mellitus

◆ Many complications are associated with diabetes mellitus

❯ Microvascular and macrovascular changes can increase the risk of heart disease, accelerate atherosclerotic disease, and cause cerebrovascular accidents, hypertension, and peripheral vascular disease

❯ Microvascular changes can thicken capillary basement membranes and cause changes in the vessels of the kidneys and eyes

❯ Motor and sensory neuropathies may result in weakness, hyperesthesia, hypoesthesia, and pain; autonomic neuropathy generally occurs after many years and may cause cardiac abnormalities, diabetic diarrhea, gastroparesis, impotence, and urine retention

❯ Infections can result from accumulation of serum glucose in the skin and poorly functioning white blood cells

◆ With diabetes mellitus, hyperglycemia results from insulin deficiency or insulin resistance, which makes insulin unavailable to cells; the discrepancy between the amount of insulin available to tissues and the amount needed leads to impaired carbohydrate, protein, and fat metabolism

■ Signs and symptoms

Treatments for diabetes mellitus

A patient with diabetes mellitus commonly follows a regimen that requires medications (an oral antidiabetic or insulin), diet, and physical activity.

Oral antidiabetics

An oral antidiabetic may be prescribed alone or in combination with another drug and/or insulin for a patient with type 2 diabetes mellitus. A sulfonylurea (such as acetohexamide, chlorpropamide, glimepiride, glipizide, glyburide, tolazamide, and tolbutamide) works by stimulating the pancreas to release insulin but doesn't lead to hypoglycemia. Metformin, a biguanide, works by reducing the production of glucose in the liver and by making the tissues more sensitive to insulin; the drug may cause hypoglycemia. Acarbose and miglitol, alpha-glucosidase inhibitors, reduce glucose levels by interfering with glucose absorption in the small intestine; when used alone, these drugs don't cause hypoglycemia. Repaglinide, a benzoic acid derivative, stimulates beta cells to produce insulin; because the drug is quickly metabolized and is short acting, it's less likely to cause hypoglycemia. Troglitazone, a thiazolidinedione, increases insulin sensitivity by activating genes involved in fat synthesis and carbohydrate metabolism; when used alone, the drug doesn't cause hypoglycemia.

Insulin

Insulin therapy may be prescribed for other diabetic patients. Regular, lispro (Humalog) and aspart (Novolog) insulins are appropriate for short-acting therapy. Their action begins in less than 1 hour, peaks in 2 to 4 hours, and lasts 3 to 6 hours. Neutral protamine Hagedorn (NPH) or Lente insulin is used for intermediate-acting therapy. Each of these drugs begins to act in 1 to 4 hours, produces peak action in 6 to 12 hours, and pro-

duces effects for 12 to 24 hours. Protamine zinc or Ultralente insulin can be used for long-acting therapy. For these drugs, onset occurs in 4 to 8 hours, action peaks in 16 to 18 hours, and action lasts up to 30 hours. Glargine insulin is used as basal therapy. It has an onset of 2 to 4 hours, has no peak effectiveness period, and lasts 20 to 24 hours. An insulin pump may be used to deliver rapid-acting insulin to meet both basal and bolus needs; the pump can be implanted under the skin or worn externally.

Diet

Diet therapy is individualized based on metabolic, nutritional, and lifestyle requirements. Emphasis is placed on achieving glucose, lipid, and blood pressure control. The following restrictions are recommended: Fat intake should equal 20% to 30% of total calories; protein intake, 10% to 20% of total calories; carbohydrate intake, 50% to 60% of calories; cholesterol intake, 300 mg or less; fiber intake, 20 to 30 g daily; and sodium intake, 2 to 3 g daily.

Physical activity

Exercise lowers blood glucose levels, maintains normal cholesterol levels, helps blood vessels perform more effectively, and may reduce the amount of insulin needed. Therefore, the patient should follow a consistent exercise program, engaging in activity when glucose levels are high. (Carbohydrate intake must be increased if the patient exercises when glucose levels are low.)

◆ The classic signs and symptoms are polydipsia, polyphagia, polyuria, and weight loss
◆ Other effects may include fatigue and somnolence
■ Diagnosis and treatment
◆ Diagnosis may be based on symptoms of diabetes mellitus and a casual plasma glucose level greater than 200 mg/dl, an 8-hour fasting plasma glucose level greater than 126 mg/dl, or a 2-hour postload glucose level greater than 200 mg/dl during an oral glucose tolerance test; testing must be confirmed on a subsequent day
◆ Hemoglobin A_{1C} levels reflect the plasma glucose level during the past 2 to 3 months
◆ The first goal of treatment is to maintain a normal blood glucose level through oral antidiabetic or insulin therapy, diet control, and physical activity (see *Treatments for diabetes mellitus*)

◆ The second goal of treatment is to prevent or delay the complications
  ▶ Hypoglycemia (insulin shock) is a condition in which the blood glucose level falls below the level required to sustain homeostasis (usually under 60 mg/dl); it may result from too little food, too much insulin or oral antihypoglycemics, or too much exercise and can cause permanent neurologic damage or rebound hyperglycemia
    • Onset occurs in minutes to hours, but most often before meals, especially if meals are delayed or snacks omitted
    • Severe signs and symptoms may include bladder spasms; a blood glucose level under 60 mg/dl; bradycardia; bradypnea; confusion; cool, moist skin; hallucinations; light-headedness; memory loss; nausea; seizures or coma; slight respiratory acidosis; vision disturbances; and vomiting
    • Milder signs and symptoms may include sweating, tremor, tachycardia, palpitations, and hunger
    • Hypoglycemia is treated with candy or orange juice if the patient's awake, followed by a snack of protein and starch within 20 to 60 minutes; it's treated with an I.V. bolus of 50% dextrose solution, if the patient is unconscious, 1 mg glucagon may be given I.V., I.M., or subcutaneously and, when awake, give a simple sugar followed by a snack
  ▶ Hyperglycemia is a condition in which the blood glucose level exceeds 120 mg/dl
    • When blood glucose exceeds 180 mg/dl, glucose is excreted in urine along with large amounts of water and electrolytes; excessive thirst, hunger, and ketosis also occur
    • Hyperglycemia is treated with short-acting insulin and exercise to lower blood glucose levels
  ▶ Diabetic ketoacidosis (DKA) results from too little insulin, which prevents glucose from entering cells and causes it to accumulate in the blood
    • DKA is treated with regular I.V. insulin, I.V. fluids to supplement intravascular volume, potassium replacement, and sodium bicarbonate if the pH is less than 7.0
  ▶ Hyperosmolar hyperglycemic nonketotic syndrome (HHNS) resembles DKA, but ketoacidosis doesn't occur; the patient has enough insulin to inhibit lipolysis (see *Understanding the difference between DKA and HHNS*)
    • HHNS can be precipitated by infection, myocardial infarction, stroke, pancreatitis, a severe burn treated with a high concentration of sugar, stress, or therapy with thiazide diuretic, a mannitol steroid, phenytoin, or total parenteral nutrition
    • It occurs most frequently in persons ages 50 to 70 who have no history of diabetes or mild type 2 diabetes
    • It's treated with insulin, I.V. fluids with half-normal saline solution or normal saline solution, and potassium replacement when urine output is adequate
■ Nursing interventions

Understanding the difference between DKA and HHNS

Diabetic ketoacidosis (DKA) and hyperosmolar hyperglycemic nonketotic syndrome (HHNS), both acute complications associated with diabetes, share some similarities, including changes in level of consciousness and extreme volume depletion, but they're two distinct conditions. The following chart helps determine which condition your patient is experiencing.

	Associated with	Onset	Symptoms
DKA	Type 1 diabetes mellitus	Rapid	• Hyperventilation (Kussmaul's respirations) • Acetone breath odor • Blood glucose level above normal (200 to 800 mg/dl) • Mild hyponatremia • Positive or large serum ketones • Serum osmolality slightly elevated • Hyperkalemia initially, then hypokalemia • Metabolic acidosis
HHNS	Type 2 diabetes mellitus	Slow	• Slightly rapid respirations • No breath odor • Blood glucose level markedly elevated (above 600 mg/dl) • Hypernatremia • Negative or small serum ketones • Serum osmolality markedly elevated • Normal serum potassium • Lack of acidosis

◆ Protect the patient from infection and injury related to circulatory compromise and possible nerve impairment
  ▶ Report wounds to the practitioner for treatment
  ▶ Apply lanolin to the feet and ankles
  ▶ Carefully dry the feet, especially between the toes
  ▶ Encourage the use of cotton socks to reduce moisture, and wear well-fitting shoes
  ▶ Have toenails clipped by a podiatrist
  ▶ Teach the patient and family about good skin care
  ▶ Tell the patient to avoid heating pads and to exercise caution when near open fires because burns are more difficult to treat in diabetic patients
  ▶ Treat fluid loss caused by hyperglycemia
  ▶ Rapidly infuse I.V. isotonic (normal) or hypotonic (half-normal) saline solution
  ▶ When blood glucose level falls below 250 mg/dl, administer I.V. dextrose 5% in water to prevent hypoglycemia and cerebral edema
  ▶ Check urine output and ketone levels hourly
  ▶ Monitor potassium level, and replace potassium as needed
◆ Help the patient maintain good nutritional habits
  ▶ Obtain a diet history, and note the impact of lifestyle and culture on food intake
  ▶ Encourage the patient to follow the American Diabetes Association's calculated diet plan; encourage the obese patient to lose weight

▶ Explain the importance of exercise and a balanced diet
◆ Teach the patient and his family about the disease, complications, and treatment
▶ Discuss blood glucose self-testing, skin care, and treatment of minor injuries; discuss which injuries should be reported to a practitioner
▶ Make sure the patient and his family know the signs of hyperglycemia and hypoglycemia
▶ Make sure the patient and family know how to adjust insulin doses for changes in diet, exercise, and stress level
▶ Have the patient or a family member demonstrate the technique for drawing up and administering insulin
▶ Teach the patient how to adjust doses if an insulin-infusion pump is used
▶ Educate the patient and his family about care during illness; tell the patient to monitor blood glucose levels more frequently, to increase fluid intake, and not to stop taking his antidiabetic without consulting with the practitioner
◆ Provide care for a diabetic patient with peripheral neuropathy
▶ Discuss causes of aching or burning sensation in legs
▶ Provide foot cradles to prevent contact with bed linens for a patient in severe pain
▶ Encourage exercise as tolerated, which may help to relieve pain
◆ Provide care for a diabetic patient with altered bowel and bladder elimination related to neuropathy by providing psychological support, administering prescribed drugs such as metoclopramide hydrochloride, and discussing the signs of bladder infection with the patient and family
◆ Provide care for a diabetic patient with retinopathy by encouraging independence, providing a safe environment, and eliciting the support of community agencies
◆ Provide care for a patient with diabetes who has a sexual dysfunction related to neuropathy by encouraging expression of feelings; exploring options such as a penile prosthesis; and recommending professional counseling as needed

❖ Hyperthyroidism

■ Description
◆ Hyperthyroidism is the excessive production of thyroid hormone resulting in a hypermetabolic state
◆ Severe hyperthyroidism can precipitate a thyroid storm or crisis, which is a life-threatening emergency; the crisis can be triggered by minor trauma or stress
◆ The two types of spontaneous hyperthyroidism are Graves' disease and toxic nodular goiter; signs and symptoms vary with the type and severity of the disease (see *Signs and symptoms of hyperthyroidism*)
▶ Graves' disease commonly occurs in the third or fourth decade of life; it's more common in women than in men, it has a familial predisposition, and it may cause extrathyroidal symptoms, goiter, and symptoms of hypermetabolism and sympathetic nervous system hyperactivity

Signs and symptoms of hyperthyroidism

Different forms of hyperthyroidism can produce various signs and symptoms as summarized below.

Graves' disease
(Signs and symptoms of hypermetabolism and sympathetic overactivity)

- Brittle hair and friable nails
- Emotional lability, anxiety, and irritability
- Fatigue
- Heat intolerance
- Increased respiratory rate and shortness of breath
- Increased sweating
- Loss of pubic hair in women; premature graying in men
- Muscle weakness and atrophy
- Tachycardia with palpitations
- Tremor
- Warm, moist skin
- Weight loss with increased appetite

Graves' disease
(Extrathyroid signs and symptoms)

- Exophthalmos
- Eyelid lag, or a slowed movement of the lid in relation to the eyeball
- Periorbital edema
- Pretibial myxedema that produces raised, thickened skin that may be hyperpigmented, itchy, and well-demarcated from normal skin; lesions that appear plaquelike or nodular
- Staring with decreased blinking

Toxic nodular goiter

- Arrhythmias that don't respond to digoxin therapy
- Muscle wasting with weakness
- Staring with decreased blinking
- Weight loss

Thyroid storm or crisis

- Fever, which usually precedes thyroid storm
- Increased blood pressure
- Severe tachycardia
- Altered mental state — delirium and coma
- General worsening of all symptoms

◗ Toxic nodular goiter typically occurs in elderly people; its slow onset causes less severe symptoms than Graves' disease
◆ Hyperthyroidism can result from discontinuation or excessive use of antithyroid medication, tumors that stimulate thyroid secretion, or deterioration of preexisting hyperthyroid state due to DKA, infection, toxemia, trauma, or excessive iodine intake
■ Diagnosis and treatment
◆ Laboratory tests show increased levels of thyroid hormones (triiodothyronine [T_3] and thyroxine [T_4]), decreased thyroid-stimulating hormone (TSH) level, and an increased blood glucose level resulting from impaired insulin secretion
◆ Electrocardiography shows atrial fibrillation, P- and T-wave alterations, and tachycardia; thyroid scan shows increased uptake of radioactive iodine
◆ The principal goal of treatment is to reduce thyroid hormone levels
◗ Antithyroid medications are generally used for pretreating patients who are elderly or who have cardiac disease before starting radioactive iodine; methimazole and propylthiouracil are slow-acting drugs that block thyroid synthesis and typically produce improvement after 2 to 4 weeks of therapy; a beta-adrenergic blocker such as propranolol may be used as an adjunct to control activity of the sympathetic nervous system
◗ Surgery (subtotal thyroidectomy) is reserved for patients with a very large gland, or who can't undergo other treatments, or who have

thyroid cancer; before surgery, the patient receives antithyroid medication to reduce hormone levels and saturated solution of potassium iodide to decrease surgical complications

▶ Radioactive iodine therapy also is the standard for treating hyperthyroidism; dosing is based on the patient's symptoms; it's contraindicated during pregnancy or breastfeeding, and many patients who receive radioactive iodine become euthyroid or hypothyroid, requiring levothyroxine treatment

◆ The second goal of treatment is to prevent thyroid storm

▶ The patient is taught to take medication (including an antipyretic) only as prescribed and to seek care for infection

▶ Fluids are replaced as needed to prevent the condition from worsening

■ Nursing interventions

◆ Maintain normal fluid and electrolyte balance to prevent arrhythmias

◆ Tell the patient to avoid caffeine, which can stimulate the sympathetic nervous system

◆ Provide a high-calorie, high-protein diet through several small, well-balanced meals

◆ Ensure adequate hydration

◆ Conserve the patient's energy to help decrease metabolism needs

◆ Prevent thyroid crisis by using a cooling mat to achieve normal temperature, keeping the patient's room cool, establishing a calm environment, using relaxation techniques, administering drugs as prescribed, identifying and treating precipitating factors, and teaching the patient and family how to prevent thyroid storm

◆ If the patient has exophthalmos, administer eyedrops or ointment, and encourage the use of sunglasses for comfort and to protect his eyes

◆ If the patient has diaphoresis, keep his skin dry with powders that contain cornstarch, and frequently change his bed linens

◆ If the patient underwent a thyroidectomy, keep him in Fowler's position to promote venous return from the head; assess for signs of respiratory distress and vocal changes; keep a tracheotomy tray at the bedside; monitor him for signs of hemorrhage; assess for hypocalcemia (such as tingling and numbness of the extremities, muscle twitching, laryngeal spasm, and positive Chvostek's and Trousseau's signs), which may occur if parathyroid glands are damaged; assess for signs of thyroid storm (such as tachycardia, hyperkenesis, fever, vomiting, and hypertension); and keep calcium gluconate available for emergency I.V. administration

❖ Hypothyroidism

■ Description

◆ Hypothyroidism is the diminished production of thyroid hormone, leading to thyroid insufficiency

◆ Primary hypothyroidism is caused by thyroid gland dysfunction; secondary hypothyroidism, from insufficient secretion of TSH by the pituitary gland

◆ Hypothyroidism occurs as myxedema in adults, as juvenile hypothyroidism in young children, or as congenital hypothyroidism

◆ Thyroid insufficiency causes decreased consciousness, hypometabolism, hypothermia, and hypoventilation

◆ Unrecognized and untreated congenital hypothyroidism — cretinism — can result in mental and physical retardation

◆ Hypothyroidism may be caused by worsening of a preexisting hypothyroid condition; insufficient thyroid hormone replacement therapy for hyperthyroidism; pituitary gland dysfunction due to infection, surgery, trauma, or tumor; autoimmune disease; iodine deficiency; and drugs (such as lithium and amiodarone)

■ Signs and symptoms

◆ Vital sign measurements may reveal bradycardia, decreased respiratory rate with shallow inspirations, hypotension, and hypothermia

◆ Hoarseness, impaired hearing, myxedema (nonpitting edema), and a puffy face, hands, and tongue may result from swelling

◆ Crackles may stem from pleural effusion

◆ Other effects may include intolerance to cold; dry, coarse skin; lethargy, stupor, coma; menstrual irregularities; fatigue; alopecia; and brittle nails

■ Diagnosis and treatment

◆ Diagnostic tests may include measurement of serum TSH, T_3, and T_4, and free T_4 levels; T_3 resin uptake test; and radioisotope thyroid uptake test

◆ Laboratory studies may show a decreased blood glucose level, decreased plasma osmolality, a decreased TSH level (with a pituitary or hypothalamic defect) or an increased TSH level (with a thyroid defect), and hyponatremia

◆ The primary treatment is lifelong replacement of the deficient hormone; synthetic levothyroxine sodium is the preferred thyroid hormone replacement and typically relieves symptoms in 2 to 3 days

◆ If myxedema coma develops, immediate I.V. administration of a corticosteroid, glucose, and levothyroxine sodium can reverse this life-threatening condition

■ Nursing interventions

◆ Administer replacement therapy as prescribed

◆ Avoid sedating the patient, which may further decrease respirations

◆ Recognize that slower metabolism may slow drug absorption and excretion

◆ Provide frequent skin care to prevent breakdown and decrease the risk of infection

◆ Administer fluids as prescribed; correct imbalances without causing fluid overload

◆ Monitor fluid intake and output, and weigh the patient daily to check for fluid retention

◆ If the patient has hypothermia, increase body temperature gradually by using warm blankets or increasing the room temperature

◆ Encourage coughing and deep breathing, and administer oxygen as prescribed
◆ Ask the patient and his family to demonstrate their understanding of the medication schedule
◆ Give the patient and his family opportunities to ask about the disease and its treatment
◆ Provide supportive care for a patient in myxedema coma; maintain a patent airway, monitor vital signs closely, and administer oxygen and I.V. fluid replacement until the patient begins to recover from the coma

Review questions

1. A 28-year-old woman is scheduled for a glucose tolerance test. She asks the nurse what results indicate diabetes mellitus. The nurse should respond that the minimum parameter for indication of diabetes mellitus is a 2-hour blood glucose level greater than:

○ **A.** 120 mg/dl.

○ **B.** 150 mg/dl.

○ **C.** 200 mg/dl.

○ **D.** 250 mg/dl.

Correct answer: C   A glucose tolerance test indicates a diagnosis of diabetes mellitus when the 2-hour blood glucose level is greater than 200 mg/dl. Confirmation occurs when at least one subsequent result is greater than 200 mg/dl. Options A and B are incorrect because they're below the minimum parameter; option D is incorrect because it's above the minimum parameter.

2. A patient is diagnosed with hyperthyroidism. The nurse should expect clinical signs and symptoms similar to:

○ **A.** hypovolemic shock.

○ **B.** sympathetic nervous system stimulation.

○ **C.** benzodiazepine overdose.

○ **D.** Addison's disease.

Correct answer: B   Hyperthyroidism is a hypermetabolic state characterized by such signs and symptoms as anxiety, increased blood pressure, and tachycardia—all seen in sympathetic nervous system stimulation. Symptoms of hypovolemic shock (option A), benzodiazepine overdose (option C), and Addison's disease (option D) are more similar to a hypometabolic state.

3. A patient with thyroid cancer undergoes a thyroidectomy. After surgery, the patient develops peripheral numbness and tingling and muscle twitching and spasms. The nurse should expect to administer:

 ○ **A.** a thyroid supplement.

 ○ **B.** an antispasmodic.

 ○ **C.** a barbiturate.

 ○ **D.** I.V. calcium gluconate.

Correct answer: D   Damage to the parathyroid glands during thyroidectomy can cause hyposecretion of parathyroid hormone, leading to calcium deficiency. Symptoms of calcium deficiency include muscle spasms, numbness, and tingling. Treatment includes immediate I.V. administration of calcium gluconate. Thyroid supplementation (option A) is necessary following thyroidectomy but isn't specifically related to the identified problem. An antispasmodic (option B) doesn't treat the problem. A barbiturate (option C) isn't indicated.

4. A patient with intractable asthma develops Cushing's syndrome. Development of this complication can most likely be attributed to long-term or excessive use of:

 ○ **A.** prednisone.

 ○ **B.** theophylline.

 ○ **C.** metaproterenol (Alupent).

 ○ **D.** cromolyn (Intal).

Correct answer: A   Cushing's syndrome results from long-term or excessive use of a glucocorticoid such as prednisone. Theophylline (option B), metaproterenol (option C), and cromolyn (option D) don't cause Cushing's syndrome.

5. Which nursing diagnosis is most likely for a patient with an acute episode of diabetes insipidus?

 ○ **A.** Imbalanced nutrition: More than body requirements

 ○ **B.** Deficient fluid volume

 ○ **C.** Impaired gas exchange

 ○ **D.** Ineffective tissue perfusion: Cardiopulmonary

Correct answer: B   Diabetes insipidus causes a pronounced loss of intravascular volume; therefore, the most prominent risk to the patient is deficient fluid volume. The patient is at risk for imbalanced nutrition, impaired gas exchange, and ineffective tissue perfusion (options A, C, and D), but these risks stem from the deficient fluid volume.

Renal and urinary tract disorders

❖ Introduction

- ■ The urinary system forms and stores urine, regulates body fluids and electrolytes, and controls urine elimination
- ■ Urinary tract infections (UTIs) and obstructions may cause permanent loss of renal function
- ■ Acute and chronic renal failure are both serious and potentially life-threatening conditions
  - ◆ In a patient with *renal impairment* or *diminished renal reserve*, the healthier kidney compensates for the impaired kidney and continues to clear metabolic waste unless it meets with increased demand or unusual stress; as a result, the patient is asymptomatic, and specific concentration and dilution tests are needed to detect reduced renal function
  - ◆ In a patient with *renal insufficiency*, compensation begins to fail, and metabolic wastes build up; the degree of insufficiency can be mild, moderate, or severe and is measured by the decreasing glomerular filtration rate (GFR)
  - ◆ In a patient with *end-stage renal disease*, the kidneys can't perform their normal homeostatic functions or meet normal body demands
    - ▶ Excess nitrogenous wastes build up in the blood
    - ▶ Fluid, electrolyte, and acid-base abnormalities occur
    - ▶ Dialysis or kidney transplantation is necessary to sustain life
- ■ Nursing history
  - ◆ The nurse asks the patient about the *chief complaint*
    - ▶ A patient with a renal or urinary tract disorder may be experiencing output changes, such as polyuria, oliguria, or anuria; he may also note voiding pattern changes, such as hesitancy, frequency, urgency, nocturia, or incontinence; urine color changes; or pain
    - ▶ The patient may also see changes in voiding pattern, such as hesitancy, frequency, urgency, nocturia, or incontinence; urine color changes; or pain
  - ◆ The nurse then questions the patient about his *present illness*
    - ▶ Ask the patient about his symptom, including when it started, associated symptoms, location, radiation, intensity, duration, frequency, and precipitating and alleviating factors
    - ▶ Ask about the use of prescription and over-the-counter drugs, herbal remedies, and vitamin and nutritional supplements
  - ◆ The nurse asks about *medical history*

   ▶ Question the patient about other renal and urinary disorders, such as UTIs, kidney trauma, and kidney stones
   ▶ Ask about a history of other chronic illnesses that may affect the renal system, such as diabetes mellitus or hypertension
   ◆ The nurse then assesses the *family history*
   ▶ Ask about a family history of chronic illnesses that can affect the renal system, such as hypertension, diabetes mellitus, coronary artery disease, vascular disease, or hyperlipidemia
   ▶ Determine whether the family history suggests a genetic predisposition to certain renal diseases such as polycystic kidney disease
   ◆ The nurse obtains a *social history*
   ▶ Ask about work, exercise, diet, use of recreational drugs and alcohol, and hobbies
   ▶ Also ask about stress, support systems, and coping mechanisms
■ Physical assessment
   ◆ Nurse begins with *inspection*
   ▶ Observe the patient's overall appearance; note his mental status and behavior
   ▶ Examine his skin for color, turgor, intactness, edema, and texture
   ▶ Inspect his abdomen for size and shape, noting any abnormal markings
   ◆ Next, the nurse uses *palpation*
   ▶ Palpate the bladder for distention
   ▶ Note any areas of tenderness
   ◆ Then the nurse uses *percussion*
   ▶ Percuss for costovertebral tenderness
   ▶ Percuss the bladder to elicit tympany or dullness
   ◆ The nurse then uses *auscultation*
   ▶ Listen for renal artery bruits
   ▶ Note any bruits over the aorta, iliac, and femoral arteries

❖ Acute renal failure

■ Description
   ◆ Acute renal failure is a sudden and almost complete loss of kidney function characterized by rising levels of blood urea nitrogen (BUN) and serum creatinine and an inability of the kidneys to regulate fluid and electrolyte balance; it occurs over several hours to several days
   ◆ Acute renal failure may be reversible — or it may lead to death
   ◆ *Prerenal failure*, or prerenal azotemia, occurs when blood flow to the kidneys is disrupted, which causes ischemia and nephron damage
   ▶ It can result from a condition that decreases blood flow and kidney perfusion, such as hypovolemia, hemorrhage, or burns; a condition that decreases cardiac output, such as a myocardial infarction (MI) or an arrhythmia; vascular failure related to sepsis, anaphylaxis, or severe acidosis; or an occlusion that obstructs renal arteries
   ▶ It generally can be reversed by treating the cause and restoring normal intravascular volume

◆ *Intrarenal failure* occurs when the renal parenchyma is damaged; when this occurs, the kidneys can't concentrate urine or excrete nitrogenous wastes

▶ Intrarenal failure can be caused by nephron damage resulting from acute tubular necrosis, acute glomerulonephritis, or a related disorder or from exposure to a nephrotoxic drug or chemical, such as certain antibiotics, an antineoplastic, a fluorinated anesthetic, a heavy metal, or a radiographic contrast dye

▶ Other causes include trauma, neoplasms, hypertension, systemic lupus erythematosus, toxemia of pregnancy, and hypercalcemia

◆ *Postrenal failure*, or postrenal azotemia, occurs when urine flow from the collecting ducts in the kidney to the external urethral orifice is obstructed or when venous blood flow from the kidney is obstructed

▶ Renal calculi, tumors, clots, benign prostatic hyperplasia, strictures, trauma, bilateral renal vein thrombosis, and congenital malformation can all cause urinary obstruction

▶ Postrenal failure is usually reversible

◆ Acute renal failure can lead to hyperkalemia or can cause uremia that compromises the immune system

■ Signs and symptoms

◆ Acute renal failure typically progresses through three phases: an oliguric or anuric phase, a diuretic phase, and a recovery phase; signs and symptoms vary from phase to phase

◆ The oliguric phase produces a BUN level of 25 to 30 mg/dl, a serum creatinine level of 1.5 to 2 mg, sudden oliguria (urine output less than 400 ml daily) or anuria (rare), and reduced GFR

◆ The diuretic phase causes a gradual return of renal function; normal or high urine output (1 to 5 L daily); potentially life-threatening loss of sodium, potassium, and magnesium; and increased azotemia (elevated BUN and serum creatinine levels)

◆ The recovery phase is associated with decreasing BUN and serum creatinine levels; it continues until normal renal tubular function is established

◆ High-output renal failure, a type of acute nonoliguric renal failure, occasionally occurs; it commonly results from the use of a nephrotoxic antibiotic

▶ Although symptoms of acute renal failure may develop, fluid overload generally isn't a problem

▶ If high-output renal failure is recognized early, and the antibiotic is discontinued, normal renal function gradually returns

■ Diagnosis and treatment

◆ Diagnosis of acute renal failure is based on patient history and abnormal laboratory findings (see *Understanding acute renal failure*), assessment of fluid balance, preexisting disorders, precipitating events, and current health status

◆ Other diagnostic tests may include abdominal X-ray, ultrasonography, or computed tomography (CT); excretory urography or cystoscopy with retrograde pyelography; renal angiography; and renal biopsy

Understanding acute renal failure

The pathophysiologic processes of acute renal failure (ARF) determine the patient's signs, symptoms, and laboratory test result changes.

Pathophysiologic process	Signs and symptoms	Laboratory test results
Inability to excrete nitrogenous wastes	• Nausea, vomiting, GI bleeding • Drowsiness, confusion, delirium, coma • Pericarditis • Asterixis	• Elevated blood urea nitrogen • Elevated creatinine
Decreased urine volume	• Edema, heart failure, pulmonary edema, interstitial infiltrates in lungs • Hypertension	• In prerenal ARF, increased urine specific gravity and osmolarity and decreased urine sodium level • In intrarenal ARF, decreased urine specific gravity and osmolarity and increased urine sodium level • In postrenal ARF, possibly normal urine osmolarity and urine sodium level
Inability to regulate electrolytes	• Electrocardiogram (ECG) changes (peaked, tent-like T waves; widened QRS complex; and arrhythmias); neuromuscular changes (weakness and paralysis) • Dyspnea, edema, anasarca, increased jugular vein distention, crackles • Thirst, dry mouth, weakness, tachycardia, hypotension, decreased skin turgor (diuretic phase) • Weakness, paralysis, constipation, paralytic ileus, hypoventilation, prominent U waves on ECG (diuretic phase) • Muscle weakness, hypoventilation, hypotension, flushing • Tremors, seizures	• Hyperkalemia • Hypernatremia • Hyponatremia • Hypokalemia • Hypermagnesemia • Hyperphosphatemia and hypocalcemia
Inability to maintain acid-base balance	• Hyperventilation, Kussmaul's respirations, weakness	• Metabolic acidosis (decreased pH and bicarbonate levels)
Uremic syndrome	• Early manifestations: anorexia, nausea, vomiting • Later manifestations: bleeding, uremic pneumonitis, pericarditis, colitis, pericardial effusion • Other manifestations: increased susceptibility to infection; dry, itchy skin	• Altered platelet function, anemia

◆ Laboratory tests include serum creatinine and BUN levels (the normal ratio of BUN to creatinine ranges from 10:1 to 15:1), electrolyte and hemoglobin levels, hematocrit, urinalysis, and creatinine clearance; laboratory changes can help differentiate among prerenal, intrarenal, and postrenal acute renal failure

▶ With prerenal acute renal failure, the BUN-creatinine ratio is greater than 15:1; urine specific gravity and osmolarity are increased, and the urine sodium level is decreased

▶ With intrarenal acute renal failure, urine specific gravity and osmolarity fall to levels similar to those in serum or plasma, and the urine sodium level may exceed 30 mEq/L

▶ With postrenal acute renal failure, urine osmolarity and sodium levels may be normal; if the condition isn't quickly diagnosed and treated, the patient may develop urinary system changes similar to those of intrarenal acute renal failure

◆ Treatment aims to identify and eliminate or control the underlying cause, restore normal fluid and electrolyte balance, and prevent uremic complications while the kidneys repair themselves

◆ Reduced intravascular volume is treated early with aggressive fluid therapy to restore urine output and prevent acute tubular necrosis

▶ A therapeutic fluid challenge (500 ml over 30 minutes) may be used to differentiate prerenal from intrarenal causes of oliguria

▶ If urine output improves after the fluid challenge, I.V. fluids are continued at a rate that maintains adequate hourly urine volume

▶ If the fluid challenge is unsuccessful, a diuretic—such as mannitol (Osmitrol), bumetanide (Bumex), furosemide (Lasix), or ethacrynic acid (Edecrin)—may be used to restore urine output

◆ A patient with hypervolemia and fluid overload, hyperkalemia, metabolic acidosis, severe hyponatremia, encephalopathy, or pericarditis may require dialysis (see *Comparing types of dialysis*)

◆ Hyperkalemia is aggressively treated with I.V. hypertonic glucose and insulin (to shift extracellular potassium into cells), oral or rectal administration of the cation-exchange resin sodium polystyrene sulfonate (to exchange sodium for potassium ions in the GI tract), and dialysis (to maintain normal potassium levels)

◆ Hypotension is commonly treated with volume replacement, although a vasopressor may be needed

◆ Hypertension is treated with restriction of fluid intake to prevent fluid overload, restriction of dietary sodium, and antihypertensive therapy

◆ Diet therapy helps manage acute renal failure; the recommended diet is high in calories and carbohydrates, is low in potassium, and may restrict protein (depending on the degree of azotemia and the frequency of dialysis); protein in the diet must provide essential amino acids while minimizing the degree of nitrogenous waste products

■ Nursing interventions

◆ Monitor for signs of acute renal failure and its complications

Comparing types of dialysis

Peritoneal dialysis, hemodialysis, and continuous renal replacement therapy (CRRT) may be used to treat acute renal failure. They vary in several ways.

Selection criteria

Peritoneal dialysis typically is used for patients with cardiovascular instability because it doesn't have the same effect on cardiac output as hemodialysis. It also may be used for patients with recent cerebral bleeding, GI bleeding, or blood dyscrasias because it requires no heparinization.

Hemodialysis is more appropriate for patients who have had recent abdominal surgery or who have abdominal adhesions because these conditions interfere with the clearance ability of the peritoneal membrane used as the dialyzable surface in peritoneal dialysis. Hemodialysis also is more commonly used for patients with severe catabolism, fluid overload, or hyperkalemia because it removes wastes and fluids more rapidly than peritoneal dialysis.

CRRT may be used for critically ill patients with acute renal failure who can't tolerate hemodialysis or peritoneal dialysis because of hemodynamic instability. CRRT is used 24 hours per day, over several days, to slowly remove fluid and solutes.

Advantages and disadvantages

Hemodialysis is a complex procedure that requires expensive equipment and skilled personnel. Consequently, it may not be available in a convenient location. Peritoneal dialysis is less complex and less expensive and is available in a wider variety of settings. Home dialysis is possible with both procedures, but peritoneal dialysis is less expensive and requires a shorter training period.

Peritoneal dialysis allows the patient to be more independent, promotes more steady blood chemistry levels, and permits the patient to eat a less-restricted diet. Techniques developed by Popovich in the late 1970s, along with Tenckhoff's development of a permanent peritoneal catheter, have contributed to the increased use of peritoneal dialysis in patients with chronic renal failure.

CRRT removes fluid and solutes slowly, making it more suitable for critically ill patients with unstable conditions. However, it requires a highly trained staff. Types of CRRT include continuous arteriovenous hemofiltration, continuous venovenous hemofiltration, continuous arteriovenous hemodialysis, and continuous venovenous hemodialysis.

Types of peritoneal dialysis

Continuous ambulatory peritoneal dialysis (CAPD) can be performed independently by the patient in any location and frees him from dependence on a machine or dialysis center. With CAPD, dialysis fluid is continuously present in the peritoneum but is drained and replaced with fresh fluid three to five times per day based on his clearance needs. This technique closely resembles normal renal function, avoiding extreme shifts in blood chemistries and fluid that occur with hemodialysis.

In *continuous cyclic peritoneal dialysis* (CCPD), a cycling machine performs frequent exchanges while the patient sleeps. After the last exchange in the morning, fresh dialysate is left in the peritoneum until nighttime. CCPD generally is performed 6 or 7 days a week.

With *intermittent peritoneal dialysis* (IPD), frequent fluid changes are performed over 8 to 10 hours, 3 to 5 days a week. Dialysate isn't left in the peritoneum between dialysis periods. Although IPD can be done manually by a trained nurse, an automated cycling machine is commonly used. IPD is performed in a hospital, dialysis center, or at home, usually at night.

◆ Monitor fluid intake and output, weigh the patient daily, and administer fluids carefully; monitor electrolyte levels, and maintain proper electrolyte balance
◆ Prevent infection by frequently washing your hands; using aseptic technique with incisions, wound care, and care of I.V. and central venous catheters; assisting the patient with hygiene, including oral hygiene; frequently turning and positioning him; encouraging deep breathing, coughing, and ambulation (if possible); and avoiding use of an indwelling urinary catheter
◆ Monitor the patient for signs of infection, such as fever, local redness, swelling, heat, drainage, and elevated white blood cell (WBC) count;

watch for signs and symptoms of pericarditis, including pleuritic chest pain, tachycardia, and pericardial friction rub
◆ Provide a diet high in calories and low in potassium, protein, and sodium
◆ Monitor the patient's response to medications; because many drugs are excreted by the kidneys, the type of drug, dosage, or administration interval may need to be adjusted, based on the patient's renal function (as evidenced by GFR and other indicators)
◆ Teach the patient and family the reasons for interventions and the importance of infection prevention measures; because the patient may be acutely ill and have a decreased level of consciousness, information should be given verbally (briefly) and in writing
◆ Encourage the patient and family to express their concerns

❖ Chronic renal failure
■ Description
◆ Chronic renal failure is a slow, insidious, irreversible deterioration in renal function
◆ It typically progresses through four stages:
▶ Reduced renal reserve: GFR of 60% to 89% of normal
▶ Renal insufficiency: GFR of 30% to 59% of normal
▶ Renal failure: GFR of 15% to 29% of normal
▶ End-stage renal disease: GFR less than 15% of normal
◆ Diseases that contribute to chronic renal failure include diabetic, gouty, and hypertensive nephropathies; chronic glomerulonephritis; pyelonephritis; urinary tract obstruction; cystic kidney disease; renal cell carcinoma; renovascular disease; lupus nephritis; multiple myeloma; amyloidosis; chronic hypercalcemia and hypokalemia; renal tuberculosis; and sarcoidosis
◆ Chronic renal failure begins with a functional loss of nephrons that's asymptomatic, except for decreased urinary creatinine clearance; creatinine clearance normally ranges from 85 to 135 ml/minute; in patients with mild renal failure, it ranges from 50 to 84 ml/minute; in patients with moderate renal failure, from 10 to 49 ml/minute; and in patients with severe renal failure, 10 ml/minute or less
◆ Next, renal insufficiency occurs as more nephrons cease to function; insufficiency may be mild, moderate, or severe
▶ At first, the patient experiences no physical limitations in daily activity, although laboratory changes—such as azotemia, anemia, and loss of the ability to concentrate urine—are detectable
▶ As renal deterioration continues, the kidneys' ability to function under stress (for example, during dehydration, salt depletion, or heart failure) is impaired; renal insufficiency may progress to renal failure during periods of stress
▶ Once renal failure develops, the patient must limit daily activities; he'll eventually develop overt signs of renal failure and uremia, beginning with fluid, electrolyte, and metabolic abnormalities (including

azotemia, anemia, metabolic acidosis, hypertension, and hypocalcemia)

▶ End-stage renal disease occurs when most of the nephrons have been irreversibly damaged; the GFR falls below 100 ml/minute, and the patient requires long-term dialysis or kidney transplantation

■ Signs and symptoms

◆ Altered fluid, electrolyte, and acid-base balances may include dehydration (early) or overhydration (later in the disease), hypocalcemia and hyperkalemia, and metabolic acidosis (as evidenced by low arterial blood pH and decreased bicarbonate levels)

◆ Skin changes may include gray-bronze or yellow skin color related to uremia or pallor related to anemia, dry skin, uremic frost (white, dustlike deposits of urea and phosphate crystals on the face, nose, forehead, and upper trunk), pruritus, excoriations, ecchymosis, purpura, or infections; related changes may include thin, brittle nails and a whitened proximal section with a darker distal edge and nail ridges

◆ Cardiovascular effects may include hypertension, acceleration of atherosclerosis, increased risk of MI and cerebrovascular accident, left ventricular hypertrophy, heart failure, pericarditis (which may cause a fever and pericardial friction rub and, rarely, chest pain and hypotension), pericardial effusion (which causes disappearance of any friction rub and appearance of a paradoxical pulse), cardiac tamponade (which causes hypotension, muffled heart sounds, narrowed pulse pressure, weak peripheral pulses, and bulging neck veins), life-threatening cardiac arrhythmias, and cardiac arrest

◆ Respiratory effects may include thick, tenacious sputum and a depressed cough reflex, which increase the risk of pulmonary infections and complications; Kussmaul's respirations; uremic breath odor; increased incidence of infections, including tuberculosis; pulmonary edema; pleural effusion; and uremic pneumonitis

◆ Hematologic effects may include normochromic, normocytic anemia (which causes fatigue, weakness, pallor, exertional dyspnea, and intolerance of activity and cold); platelet dysfunction (which causes prolonged bleeding time, clotting abnormalities, easy bruising, purpura, and bleeding from mucous membranes and other body parts); changes in the immune system and granulocytic function (which decrease cellular and humoral immunity and the inflammatory response)

◆ GI effects may include metallic or ammonia-like taste in the mouth, stomatitis, ammonia or fishy breath odor, increased incidence of oral infections and tooth decay, anorexia (especially for high-protein foods), nausea, vomiting, GI bleeding, increased gastric acid production, diarrhea or constipation, fecal impaction, and increased incidence of diverticulosis

◆ The patient may develop hepatitis (see chapter 12, Gastrointestinal disorders, for information about this disease)

◆ Metabolic dysfunction may include carbohydrate intolerance (with abnormal glucose clearance), accumulation of end products of protein me-

tabolism (which causes lethargy, headache, fatigue, irritability, and depression), and hyperlipidemia
◆ Central nervous system effects may include decreased attention span, memory problems, inability to think clearly (progressing to actual confusion), flattened affect, depression, irritability, lability, stupor, coma, and seizures
◆ Peripheral nervous system effects may include peripheral neuropathies (numbness, tingling, or pain of the feet and hands; weakness of the feet; and atrophy of leg muscles), footdrop, loss of motor function, and "burning feet" syndrome (swelling, redness, and extreme tenderness of the soles and dorsum of the feet)
◆ Autonomic nervous system effects may include loss of the ability to compensate for a change in blood pressure through reflex tachycardia or bradycardia, which leads to poor blood pressure control
◆ Musculoskeletal effects may include impaired physical mobility, loss of muscle mass and muscle strength, osteomalacia, osteoporosis, and osteitis fibrosa cystica
◆ Reproductive effects may include impotence in men, amenorrhea and infertility in women, and markedly decreased libido in both sexes
■ Diagnosis and treatment
◆ Laboratory tests, X-rays, and other diagnostic tests for chronic renal failure are the same as those for acute renal failure; renal biopsy establishes percentage of functioning nephrons
◆ Treatment has several goals: to preserve current renal function and prevent or delay further deterioration of function, to treat symptoms of uremia, to postpone or eliminate the need for long-term dialysis or kidney transplantation, to prevent complications of uremia, and to promote comfort and improve the patient's quality of life
◆ Most patients with chronic renal failure can be managed successfully with diet and fluid therapy; long-term dialysis or kidney transplantation is unnecessary until the GFR falls to 10% to 15% of the normal rate
◆ Strict adherence to a low-protein diet can delay progression to end-stage renal disease
▶ A high-protein load causes the kidneys to dilate from increased blood flow and increased GFR in an attempt to clear the by-products of protein metabolism; this increased vasodilation accelerates the deterioration of renal function
▶ For adult patients, a protein intake of about 50 g daily appears to have a therapeutic effect without contributing to malnutrition; most of the protein must be of high biological value to supply sufficient essential amino acids; protein of low biological value increases the waste load to the kidneys
◆ Depending on the stage of the disease and on fluid and electrolyte alterations, fluid intake may need to be restricted
▶ If urine output is decreased, and fluid overload becomes a problem, fluid intake typically is restricted to the previous day's urine output plus 500 ml for insensible loss

▶ If excessive fluid is lost—for example, because of fever, vomiting, or diarrhea—fluid requirements may increase

◆ Sodium, potassium, and phosphorus also may be restricted

▶ Sodium restriction may be warranted if the patient develops hypertension, edema, or heart failure

▶ Dietary potassium generally isn't restricted if the urine output exceeds 1,000 ml daily; it's restricted if the serum potassium level exceeds 5.5 mEq/L

◆ Supplements of B-complex vitamins, folic acid, and vitamin C may be needed to compensate for deficiencies that result from a restrictive diet or dialysis; iron and zinc supplements also may be prescribed

◆ Once long-term dialysis begins, a more liberal protein intake is allowed, and the fluid intake is controlled to allow a weight gain of 2 to 2.5 lb (0.9 to 1.1 kg) between dialysis treatments

◆ Despite anorexia, nausea, and taste changes, the patient must consume sufficient calories to prevent catabolism and muscle breakdown

◆ Disturbances in calcium metabolism may be managed with calcium supplements, dietary restriction of phosphorus, and phosphate binders, such as aluminum hydroxide gels (Amphojel), which are given at mealtimes; a patient receiving hemodialysis may receive calcium carbonate instead of a phosphate binder, which can exacerbate bone disease and promote faulty mineralization

◆ When end-stage renal disease develops, and diet, fluid restrictions, and drugs are no longer effective, the patient may undergo long-term dialysis (peritoneal dialysis or hemodialysis) or kidney transplantation; peritoneal dialysis and hemodialysis achieve the same results but in different ways

■ Nursing interventions

◆ Monitor physiologic changes and fluid and electrolyte changes

◆ Consult the dietitian about ways to ensure that the patient consumes sufficient calories while adhering to dietary restrictions

◆ Teach the patient how to relieve uremic skin symptoms; dry, itchy skin contributes to discomfort, irritability, restlessness, and frustration, and scratching increases the risk of infection

▶ Use tepid water and avoid soap (hot water and soap can worsen dryness and itching); use emollients, creams, and bath oils liberally to control dryness

▶ Administer antihistamines and antipruritics as needed to control itching

▶ Keep nails clean and trimmed short to reduce the risk of infection from scratching; use a soft washcloth, not fingernails, to scratch

▶ Keep hair clean and moisturized but avoid frequent shampooing to prevent dryness

◆ Teach the patient how to perform oral care; decreased salivary flow and fluid restrictions can contribute to problems in the oral mucosa

▶ Encourage frequent and gentle brushing with a soft toothbrush to decrease oral bacteria, prevent stomatitis, improve taste, and eliminate mouth odors

▶ Encourage the patient to use mouthwash and to suck on hard candy to treat dry mouth, alleviate thirst, and improve taste

◆ Teach the patient how to prevent constipation by encouraging increased intake of dietary fiber, use of stool softeners, and increased activity; advise him to avoid laxatives that contain magnesium because of the risk of magnesium toxicity

◆ Help the patient increase mobility and activity as tolerated—for example, help him plan activities to avoid fatigue, teach him how to use ambulatory aids, and refer him to a physical therapist if needed

◆ Help prevent pulmonary complications by teaching the patient how to deep-breathe, cough, and use an incentive spirometer to prevent atelectasis and infection and by preventing and treating fluid overload

◆ Teach the patient and family about the disease, its complications, and measures that can prevent further renal deterioration; refer the patient to the National Kidney Foundation

◆ Make sure the following areas are discussed with the patient and family: monitoring of fluid intake and output; signs of fluid overload and common electrolyte imbalances; therapeutic and adverse effects of prescribed drugs; methods of promoting skin integrity; methods of preventing infection, pulmonary complications, hyperkalemia, constipation, and fecal impaction; importance of controlling blood pressure; methods of maintaining mobility; need for phosphate-binders to prevent bone disease; need for dietary modifications; advantages and disadvantages of peritoneal dialysis and hemodialysis; and home dialysis

❖ Glomerulonephritis

■ Description

◆ Glomerulonephritis is an inflammation of the glomeruli

◆ Acute glomerulonephritis follows a streptococcal infection of the respiratory tract or, less commonly, a skin infection, such as impetigo, immunoglobulin A nephropathy (Berger's disease) or lipid nephrosis; most people fully recover, others may progress to chronic renal failure

◆ Chronic glomerulonephritis is a slowly progressive disease that results in sclerosis, scarring and, eventually, renal failure

■ Signs and symptoms

◆ The patient with acute glomerulonephritis may experience azotemia, dyspnea, edema, fatigue, hematuria, mild to severe hypertension, oliguria, and proteinuria

◆ Chronic glomerulonephritis develops insidiously and without symptoms, typically over many years; when it becomes suddenly aggressive, the patient may have edema and hypertension; in later stages, the patient may complain of nausea, vomiting, pruritus, dyspnea, malaise, fatigue, and mild to severe edema

■ Diagnosis and treatment

◆ Urinalysis typically reveals proteinuria, hematuria, WBCs, and casts

◆ 24-hour urine sample shows low creatinine clearance and impaired glomerular filtration

◆ Blood studies reveal rising BUN and serum creatinine levels in those with advanced renal insufficiency as well as a decrease in hemoglobin levels

◆ Renal biopsy can confirm the diagnosis and identify underlying disease

◆ Elevated antistreptolysin-O titers, elevated streptozyme and anti-Dnase B titers, and low serum complement levels verify recent streptococcal infection

◆ Treatment depends on the cause; the goals are to correct fluid overload, hypertension, and uremia

  ◗ Antibiotics are given to treat streptococcal infections
  ◗ Antihypertensives are given to control hypertension
  ◗ Diuretics may be given to reduce fluid overload
  ◗ Sodium, potassium, protein, and fluid restrictions may be instituted
  ◗ Dialysis may be necessary to correct fluid and electrolyte imbalances
  ◗ Dialysis or kidney transplantation for chronic glomerulonephritis may be needed

■ Nursing interventions

◆ Check vital signs and electrolyte levels, monitor fluid intake and output and daily weight, assess renal function daily through serum creatinine and BUN levels and urine creatinine clearance, and watch for signs of acute renal failure, including oliguria, azotemia, and acidosis

◆ Consult the dietitian to provide a diet high in calories and low in protein, sodium, potassium, and fluids

◆ Provide bed rest during the acute period of the disease

◆ Provide emotional support for the patient and family; if the patient is receiving dialysis, explain the procedure

◆ Teach the patient to report signs and symptoms of infection to the practitioner and the importance of follow-up examinations

◆ Explain any dietary restrictions to the patient and family

❖ Neurogenic bladder

■ Description

◆ Neurogenic bladder refers to all types of bladder dysfunction caused by an interruption of normal bladder innervation (see *Types of neurogenic bladder,* page 260)

◆ Subsequent complications include incontinence, residual urine retention, UTI, stone formation, and renal failure

◆ A neurogenic bladder may be described as spastic (resulting from an upper motor neuron lesion) or flaccid (resulting from a lower motor neuron lesion)

◆ Neurogenic bladder may result from an acute infectious disease; a cerebral disorder; chronic alcoholism; a collagen disease; a peripheral innervation disorder; distant effects of cancer, such as primary oat cell carcinoma of the lung; heavy metal toxicity; herpes zoster; a metabolic disturbance; sacral agenesis; spinal cord disease or trauma; a vascular disease, such as atherosclerosis; or another condition

Types of neurogenic bladder

Different types of neurogenic bladder have varied causes as summarized below.

Neural lesion	Type	Cause
Upper motor	Uninhibited	• Lack of voluntary control in infancy • Multiple sclerosis
	Reflex or automatic	• Spinal cord transection • Cord tumors • Multiple sclerosis
Lower motor	Autonomous	• Sacral cord trauma • Tumors • Herniated disk • Abdominal surgery with transection of pelvic parasympathetic nerves
	Motor paralysis	• Lesions at levels S2, S3, S4 • Poliomyelitis • Trauma • Tumors
	Sensory paralysis	• Posterior lumbar nerve roots • Diabetes mellitus • Tabes dorsalis

■ Signs and symptoms
   ◆ A patient with flaccid neurogenic bladder may experience overflow incontinence, diminished anal sphincter tone, and a distended bladder
   ◆ A patient with spastic neurogenic bladder may experience spontaneous spasms of the arms and legs, involuntary or frequent scanty urination without a feeling of bladder fullness, and increased anal sphincter tone
   ◆ Other signs and symptoms may include altered micturition, hydronephrosis, incontinence, and vesicoureteral reflux (passage of urine from the bladder back into a ureter)
   ◆ The patient may also have symptoms of a UTI or kidney stones
■ Diagnosis and treatment
   ◆ Voiding cystourethrography evaluates bladder neck function, vesicoureteral reflux, and continence
   ◆ Urodynamic studies—which consist of cystometry, uroflometry, urethral pressure profiles, and sphincter electromyography—help evaluate how urine is stored in the bladder, how well the bladder empties, and how quickly urine moves out of the bladder during voiding
   ◆ Techniques for bladder elimination include Valsalva's maneuver, indwelling urinary catheter insertion, intermittent self-catheterization, and Crede's maneuver (pressing on the suprapubic area with a downward motion to express urine from the bladder)

◆ Drug therapy may include terazosin, doxazosin, and phenoxybenzamine to facilitate bladder emptying and propantheline, flavoxate, dicyclomine, imipramine, and pseudoephedrine to aid urine storage

◆ When conservative treatment fails, surgery may be used to correct the structural impairment through transurethral resection of the bladder neck, urethral dilation, external sphincterotomy, or urinary diversion; implantation of an artificial urinary sphincter may be necessary if permanent incontinence follows surgery

■ Nursing interventions

◆ Use strict aseptic technique during insertion and maintenance of an indwelling urinary catheter; don't interrupt the closed drainage system for any reason; keep the drainage bag below the level of the bladder

◆ Assess the patient for signs and symptoms of infection

◆ Teach the patient to report signs and symptoms of infection and how to prevent UTI; encourage him to increase his fluid intake

◆ Teach dietary measures to prevent kidney stone formation

◆ Keep the patient as mobile as possible; perform range-of-motion exercises, if necessary

◆ Teach the patient techniques, such as Crede's maneuver and intermittent self-catheterization

◆ If urinary diversion procedure is to be performed, arrange for consultation with an enterostomal therapist

❖ Urinary calculi

■ Description

◆ Urinary calculi (stones) are the most common urologic problem in adults; *nephrolithiasis* is the presence of calculi in the renal parenchyma, *urolithiasis* is the presence of calculi in the urinary tract, and *ureterolithiasis* is the presence of calculi in the ureters

◆ Calculi vary in size, from the size of a grain of sand to the size of a baseball; they're more common in men than in women, more common in hot summer months, and often recur

◆ Urinary calculi vary in type and composition (see *Types of urinary calculi,* page 262)

◆ Urinary calculi may be caused by infection, urine retention, urinary stasis, immobility, dehydration, sedentary lifestyle, or persistently low urine output

◆ The exact mechanism of stone formation is unknown; it may be related to changes in urine pH, volume depletion, or use of diuretics or other drugs

◆ Calculi formed in the kidney may pass into the ureter, occlude the flow of urine, and cause urine to flow back to the kidney; this can lead to ureteral spasm, hematuria, urinary stasis, UTI, impaired renal function and, eventually, hydronephrosis (kidney enlargement)

■ Signs and symptoms

◆ Symptoms vary with the location of the calculi and the presence of obstruction, infection, and edema

Types of urinary calculi

Different types of calculi vary in chemical content, incidence, and predisposing factors.

Calculi and description	Predisposing factors
Calcium calculi Formed from calcium oxalate, calcium phosphate, or both and account for 80% to 90% of all urinary calculi	• Immobility • Hyperthyroidism • Myeloproliferative disease • Renal tubular acidosis • Hyperuricemia • Increased dietary intake of milk, alkali products (such as antacids), and vitamin D • Prolonged use of steroids
Oxalate calculi Formed from oxalate and are the second most common type of calculi	• High intake of grains • Inflammatory bowel disease • Small bowel resection • Ileostomy • Vitamin A deficiency
Uric acid calculi Formed from uric acid and account for 5% to 10% of calculi in the United States	• Hyperuricemia • Gout • High dietary intake of purine-rich foods, such as herring, sardines, organ meats, and yeast
Struvite (staghorn) calculi Formed from magnesium ammonium phosphate and account for 1% to 4% of urinary calculi	• Chronic urinary tract infections caused by urea-splitting bacteria, such as *Proteus, Pseudomonas, Klebsiella,* and *Staphylococcus*
Cystine calculi Formed from cystine and account for 1% to 4% of urinary calculi	• Genetic defect in the renal transport of cystine
Xanthine calculi Formed from xanthine and are rare	• Hereditary condition that causes xanthine oxidase deficiency

◆ Small or large nonobstructing stones in the renal calyces or renal pelvis may cause no symptoms

◆ Obstructing stones in the renal calyces or renal pelvis can cause recurrent infection, flank pain (described as a constant, intense, deep, dull ache), hematuria, and hydronephrosis; pyelonephritis and gram-negative septicemia may occur

◆ Renal calculi that pass into the ureter or become lodged at the ureteropelvic junction result in severe, sometimes excruciating, colicky pain in the lumbar area; microscopic or gross hematuria occurs

◆ Extremely small renal calculi may pass through the urinary system without causing noticeable symptoms

◆ Bladder calculi usually cause irritation and inflammation or, if they obstruct the urethra, urine retention and urinary obstruction

◆ Diarrhea, nausea, vomiting, and costovertebral tenderness commonly accompany colicky pain

■ Diagnosis and treatment

◆ Abdominal X-ray or X-ray of the kidneys, ureters, and bladder can detect calculi; ultrasonography, nephrotomography, and excretory urography also may be used

◆ Other diagnostic tests may include urinalysis and urine culture; serum calcium, phosphorus, creatinine, uric acid, and electrolyte levels; urine pH; and tests for hypercalciuria, hyperuricuria, urinary oxalate, citrate, and cystine (using 24-hour urine specimen)

◆ Because the causes and treatment of urinary calculi are based on their chemical composition, recovered stones are usually analyzed

◆ The main goals of treatment are to relieve pain, prevent nephron destruction, eliminate calculi, and prevent recurrence

▶ Opioids, such as morphine sulfate and meperidine, and antispasmodics, such as oxybutynin chloride and propantheline bromide, are used to control severe pain; antiemetics are used when pain is accompanied by nausea and vomiting

▶ Nephron destruction is prevented by controlling infection and by removing obstructions to urine flow to prevent backflow; urosepsis (septicemia related to UTI) is prevented with prophylactic antibiotic therapy

▶ Because almost 90% of urinary calculi pass spontaneously, calculi that aren't causing renal damage, obstruction, or infection are left in place for several months in the hope that they'll pass spontaneously

▶ Depending on the underlying causes and chemical composition of the calculi, dietary modifications and drug therapy may be used to help prevent recurrence; a fluid intake of 3 to 4 qt (3 to 4 L) daily is recommended, regardless of the type of calculi

◆ Procedures to remove renal calculi include extracorporeal shock-wave lithotripsy, ureteroscopic stone removal, and percutaneous nephrolithotomy

▶ Extracorporeal shock-wave lithotripsy is the most commonly used procedure to treat urinary calculi

● In this procedure, ultrasonic shock waves pulverize the calculi into many small fragments that pass through the urinary tract over several months

● The procedure has reduced the need for surgery and endoscopy to treat urinary calculi

▶ Percutaneous nephrolithotomy is used for removing large or inaccessible stones

● A nephroscope is inserted through an incision to the kidney, where the stone is removed

● Ultrasound may be needed to break up larger stones

▶ Ureteroscopic stone removal may be used for stones in the ureters

● A fiber-optic ureteroscope is passed through the urethra and bladder into the ureters

● The calculi is then removed or treated with shock waves

■ Nursing interventions
  ◆ Promote comfort for the patient with renal calculi
    ▶ Administer opioid analgesics, antispasmodics, and antiemetics, as prescribed
    ▶ Give hot baths or apply warm, moist packs to promote relaxation
    ▶ Administer 3 to 4 L of fluids daily to help calculi passage; use I.V. fluids if the patient can't tolerate oral fluids
    ▶ Encourage the patient to participate in usual activities and to ambulate frequently; these actions promote calculi passage
  ◆ Prevent urinary obstruction and infection
    ▶ Teach the patient the importance of monitoring urine output for changes in voiding pattern or amount and for cloudiness, foul odor, and blood
    ▶ Tell the patient to promptly report signs of UTI and flank, lumbar, and abdominal pain to the practitioner
    ▶ Teach the patient the importance of completing the full course of antibiotic therapy and the need to maintain fluid intake at 2 to 3 qt (2 to 3 L) daily to promote dilution and rapid drug excretion
    ▶ Encourage the patient to increase daily fluid intake to 3 qt (3 L) or more to promote urine flow, dilute crystalloids in the urine, and prevent precipitation of crystalloids into stones
    ▶ Encourage the patient with calcium-containing calculi to increase fluid intake 2 to 4 hours after meals, during heavy physical activity and dehydration, and at night; urine is more likely to be saturated with calcium at these times
  ◆ Prevent urinary calculi from recurring
    ▶ Encourage increased fluid intake to prevent urinary stasis and calculi development
    ▶ Instruct the patient to strain the urine to recover the calculi
    ▶ Teach the patient about predisposing factors, such as dehydration, low urine output, prolonged immobilization, and UTI
    ▶ Teach the patient with phosphate or uric acid stones how to monitor urine pH and alkalinize or acidify his urine
    ▶ Provide instructions about diet and prescribed drugs for a patient with calcium calculi
      • Reduce dietary intake of calcium and vitamin D, which prevents parathyroid hormone production
      • Restrict sodium intake to reduce intestinal absorption of calcium
      • Limit refined carbohydrates and animal protein to decrease hypercalciuria
      • Encourage the intake of high-fiber foods to help bind calcium
      • Suggest the use of orthophosphates to decrease the incidence of recurrent calculi formation in patients with hypercalciuria
      • Administer thiazide diuretics, as prescribed, to increase calcium reabsorption in the kidneys and reduce calcium excretion
      • Administer sodium cellulose phosphate, which binds calcium in the intestinal tract, to lower the urinary calcium level

▶ If the patient has phosphate calculi, provide instructions about diet and prescribed drugs
  ● Because phosphate stones develop in alkaline urine, encourage the intake of ascorbic acid, cranberry and prune juices, plums, meats, eggs, and fish to maintain acid urine
  ● Use an aluminum hydroxide gel, which combines with excess phosphorus and increases phosphorus excretion through the intestines
▶ If the patient has oxalate calculi, provide instructions about diet and prescribed drugs
  ● Restrict the intake of oxalate-rich foods and drinks, including apples, asparagus, beans, beer, chocolate, citrus fruits, colas, cranberries, grapes, green leafy vegetables (such as spinach and cabbage), instant coffee, peanut butter, peanuts, rhubarb, and tea
  ● Make sure the patient's urine remains diluted, to prevent more calculi from developing
  ● Administer an antacid that contains aluminum, to help bind oxalate and prevent urinary excretion
▶ If the patient has uric acid calculi, provide instructions about diet and prescribed drugs
  ● Recommend a low-purine diet that avoids fish (including shellfish), red wine, and rich foods, such as organ meats and foods with heavy sauces
  ● If the patient has gout, restrict dietary intake of protein
  ● Because uric acid stones are less likely to form in alkaline urine, encourage the use of sodium bicarbonate or sodium citrate solutions to maintain alkaline urine
▶ If the patient has struvite calculi, provide instructions about diet and prescribed drugs
  ● Make sure that the patient receives prompt treatment for UTIs and that measures are taken to reduce the incidence of infection
  ● Administer acetohydroxamic acid to inhibit the chemical reaction caused by bacteria, which may help prevent struvite calculi
▶ If the patient has cystine calculi, provide instructions about diet and prescribed drugs
  ● Restrict dietary protein intake, and encourage the use of measures to alkalinize the urine
  ● Use penicillamine to reduce cystine in the urine

❖ **Urinary tract infection**
  ■ Description
    ◆ *Urinary tract infection* is a general term used to describe infections of the upper or lower urinary tract; upper UTIs affect the kidneys, whereas lower UTIs affect the urinary bladder (cystitis) and urethra (urethritis)
    ◆ UTIs are the most common bacterial infections in all patients and are a significant source of morbidity; they're more common in women than in men, and they increase in frequency with age

◆ Factors that increase the risk of developing a UTI include female sex, increased sexual activity, pregnancy, structural and functional urinary tract abnormalities (such as strictures), obstructed urine flow, impaired bladder innervation, urinary stasis, incomplete bladder emptying, chronic health problems that alter renal tissue structure and function, urinary tract instrumentation (such as bladder catheterization and cystoscopy), and age

◆ UTIs in men and women typically develop as an ascending infection from the urethra; other pathways for infection—such as hematogenous spread, lymphatic spread, and direct extension from other organs—are rare

◆ A shorter urethra and its anatomic closeness to the vagina and rectum predispose women to ascending UTIs; besides anatomic differences that help protect men against UTIs, prostatic fluid provides an antibacterial effect

◆ Infection of the kidney by bacteria usually occurs secondary to ascending infection from the bladder; infection commonly results from ureterovesical reflux in which an incompetent valve allows urine to flow back into the ureters during voiding

◆ Gram-negative bacteria cause most bacterial UTIs; gram-negative and gram-positive bacteria may occasionally cause pyelonephritis (an infectious inflammation of the renal pelvis, tubules, and interstitial tissue that can be acute or chronic and may affect one or both kidneys)

❯ Acute pyelonephritis is seldom associated with permanent renal damage

❯ Chronic pyelonephritis is commonly associated with structural abnormalities and other conditions (such as calculi and diabetes) that contribute to repeated infection; it's more likely than acute pyelonephritis to cause permanent kidney damage and dysfunction from repeated inflammation and scarring

■ Signs and symptoms

◆ Symptoms of UTIs vary; some UTIs are asymptomatic and are diagnosed when routine urine testing detects bacteriuria

◆ Cystitis commonly causes urinary frequency, urinary urgency, and dysuria (pain and burning on urination); it also may produce microscopic to gross hematuria, urinary tenesmus (persistent desire to urinate small amounts), suprapubic and bladder spasms, and cloudy, foul-smelling urine

◆ Acute pyelonephritis typically manifests with an abrupt onset of shaking chills and moderate to high fever (101.3° to 104° F [38.5° to 40° C]), tachycardia, flank pain, malaise, nausea, vomiting, and costovertebral angle tenderness

❯ These signs and symptoms may be accompanied by symptoms of lower urinary tract involvement (dysuria and urinary frequency and urgency)

❯ Chills, fever, and signs of toxicity (such as falling blood pressure, tachycardia, and skin color changes) suggest deeper infection of the kidney

◆ Chronic pyelonephritis develops slowly and may progress to chronic renal failure

■ Diagnosis and treatment

◆ Diagnosis is usually based on the initial clinical presentation

◆ Urine culture may reveal at least 10^5 (100,000) colonies of bacteria per milliliter from a clean-catch midstream or catheterized urine specimen

▶ Urinalysis shows WBCs, casts, bacteria and, possibly, red blood cells

▶ Suprapubic needle aspiration of the bladder (if done) shows bacteria in the specimen

◆ Patients with recurrent or complicated UTIs may undergo additional diagnostic studies—such as abdominal ultrasonography, excretory urography, cystography, cystoscopy with retrograde pyelography and voiding urography, and abdominal CT—to rule out calculi or structural abnormalities of the urinary tract as the cause of recurrent infections

◆ Treatment of UTI and acute pyelonephritis has two goals: sterilizing the urine with antibacterial, antimicrobial, or urinary antiseptic drug therapy and identifying any illness or urinary tract abnormality that may be contributing to the infection

◆ Increased urine output dilutes the urine, which relieves urethral irritation and burning; a continual urine flow also discourages urinary stasis and organism growth

◆ Acute UTI symptoms may be relieved temporarily with urinary analgesics (such as an phenazopyridine [Pyridium], anticholinergics, or antispasmodics)

■ Nursing interventions

◆ If the patient has a lower UTI, administer antimicrobials, urinary analgesics, or antispasmodics, as prescribed; increase his fluid intake up to 3 L daily to help dilute his urine; and give him a warm sitz bath two or three times a day for 10 to 20 minutes to relieve local symptoms

◆ If the patient has pyelonephritis, make sure he maintains bed rest; administer antimicrobials, analgesics, antipyretics, and antiemetics, as prescribed; and maintain adequate fluid intake and output

◆ Emphasize to the patient the importance of taking his antimicrobial for the full course of therapy, even if his symptoms improve

◆ Teach the patient how to prevent urinary stasis by drinking 2 to 3 L of fluid daily, voiding every 2 to 3 hours, and emptying the bladder completely

◆ Stress to the patient the importance of emptying his bladder as soon as he has the urge to urinate; delayed urination encourages UTI by promoting urinary stasis

◆ Encourage women whose UTIs are related to sexual activity to empty their bladder before and after sexual intercourse

◆ Teach female patients how to reduce the number of pathogens in the perineal area by wiping from front to back after urination or defecation and cleaning the perineal and perianal area after each bowel movement

Review questions

1. The nurse is providing postprocedure care for a patient who underwent extracorporeal shock-wave lithotripsy for the treatment of renal calculi. The nurse should instruct the patient to:

○ **A.** limit oral fluid intake for 1 to 2 weeks.

○ **B.** report the presence of fine, sandlike particles in the urine.

○ **C.** notify the practitioner about cloudy or foul-smelling urine.

○ **D.** report bright pink urine within 24 hours after the procedure.

Correct answer: C The patient should report the presence of foul-smelling or cloudy urine. Option A is incorrect because, unless contraindicated, the patient should be instructed to drink large quantities of fluid each day to flush the kidneys. Option B is incorrect because sandlike debris is normal due to residual stone products. Option D is incorrect because hematuria is common after lithotripsy.

2. The nurse is planning a teaching session for a female patient who had a UTI. Which point should the nurse include?

○ **A.** Limit fluid intake to reduce the need to urinate.

○ **B.** Take prescribed antibiotic until symptoms subside.

○ **C.** Notify the practitioner if urinary urgency, burning, frequency, or difficulty occurs.

○ **D.** Wear only nylon underwear to reduce the chance of irritation.

Correct answer: C Urinary urgency, burning, frequency, and difficulty are all common symptoms of a UTI. The patient should notify the practitioner so that a urine culture and microscopic urinalysis can be done and appropriate treatment initiated. Option A is incorrect because women should be instructed to drink 2 to 3 qt (2 to 3 L) of fluid a day, to dilute the urine and reduce irritation on the bladder mucosa. Option B is incorrect because the patient must take the full amount of antibiotics prescribed for her UTI, despite the improvement in her symptoms. Option D is incorrect because women should wear cotton underwear, not nylon, to reduce the chance of irritation.

3. The nurse is caring for a patient with acute renal failure. The nurse should expect hypertonic glucose, insulin infusions, and sodium bicarbonate to be used to treat:

○ **A.** hypernatremia.

○ **B.** hypokalemia.

○ **C.** hypercalcemia.

○ **D.** hyperkalemia.

Correct answer: D Hyperkalemia is a common complication of acute renal failure. It's life-threatening if immediate action isn't taken to reverse it. The administration of glucose and regular insulin infusions, with sodium bicarbonate if necessary, can temporarily prevent cardiac arrest by moving potassium into the cells and temporarily reducing serum potassium levels. Hypernatremia (option A), hypokalemia (option B), and hypercalcemia (option C) don't usually occur with acute renal failure and aren't treated with glucose, insulin, or sodium bicarbonate.

4. The nurse is teaching a patient with chronic renal failure which foods to avoid. It would be most accurate for the nurse to teach the patient to avoid foods high in:

○ **A.** monosaccharides.

○ **B.** disaccharides.

○ **C.** iron.

○ **D.** protein.

Correct answer: D Proteins are typically restricted in patients with chronic renal failure because of their metabolites. Carbohydrates (options A and B) and iron (option C) aren't restricted.

5. A patient with acute renal failure is being assessed to determine whether the cause is prerenal, renal, or postrenal. If the cause is prerenal, which condition most likely caused it?

○ **A.** Heart failure

○ **B.** Glomerulonephritis

○ **C.** Ureterolithiasis

○ **D.** Aminoglycoside toxicity

Correct answer: A By causing inadequate renal perfusion, heart failure can lead to prerenal failure. Glomerulonephritis (option B) and aminoglycoside toxicity (option D) are renal causes, and ureterolithiasis (option C) is a postrenal cause.

Reproductive system disorders

❖ Introduction

- The chief function of the reproductive system is procreation and the manufacture of sex hormones
- Alterations in the reproductive system affect the ability to procreate and alter human social and emotional health
- Nursing history
  - ◆ The nurse asks the patient about the *chief complaint*
    - ▶ The female with a reproductive disorder may be experiencing pain, vaginal discharge, abnormal uterine bleeding, pruritus, or infertility
    - ▶ The male with a reproductive disorder may be experiencing penile discharge, impotence, infertility, or scrotal or inguinal masses, pain, or tenderness
  - ◆ The nurse then questions the patient about the *present illness*
    - ▶ Ask the patient about his symptoms, including when they started, associated symptoms, location, radiation, intensity, duration, frequency, and precipitating and alleviating factors
    - ▶ Ask about the use of prescription and over-the-counter drugs; herbal remedies; vitamin and nutritional supplements, including oral contraceptives and hormones; and use of any alternative therapies
  - ◆ The nurse asks about the *medical history*
    - ▶ Question the female patient about her reproductive history, endocrine disorders, human immunodeficiency virus (HIV) status, infection or cancer of the reproductive organs, and sexually transmitted disease (STD)
    - ▶ Question the male patient about his medical history, including diabetes, hypertension, mumps, HIV status, STD, endocrine disorders, and infection or cancer of the reproductive organs
  - ◆ The nurse then assesses the *family history*
    - ▶ Ask about a family history of diabetes and hypertension
    - ▶ Also question the patient about a family history of cancer of the reproductive organs, diethylstilbestrol exposure, and other reproductive disorders
  - ◆ The nurse obtains a *social history*
    - ▶ Ask about work, exercise, diet, use of recreational drugs and alcohol, and hobbies
    - ▶ Also ask about stress, support systems, and coping mechanisms

▶ Then, question the patient about the use of birth control, safe sex practices, sexual preference, number of sexual partners, and satisfaction

■ Physical assessment
   ◆ The nurse begins with *inspection*
      ▶ Observe the patient's general appearance, noting behaviors and mental status
      ▶ Inspect the external genitalia and pubic hair, noting any swelling, lumps, discharge, rashes, lesions, lice, or odors
      ▶ Observe the size and shape of the breasts, noting any nipple discharge
      ▶ Inspect the female patient's internal genitalia using a speculum
      ▶ Assess the male patient for inguinal and femoral hernias during the Valsalva maneuver and while coughing
   ◆ Next, the nurse uses *palpation*
      ▶ Palpate the external genitalia, noting any areas of swelling, tenderness, or hardness
      ▶ Palpate the breasts for lumps and nipple discharge
      ▶ Palpate the scrotal sac, noting the size and shape of the testicles and the presence of masses or tenderness
      ▶ If the patient is a male, palpate the inguinal area, and check for hernia

❖ Benign prostatic hyperplasia
■ Description
   ◆ Benign prostatic hyperplasia is prostate gland enlargement; about 50% of men older than age 50 and 75% of men older than age 70 have symptoms of such enlargement
   ◆ The cause is unknown but may be linked to hormonal changes
   ◆ As the prostate enlarges, the urethral opening narrows and obstructs or interferes with urine flow, causing urine retention or incomplete emptying; eventually, the ureters and kidneys dilate, and urinary tract infections (UTIs) result from urinary stasis
   ◆ Progressive bladder distention may cause a pouch to form in the bladder that retains urine when the rest of the bladder empties
■ Signs and symptoms
   ◆ Signs and symptoms include urinary frequency; nocturia; smaller, less-forceful urine stream; urinary hesitancy; dribbling after urination; bladder distention; cystitis; and acute urine retention
   ◆ Hematuria, bladder calculi, impaired renal function, fatigue, nausea, vomiting, anorexia, and abdominal discomfort also may occur
■ Diagnosis and treatment
   ◆ Digital rectal examination can detect the enlarged lateral lobes of the prostate; cystoscopy, urethrography, excretory urography, and hematologic and kidney function studies may be performed; prostate-specific antigen (PSA) can help to rule out prostatic carcinoma; and postvoid residual urine test and transrectal ultrasonography may also be performed

Types of prostatectomies

Four types of prostatectomy may be used to treat benign prostatic hyperplasia (BPH).

Transurethral resection of the prostate

Transurethral resection of the prostate (TURP) is the most common surgical procedure for treating BPH. The urologist passes an endoscopic instrument directly through the urethra to visualize the prostate without making an incision. Then the urologist removes the medial lobe of the gland in small pieces, leaving behind the prostatic capsule. After removing the prostate tissue, the urologist inserts a large, three-way indwelling urinary catheter with a 30-ml balloon to continuously irrigate the bladder and keep it free from clots. Traction may be placed briefly on the catheter to facilitate hemostasis at the operative site. However, prolonged traction can cause tissue necrosis.

The traction and balloon pressure cause transient postoperative bladder spasms and a continual urge to void. Postoperative complications include hemorrhage, clot retention, bladder perforation during surgery, catheter displacement, urinary tract infection, and water intoxication related to continuous bladder irrigation.

Suprapubic prostatectomy

Suprapubic prostatectomy is performed when a large mass of tissue must be removed. After making an abdominal incision, the urologist removes the prostate through the bladder. Then a suprapubic catheter, indwelling urinary catheter, and sometimes a surgical drain are put in place, and the bladder is irrigated continuously for the first 24 hours after surgery to remove clots. The suprapubic catheter is removed 3 to 4 days after surgery; the indwelling urinary catheter remains in place until the suprapubic catheter site heals.

Suprapubic prostatectomy can produce the same complications as TURP as well as complications related to abdominal surgery.

Perineal prostatectomy

Perineal prostatectomy, which is commonly performed while treating prostate cancer, removes prostate tissue through an incision made between the rectum and the scrotum. If cancer is confirmed, adjacent tissue also may be removed in a procedure called radical perineal resection. An indwelling urinary catheter and sometimes a surgical drain are put in place.

The chief postoperative complication is wound infection because of the incision's location. Urinary incontinence and impotence can result from radical perineal resection.

Retropubic prostatectomy

Retropubic prostatectomy takes an abdominal approach to excising a large prostate gland high in the pelvis. The bladder is retracted, and the prostate is removed through an incision in the prostatic capsule. An indwelling urinary catheter is put in place.

Postoperative complications are the same as suprapubic prostatectomy.

◆ Conservative treatment may include finasteride (Proscar) to decrease the size of the prostate and alpha-adrenergic blockers, such as prazosin (Minipress), doxazosin (Cardura), tamsulosin (Flomax), and terazosin (Hytrin), to relax the muscles and promote urination

◆ For acute cases, a urologist may insert a urinary catheter; a stylet may be needed to pass through the obstruction, or a suprapubic cystostomy (incision and catheter placement in the bladder through the abdomen wall) may be needed

◆ When a urinary obstruction is present, prostatectomy (surgical removal of soft tissue from the prostate) by one of four techniques is commonly performed (see *Types of prostatectomies*)

◆ Newer treatments include balloon urethroplasty, laser therapy, and intraurethral stents

◆ Other minimally invasive surgical techniques include:

❱ Transurethral needle ablation to burn away well-defined regions of the prostate, thereby improving urine flow with less risk

    ❱ Transurethral microwave treatment to destroy portions of the prostate with heat
- Preoperative nursing interventions
  - ◆ Explain the surgical procedure, perioperative experience, and expected postoperative course to help decrease the patient's anxiety
  - ◆ Allow the patient to discuss fears and concerns about postoperative urinary incontinence and impotence, but assure him that they aren't common after prostate surgery, only after radical perineal resection
- Postoperative nursing interventions
  - ◆ Evaluate the patient's pain and response to analgesia
    - ❱ Explain to the patient that after transurethral resection of prostate (TURP), bladder spasms are typical; explain to him that the sensation of needing to void is normal and that avoiding straining may decrease the frequency and intensity of bladder spasms
    - ❱ Observe and maintain the patency of the three-way irrigation system; clots can obstruct the system and cause pain and bladder spasms; if clots form, increase the flow of saline solution to dilute the urine and allow the clots to flow out
    - ❱ Check for pain at the incision site, penile inflammation at the catheter site, and pain in the flank area caused by UTI
    - ❱ Administer opioids for pain as prescribed; belladonna and opium suppositories may be prescribed for bladder spasms
  - ◆ Monitor the patient for potential complications
    - ❱ Watch for hemorrhage and shock, which can occur postoperatively because the prostate is a highly vascular gland
      - • Check urinary drainage, which initially should be reddish pink with a few small clots and then lighter pink during the first 24 hours after surgery; bright red drainage with clots indicates arterial bleeding and typically requires surgical intervention
      - • Check for hemodynamic alterations (such as tachycardia, increased respiratory rate, and decreased blood pressure) and other signs of hemorrhage, including restlessness, pallor, and cold, clammy skin
    - ❱ Monitor the patient's fluid and electrolyte status
    - ❱ Make sure that the catheter drains well; catheter obstruction by clots can cause prostatic capsule or bladder distention and hemorrhage
      - • Assess patient for bladder distention by palpating for a rounded swelling above the pubis
      - • Using aseptic technique, perform manual irrigation when needed with 50 ml of sterile normal saline solution to remove clots
      - • Carefully record the intake of irrigating solution and the output of urine and irrigating solution
    - ❱ Observe the patient for signs of cerebral edema, such as confusion and agitation; water intoxication can result when the irrigating solution is absorbed into the vascular system during surgery
    - ❱ Check for and take precautions to prevent wound infection, UTI, and epididymitis

● Use aseptic technique when performing catheter care and changing dressings and irrigation solution containers

● Avoid taking rectal temperatures and administering enemas to prevent trauma to the operative area

● Monitor the patient for signs of infection, such as fever, redness, swelling, and drainage from the incision site

● Change wet dressings frequently to prevent skin maceration

▶ After a suprapubic, perineal, or retropubic prostatectomy, monitor the patient for and take steps to prevent deep vein thrombosis (DVT) and pulmonary embolism

▶ Monitor the patient for postoperative respiratory complications

◆ Assess urinary continence after the catheter is removed

▶ Monitor urine output, and observe the patient for urine retention

▶ Explain that incontinence is normal after prostate surgery, that it's transient and will gradually improve, except after radical perineal surgery

▶ Encourage perineal exercises and voluntary interruption of the urine stream to expedite the return of bladder control

◆ Prepare the patient for discharge

▶ Follow the patient to discuss his feelings about sexual activity

● Discuss with the surgeon when the patient can resume sexual activity (usually within 3 to 8 weeks)

● Advise the patient about retrograde ejaculation to the bladder (urine may appear milky)

● Refer a patient who has had a radical prostatectomy for counseling because physiologic impotence may occur

▶ Tell the patient to avoid prolonged sitting, vigorous exercise, heavy lifting, and straining to decrease pressure on the operative area and help prevent bleeding

▶ Discuss ways to avoid constipation; provide dietary suggestions to promote soft stools and enhance wound healing

▶ Advise the patient to drink 2½ qt (2.5 L) of fluid daily to keep stools soft and prevent urinary stasis and UTI (unless contraindicated); discourage the intake of caffeine-containing and cola beverages, which can irritate the urinary system; and encourage decreased fluid intake in the evening to minimize nocturia

▶ Alert a patient who has undergone TURP of the possibility of secondary hemorrhage 2 weeks after the operation

▶ Instruct the patient to call the surgeon immediately if bleeding, decreased urinary stream, or signs of infection develop

❖ Breast cancer
■ Description

◆ Breast cancer is the most common cancer in women and the second leading cause of cancer deaths in women; it affects one of eight women in the United States, and its incidence increases with age; 1% of all breast cancer occurs in men

◆ The cause of breast cancer is unknown, but risk factors include a family history of breast cancer, inherited gene factors BRCA1 and BRCA2, obesity, hypertension, diabetes, exposure to ionizing radiation or chemical carcinogens, nulliparity or low parity, lack of breast-feeding, use of estrogen replacement therapy for menopausal symptoms, high-fat diet, and onset of menarche before age 12, menopause after age 55, and first pregnancy after age 30

◆ The lifetime risk of breast cancer for women with BRCA1 mutation is 50% to 85%, compared with a risk of 11% for women without this gene mutation

◆ The prognosis depends on the type of cancer and the stage of the disease at the time of treatment; early detection and treatment result in a more favorable prognosis

◆ Breast cancer commonly begins as atypical cells, progresses to ductal or lobular carcinoma in situ, and then enters an invasive stage; in the invasive stage, the cancer can spread quickly to regional lymph nodes and the systemic circulation

◆ Common metastatic sites include the lungs, bone, liver, brain, pelvis, and abdomen

■ Signs and symptoms

◆ A small, nontender, palpable, movable mass in the breast is an early sign of breast cancer, although it may go undetected until later signs develop; the common site for such a mass is the upper outer quadrant of the breast

◆ Late signs of breast cancer include skin dimpling or puckering, skin color changes over the lesion, nipple retraction, breast contour changes, serous or bloody nipple discharge, and palpable axillary or other lymph nodes, breast asymmetry, erythema, ridging, and prominent venous pattern

◆ Inflammatory carcinoma is a rare form of breast cancer that produces a tender, enlarged, reddened, hot breast; in advanced cases, the breast may become ulcerated, infected, and necrotic

■ Diagnosis and treatment

◆ About 90% of breast cancers are discovered by breast self-examination (BSE); BSE and annual breast examination by a health care professional may detect early disease; however, micrometastases may have disseminated by the time the tumor is palpable

◆ Mammography can detect early lesions before they're palpable; xeroradiography, ultrasonography, magnetic resonance imaging (MRI), and positron emission tomography also may be used

◆ The diagnosis of breast cancer is made by fine-needle aspiration and excisional biopsy of the tumor; the biopsied tissue is analyzed to determine whether the tumor is hormone-dependent, a factor that influences treatment

  ▶ Newer biopsy techniques include mammotone biopsy, minimally invasive breast biopsy, and advanced breast biopsy instrument

  ▶ Ductal lavage may also be performed to detect malignant cells

Types of breast surgery

Several surgical options are available for a patient with breast cancer.

- **Lumpectomy** or **tumorectomy** (simple excision of the tumor along with a margin of normal tissue) is used to treat early disease.
- **Quadrantectomy** (resection of the involved breast quadrant and dissection of axillary lymph nodes) also may be used to treat early disease.
- **Simple mastectomy** (removal of the main breast structure) may be performed for early disease or palliation in advanced, ulcerative disease. It doesn't remove the overlying skin, axillary nodes, and underlying muscles.
- **Modified radical mastectomy** (removal of the entire breast, some overlying skin and adjacent soft tissue, axillary lymph nodes, and the pectoralis major muscle) is the most common surgery for early disease.
- **Radical mastectomy** (removal of the entire breast, both pectoral muscles, and axillary nodes) is rarely used since the advent of less disfiguring procedures.

▶ Sentinel lymph node mapping, in which a radioactive substance or blue dye is injected around the biopsy site, may be performed before surgery; the sentinel node (the one most likely to contain malignant cells) is the one that contains the most radioactivity and blue dye, which then will be biopsied

◆ Treatment depends on the tumor's histopathology and aggressiveness, hormonal factors (the patient's menopausal status and the tumor's hormone dependency), extent of disease, and the patient's overall health and treatment preferences

◆ Surgery is the primary treatment for breast cancer; breast reconstruction surgery may be performed immediately after surgery or later (see *Types of breast surgery*); laser ablation is an alternative to lumpectomy in women with tumors that are smaller than ¾″ (2 cm)

◆ Radiation therapy is the primary treatment for patients who can't tolerate anesthesia or surgery or who have inflammatory carcinoma

▶ Primary radiation therapy with "boost" to the tumor site (application of additional radiation by external beam or placement of iridium needles in the former tumor site) may be used in early stages of breast cancer as a supplement to surgery and primary radiation

▶ Radiation therapy to the breast and lymph nodes followed by "boost" to the tumor site is used after breast-preserving surgery (such as lumpectomy, quadrantectomy, and simple mastectomy)

◆ Adjuvant chemotherapy is recommended after primary treatment and typically involves a combination of doxorubicin (Adriamycin), cyclophosphamide (Cytoxan), paclitaxel (Taxol), methotrexate (Amethopterin, Mexate, Folex), tamoxifen (Nolvadex), and fluorouracil (Floururacil, 5-FU, Adrucil); metastatic breast cancer is usually treated with fluorouracil, paclitaxel, or docetaxel (Taxotere), capecitabine (Xeloda), vinorelbine (Navelbine), or gemcitabine (Gemzar)

◆ Hormone therapy or surgery is indicated for patients with hormone-dependent breast cancer; antiestrogen drugs such as tamoxifen (Nolvadex) may be prescribed, and adrenalectomy, oophorectomy, or hypophysectomy may be considered

◆ Monoclonal antibodies such as trastuzumab may be used to treat metastatic breast cancer in women who have an excess amount of breast cancer cell antigen HER2

◆ Bone marrow or blood stem cell transplantation may be used to restore stem cells

■ Nursing interventions for a patient with early breast cancer

◆ Assess the patient's and family's understanding of the disease, diagnostic tests, and treatments, and intervene accordingly

◆ Encourage the patient to discuss her fears and concerns about the disease, diagnostic tests, treatments, and sexuality; clarify misconceptions, and be aware that breast cancer treatment can change the patient's body image and self-concept

◆ Evaluate the patient's support systems, and refer her to clergy members, home health care services, hospices, or support groups (such as Reach to Recovery, a group of volunteers who provide emotional and educational support during the preoperative and postoperative periods)

■ Nursing interventions for a patient undergoing mastectomy

◆ Monitor the patient for complications of general anesthesia and surgery, such as hemorrhage, wound infection, and altered respiratory status

▶ During the initial postoperative period, frequently check the dressing and Hemovac drains for excessive bleeding

▶ Check the patency of the Hemovac drains, and empty it when half full to maintain suction and prevent fluid accumulation; the drain is typically removed after 3 to 5 days

▶ Use strict aseptic technique for dressing changes

▶ Encourage the patient to perform deep-breathing and coughing exercises; administer analgesics to prevent respiratory splinting

▶ Evaluate the patient's nutritional status, and promote adequate nutritional intake to foster wound healing

◆ Evaluate the patient's level of pain and response to analgesia and comfort measures

▶ Promote comfort by elevating the head of the bed and positioning the patient on the unaffected side supported by pillows (lying on the affected side can cause severe pain)

▶ Position the affected arm on pillows to provide support and enhance circulation

▶ Encourage the patient to use her unaffected arm to help change position or get out of bed

◆ Monitor the patient for lymphedema, and take steps to prevent it

▶ Never perform blood pressure readings, venipuncture, or injections on the affected arm

▶ Check for edema in the affected arm; diuretics may be prescribed in the acute phase, and an elastic sleeve may be used during the chronic phase

▶ Elevate, massage, and exercise the affected arm to improve circulation and prevent edema; teach the patient to do this at home

▌ Teach the patient other techniques for preventing lymphedema, such as avoiding sun exposure, applying cream several times a day, using a thimble while sewing, using gloves while cleaning or gardening, wearing medical identification at all times, avoiding restrictive jewelry and clothing, not carrying heavy objects with the affected arm, and elevating the arm above the right atrium to promote circulatory and lymphatic flow

◆ Teach the patient arm exercises to prevent muscle shortening, stiffening, and contracture and to preserve muscle tone

◆ Encourage early and frequent ambulation; help the patient from her unaffected side, and help her maintain posture

◆ Provide rest periods between activities to avoid tiring the patient

◆ Prepare the patient for discharge by providing verbal and written instructions about pain medications, activity restrictions, arm exercises, lymphedema prevention, follow-up treatments, referrals to postdischarge support services, and information about prostheses; also provide an opportunity to discuss the effect of surgery on sexuality

■ Nursing interventions for a patient receiving chemotherapy after a mastectomy

◆ Monitor for and teach the patient about the adverse effects and toxicity of chemotherapeutic agents (see Nursing implications in oncology care, page 351)

◆ Follow guidelines for handling chemotherapeutic agents to prevent personal risks associated with repeated exposure to these drugs

◆ Monitor the patient for adverse effects of hormone therapy such as fluid retention

■ Nursing interventions for a patient receiving breast-preserving surgery and radiation therapy

◆ Follow postoperative nursing interventions for a patient undergoing mastectomy

◆ Monitor the patient for complications of radiation therapy, such as nausea, dyspepsia, esophagitis, transient pneumonitis, cough, fatigue, depression, and altered skin integrity at the surgical site and iridium needle site

◆ Provide emotional support to the patient and family during "boost" therapy with an internal interstitial implant because radiation precautions require a private room and restricted visitation while the implant is in place (about 2 days) because of gamma ray emissions

■ Nursing interventions for a patient with advanced breast cancer

◆ Develop an individualized plan of care based on the patient's treatment: radiation therapy, chemotherapy, hormone therapy, oophorectomy, adrenalectomy, or hypophysectomy

◆ Evaluate the patient's pain and response to pain-control and comfort measures; inform the practitioner and other health care team members if pain-control measures are ineffective

◆ Promote comfort by positioning the patient, applying heat or cold, using massage, providing pillows and a firm mattress, and teaching the patient relaxation techniques and guided imagery

◆ Promote adequate nutritional intake, particularly protein
  ▶ Collaborate with the dietitian to improve nutrition; assess the need for supplements
  ▶ Administer antiemetics as prescribed, and provide meticulous oral hygiene to improve the patient's ability and desire to eat
◆ Prevent alterations in skin integrity
  ▶ Observe the patient's skin and mucous membranes for signs of impaired skin integrity; radiation therapy, chemotherapy, inadequate nutrition, and impaired mobility can lead to skin breakdown and mucous membrane irritation
  ▶ Provide oral and skin care; applying lip gloss or petroleum jelly to the lips may be helpful
  ▶ Promote activity and position changes to prevent prolonged pressure and tissue necrosis
  ▶ Ensure adequate nutrition

❖ Cervical cancer
■ Description
  ◆ Cervical cancer is the most common cancer of the female reproductive system; it's most common in women between ages 30 and 50 and among Black, Hispanic, and Native American women
  ◆ The most important risk factor for cervical cancer is infection with human papillomavirus (HPV); 90% of all cervical cancers are attributed to certain HPV types
  ◆ Risk factors include first intercourse at a young age, multiple male sex partners, long-term oral contraceptive use, long-term cigarette smoking, and having a weakened immune system
  ◆ About 95% of cervical cancers are squamous cell carcinomas, which affect the epidermal layer of the cervix; the precursor of this type of carcinoma is called dysplasia or cervical intraepithelial neoplasia
  ◆ About 5% of cervical cancers are adenocarcinomas, which arise from the mucus-producing gland cells of the cervix; these cancers have no precursor
  ◆ Cervical cancer is categorized according to the extent of the primary tumor, lymph node involvement, and metastasis
  ◆ The prognosis depends on the stage of the disease and the treatment required; cure rates are as high as 100% in the early stages
■ Signs and symptoms
  ◆ Early stages of cervical cancer are asymptomatic
  ◆ Later stages may cause vaginal discharge (leukorrhea) that gradually increases in amount and changes from watery to dark and foul-smelling; irregular vaginal bleeding or spotting between menstrual periods or after menopause may occur; spotting or bleeding may occur after intercourse, douching, or bowel movements
  ◆ Advanced invasive disease is associated with chronic infections, ulcers, pelvic pressure or pain, or abscesses at the tumor site; severe back and leg pain; anorexia; and anemia
■ Diagnosis and treatment

◆ The Papanicolaou (Pap) test is used to screen for cervical cancer

◆ If cervical neoplasia or cancer is detected on a Pap test, then colposcopy, punch biopsy, or endocervical curettage may be performed; lymphangiography, computed tomography (CT), and MRI also may be performed

◆ The treatment of cervical cancer depends on the patient's health and age and the presence of other complications

◆ Dysplasia and noninvasive cervical cancer (carcinoma in situ) may be removed by cryotherapy, carbon dioxide laser therapy, or conization (removal of a cone-shaped section of the cervix); these procedures maintain fertility but require frequent follow-up to detect recurrence

◆ Noninvasive cervical cancer may be treated with a simple hysterectomy (removal of the cervix and uterus) in women who don't want future pregnancies

◆ Invasive cervical cancer may be treated by radiation therapy, radical surgery, or chemotherapy (see *Treatments for invasive cervical cancer*)

■ Nursing interventions for a patient with early cervical cancer

◆ Assess the patient's and family's understanding of the disease, diagnostic tests, and treatments, and intervene accordingly

◆ Allow the patient to discuss her fears and concerns about the disease, diagnostic tests, treatments, and sexuality; clarify misconceptions and be aware that cervical cancer can change the patient's body image and self-concept

◆ Evaluate the patient's support systems, and refer her to clergy members, home health care services, hospices, or support groups as needed

■ Nursing interventions for a patient undergoing cryotherapy, carbon dioxide laser therapy, or cervical conization

◆ During the immediate postoperative period, monitor the patient for complications of anesthesia — typically a local anesthesia — and hemorrhage

◆ Before discharge, provide verbal and written instructions about activity restrictions, and tell the patient to avoid using tampons and douching and to watch for and report increased vaginal bleeding or discharge and fever

■ Nursing interventions for a patient undergoing hysterectomy

◆ Administer an enema and a douche preoperatively as prescribed

◆ Monitor the patient for complications after general anesthesia and major abdominal surgery — and take steps to prevent them

▶ Monitor the patient for hemorrhage by assessing vital signs, wound drainage, and vaginal drainage; she may have surgical drains connected to a Hemovac

▶ Initiate leg exercises and early ambulation to prevent venous stasis and thrombophlebitis

▶ Monitor bowel sounds and encourage early ambulation to expedite the return of bowel function; a nasogastric tube may be in place for the first 24 hours after surgery

Treatments for invasive cervical cancer

Radiation therapy, radical surgery, or chemotherapy may be used to treat invasive cervical cancer.

Radiation therapy

Radiation therapy, which uses whole pelvic irradiation and intracavitary implants, causes ovarian function to cease. Before treatment, the patient follows a low-residue diet, receives enemas, and has an indwelling urinary catheter inserted to prevent bowel and bladder distention. These procedures allow more room for the implant and may protect the bowel and bladder from radiation. Complications of radiation therapy include nausea, vomiting, diarrhea, malaise, fever, hemorrhage, cystitis, proctitis, phlebitis, vesicovaginal fistulas, and ureterovaginal fistulas.

Surgery

Radical hysterectomy removes the uterus and proximal vagina through an abdominal incision. Pelvic lymph node dissection may be performed for stage I and early stage II disease; a salpingo-oophorectomy also may be performed. Surgical drains are placed below the incision

site to drain excess fluid. An indwelling urinary catheter is placed preoperatively to prevent bladder trauma during surgery and to allow for postoperative urine drainage. (In the immediate postoperative period, the bladder may be atonic.)

Pelvic exenteration is used for advanced or recurrent cervical cancer confined to the pelvis. Total exenteration removes the bladder, rectosigmoid, and all reproductive organs and nodes. The bladder and sigmoid may be preserved if disease isn't evident in these structures.

For either type of surgery, complications include abdominal distention, paralytic ileus, thrombophlebitis, wound infection, atelectasis, and other complications of general anesthesia and major abdominal surgery.

Chemotherapy

Chemotherapy commonly includes fluorouracil, ifosfamide, and cisplatin alone or in combination to treat metastatic or nonresectable disease.

  ❱ Observe the patient for altered urinary elimination; because the surgery is performed near the bladder, it can cause nerve damage and trauma to the ureter and bladder
 ◆ Assess the patient's pain and response to analgesia
  ❱ If possible, administer analgesics using patient-controlled analgesia
  ❱ Ensure adequate pain relief, which encourages the patient to perform leg exercises, deep-breathing and coughing exercises, and early ambulation
 ◆ Provide written and oral discharge instructions, and instruct the patient to take showers instead of baths to prevent vaginal inflammation and infection; explain activity restrictions; encourage her to avoid sitting for prolonged periods, lifting and straining until the first postoperative checkup, and intercourse for 4 to 6 weeks; instruct her to notify the practitioner if vaginal discharge, bleeding, or fever develop; and teach her about the therapeutic and adverse effects and dosing schedule of prescribed medications
■ Nursing interventions for a patient undergoing radiation therapy
 ◆ Assess the patient's comfort level and response to analgesia; administer opioids at regularly scheduled intervals
  ❱ Position the patient for comfort, using pillows for support; strict bed rest in the supine position is maintained while the implant is in place
  ❱ Advise the patient that cell destruction by radiation causes foul-smelling vaginal discharge; minimize these effects with meticulous

perineal care, a room deodorizer, and reassurance that the discharge is a temporary result of treatment

◆ Monitor the patient for local and systemic complications of radiation therapy

◆ Promote adequate nutritional and fluid intake to maintain skin integrity, promote tissue healing, and prevent urinary complications

◆ Follow the facility's radiation precautions; provide emotional support to a patient who feels isolated because of restricted visitation

◆ Prepare the patient for discharge by providing verbal and written instructions about medications, wound care, activity restrictions (including sexual activity), and follow-up appointments; also advise her that she must douche twice daily as prescribed, that vaginal drainage and bleeding should diminish gradually over 1 to 3 months, and that she should contact the practitioner if fever, increased pain, increased drainage, or altered urinary or bowel elimination occurs

■ Nursing interventions for a patient undergoing pelvic exenteration

◆ Implement the same preoperative and postoperative nursing interventions as for a patient undergoing hysterectomy

◆ Be sensitive to the fact that this procedure exacts a tremendous physical, psychosocial, and emotional toll on the patient and requires a multidisciplinary approach to patient care, involving an enterostomal therapist, a social worker, and a dietitian

◆ Refer the patient for support to help her cope with the resulting changes in lifestyle, body image, and sexuality

■ Nursing interventions for a patient whose ovaries have been removed or undergoing radiation therapy

◆ A premenopausal woman whose ovaries have been removed or irradiated will experience menopause

◆ Discuss the physiologic changes of menopause and self-care practices to promote optimal health and a feeling of well-being; recommend regular exercise, calcium and vitamin E and B-complex supplements, a calcium-rich diet, vaginal lubricants, and hormone therapy (controversial) to relieve various menopausal symptoms

❖ Endometrial cancer

■ Description

◆ Endometrial cancer is the most commonly diagnosed gynecologic cancer

◆ Risk factors include early menarche, late menopause, infertility, extended use of tamoxifen or unopposed estrogens, obesity, diabetes, advancing age, high-fat diet, history of breast and ovarian cancers, previous pelvic radiation, and family history

◆ Most endometrial cancers are adenocarcinomas and are slow to grow and metastasize; common sites for metastasis are the lungs, liver, and bone

■ Signs and symptoms

◆ The woman may report abnormal vaginal bleeding, especially after menopause

◆ Difficult or painful urination, pain during intercourse, and pelvic pain may also occur

◆ In advanced cases, lymph node enlargement, pleural effusion, abdominal masses, or ascites may be present

■ Diagnosis and treatment

◆ Diagnosis is based on a physical examination and history

◆ Other diagnostic tools include transvaginal ultrasound, endometrial biopsy, CA-125 blood test, CT scan, MRI, cystoscopy, proctoscopy, and Pap test

◆ The primary treatment for endometrial cancer is hysterectomy; a bilateral salpingo-oophorectomy may also be performed

◆ Progesterone therapy may be indicated for patients with recurrent disease

◆ Women with metastatic disease may receive combination chemotherapy that may include doxorubicin, cisplatin, paclitaxel, etoposide, and dactinomycin

◆ Radiation therapy may be indicated before, after, or instead of surgery in some women; radioactive implants may be used

■ Nursing interventions

◆ Assess the patient's and family's understanding of the disease, diagnostic tests, and treatments, and intervene accordingly

◆ Provide analgesics and comfort measures as needed

◆ Encourage the patient to discuss her feelings regarding self-esteem and body image disturbance

■ Nursing interventions for a patient undergoing other treatments

◆ Provide care related to abdominal hysterectomy and bilateral salpingo-oophorectomy and pelvic radiation therapy (see "Cervical cancer," page 279)

◆ Provide care related to systemic chemotherapy (see Nursing implications in oncology care, page 351)

❖ Endometriosis

■ Description

◆ Endometriosis is a benign condition in which the endometrial cells that normally line the uterus are dispersed throughout the pelvis; the most common ectopic tissue sites are the ovaries, fallopian tubes, uterosacral ligaments, cul-de-sac of Douglas, pelvic peritoneum, rectovaginal septum, and cervix

◆ The misplaced endometrial cells respond to normal ovarian hormone stimulation; during menstruation, the ectopic endometrial tissue grows, becomes secretory, and bleeds, which causes pressure and inflammation at the involved site and creates fibrosis, adhesions, and cysts

◆ Endometriosis may result from transfer of endometrial cells by blood flow, lymphatic flow, or retrograde menstrual flow or from autoimmune or congenital factors

◆ Risk factors for endometriosis include family history, delayed childbearing, retroflexed uterus, use of intrauterine devices, polymenorrhea, hypermenorrhea, menstrual periods that last longer than 5 days, spotting, and being of Asian descent

◆ Endometriosis can occur in any woman of childbearing age but usually begins between ages 30 and 40; it's responsible for 30% to 45% of female infertility

■ Signs and symptoms

◆ The chief symptom of endometriosis is painful menstruation (dysmenorrhea) or menstrual cramps

◆ Many women with advanced disease are asymptomatic; the disease is discovered when they undergo testing related to infertility

◆ Other symptoms of endometriosis include dyspareunia, painful defecation, rectal pressure, and abnormal uterine bleeding (menstrual cycles of less than 27 days; menses that last longer than 7 days)

◆ The pelvic examination may reveal bluish lesions on the labia, perineal area, cervix, or vaginal wall; tender nodules in the posterior vaginal fornix of the vagina, along the uterosacral ligaments, and along the cul-de-sac; adnexal thickening and nodules; tender, enlarged, and fixed ovaries; and a fixed, retroverted uterus that's painful when moved

■ Diagnosis and treatment

◆ The diagnosis of endometriosis is determined by patient history and physical examination; biopsy—using laparoscopy—of the endometrial tissue is required to confirm the diagnosis

◆ Vaginal ultrasonography, complete blood count, cultures and blood tests for STDs, Pap test, urinalysis, and a pregnancy test may be performed

◆ Treatment of endometriosis depends on the patient's age, symptoms, stage of disease, and desire to have children

◆ Drugs may be used to treat endometriosis (see *Drug therapy for endometriosis*)

◆ Laparoscopy, under general anesthesia, may be used to diagnose and treat endometriosis; after inserting a scope into the peritoneal cavity through a small abdominal incision, the surgeon insufflates carbon dioxide into the abdominal cavity to separate the intestines from the pelvic organs and to improve visualization; after determining the extent of the disease, the surgeon uses fulguration or laser surgery to treat lesions and adhesions

◆ Women with severe, symptomatic, painful endometriosis may decide to undergo bilateral salpingo-oophorectomy and total abdominal hysterectomy; laser surgery may also be used

◆ In some women, endometriosis may disappear without treatment; in others, pregnancy causes remission of the disease

■ Nursing interventions

◆ Teach the patient about reproductive anatomy and physiology, the disease, and the medications used to treat it

◆ Teach the patient about activities that may promote comfort and help relieve symptoms: regular exercise, sexual excitement and orgasm, increased intake of natural diuretics (such as watermelons, cranberry juice,

Drug therapy for endometriosis

Various types of drugs are prescribed to manage endometriosis.

- Analgesics, nonsteroidal anti-inflammatory drugs, and diuretics are prescribed to relieve pain, inflammation, and fluid retention.
- Oral contraceptives interrupt ovulation and produce endometrial atrophy, thereby decreasing endometrial flow in the peritoneal cavity. Their adverse effects include nausea, vomiting, weight gain, depression, fatigue, breast tenderness, and recurrent vaginitis.
- Danazol (Danocrine), a synthetic androgen, may be prescribed for 6 months to suppress ovarian activity and cause ectopic endometrial atrophy. The most effective drug for endometriosis, danazol relieves pain in about 90% of patients. Because endometriosis recurs in 5% to 20% of patients, repeated 6-month courses of therapy may be needed. Adverse effects include acne, decreased breast size, voice deepening, depression, hirsutism, hot flashes, oily skin, vaginal dryness, and weight gain.
- Nasally administered nafarelin, a gonadotropin-releasing hormone (GnRH) agonist, creates a reversible "pharmacologic oophorectomy" to control ectopic endometrial activity. Nafarelin causes fewer adverse effects than danazol; nafarelin's adverse effects may include depression, hot flashes, insomnia, and vaginal dryness.
- Medroxyprogesterone, a progestin, reduces dysmenorrhea and pelvic pain. Adverse effects include breakthrough bleeding, emotional lability, blood clots, myocardial infarction, pulmonary embolism, nausea, vomiting, depression, headache, and fatigue.
- Leuprolide (Lupron) and goserelin (Zoladex), GnRH agonists, block the production and release of luteinizing hormone and follicle-stimulating hormone, thereby reducing estrogen production and leading to decreased pelvic pain and shrinking of endometrial implants. Treatment is limited to 6 months because long-term use can cause bone loss. Common adverse effects may mimic symptoms of menopause, including hot flashes, vaginal dryness, decreased libido, headache, and mood swings.

peaches, and asparagus), decreased intake of salt and high-sodium foods, increased intake of iron-rich foods, application of heat to the pelvic area and lower back, relaxation techniques, and guided imagery

◆ Allow the patient to discuss feelings about how the disease affects her lifestyle, body image, and self-concept

◆ Provide additional emotional support to a patient who is infertile; also refer the patient for infertility testing and counseling

◆ Provide postoperative care for a patient undergoing laparoscopy; monitor her for complications of general anesthesia and hemorrhage, and provide verbal and written discharge instructions to ensure that she understands self-care measures and follow-up treatment

  ▶ Teach the patient and family about wound care
  ▶ Advise the patient to expect several days of gaslike pain in the abdomen and referred shoulder pain from carbon dioxide insufflation; recommend analgesics, local heat application, and a light diet to enhance comfort
  ▶ Inform the patient about pain medications, activity restrictions (including sexual activity), and follow-up treatment

◆ Provide postoperative care for a patient undergoing hysterectomy, oophorectomy, or bilateral salpingectomy; this care is the same as that for a patient with cervical cancer who undergoes these procedures (see "Cervical cancer," page 279)

❖ Ovarian cancer

- ■ Description
  - ◆ Ovarian cancer is the most common fatal gynecologic cancer and the fifth leading cause of cancer death in women; principal sources include the epithelial cells (serous, mucous, or endometrial cells), germ cells (in cases of teratoma or dysgerminoma), mesenchymal cells (in cases of fibroma, lymphoma, or sarcoma), and gonadal stroma (granulosa, theca, Sertoli's, or Leydig's cells)
  - ◆ Although unconfirmed, risk factors for ovarian cancer may include nulliparity; infertility or history of difficulty becoming pregnant; family history; previous breast, endometrial, or colon cancer; exposure to environmental carcinogens; lack of breast-feeding; use of fertility drugs; or use of talcum powder in the genital area
  - ◆ Ovarian cancer can occur at any age but is most common between ages 50 and 60
  - ◆ The 5-year survival rate for stage I ovarian cancer is 55% to 90%; stage II, 0% to 40%; and stages III and IV, 0% to 30%
- ■ Signs and symptoms
  - ◆ Ovarian cancer typically doesn't produce any signs or symptoms until the advanced stages of the disease
  - ◆ It should be suspected in women with irregular menses, early menopause, uterine bleeding before puberty or after menopause, or other signs of endocrine dysfunction, such as infertility and masculinization
  - ◆ GI signs and symptoms—such as abdominal discomfort and feeling of fullness, abdominal distention, nausea, vomiting, dyspepsia, flatulence, and constipation—may occur as the tumor enlarges
  - ◆ Ovarian enlargement (or palpable ovaries before menarche or after menopause) suggests ovarian cancer
  - ◆ Other signs and symptoms include urinary frequency and weight loss
- ■ Diagnosis and treatment
  - ◆ No early screening tests exist for ovarian cancer; Pap tests are abnormal in about 30% of women with ovarian cancer
  - ◆ Because the ovaries are located deep in the abdomen, pelvic examination may not detect early disease; diagnosis is made after biopsy of the tumor, during exploratory laparotomy
  - ◆ CA-125 is a tumor marker specific to epithelial ovarian cancer; significantly elevated CA-125 levels are usually found in patients with ovarian cancer
  - ◆ Other diagnostic tools include transvaginal ultrasonography, urine estrogen levels, pregnanediol, CT scan, and pelvic X-rays
  - ◆ Treatment depends on the cancer's stage, which is determined during exploratory laparotomy; during this procedure, a total abdominal hysterectomy and bilateral salpingo-oophorectomy are performed to remove as much of the tumor as possible along with affected lymph nodes and other peritoneal structures
  - ◆ Radiation therapy or chemotherapy is usually recommended with surgery, for all stages of the disease

▶ Radiation therapy techniques include external pelvic irradiation or intraperitoneal instillation of radioactive phosphorus

▶ Combination chemotherapy commonly consists of carboplatin and paclitaxel

◆ Patients may undergo a "second-look" laparotomy after treatment of the early stages, to detect persistent disease

◆ Treatment of advanced ovarian cancer is usually palliative

■ Nursing interventions for a patient with early ovarian cancer

◆ Assess the patient's and family's understanding of the disease, diagnostic tests, and treatments, and intervene accordingly

◆ Encourage the patient to discuss her fears and concerns; be aware that treatment for ovarian cancer can change the patient's body image and self-concept and that the diagnosis may come at a time of life when the patient is experiencing difficulty with the physical and sociocultural aspects of aging

◆ Evaluate the patient's support systems, and refer her to clergy members, home health care services, hospices, or support groups as needed

■ Nursing interventions for a patient with advanced ovarian cancer

◆ Administer analgesics, as indicated

◆ Position and support the patient to promote comfort; also apply heat or cold, massage painful areas, use pillows, and teach the patient relaxation techniques and guided imagery

■ Nursing interventions for a patient with early or advanced ovarian cancer

◆ Promote adequate nutritional intake by collaborating with the dietitian to determine what type of food the patient should eat, how much, and how often; assessing the need for supplements; administering antiemetics as prescribed; and providing meticulous oral hygiene to improve the patient's ability and desire to eat

◆ Prevent alterations in skin integrity

▶ Observe the patient's skin and mucous membranes for signs of impaired skin integrity; radiation therapy, chemotherapy, inadequate nutrition, and impaired mobility can increase the risk of skin breakdown and mucous membrane irritation

▶ Provide oral hygiene and skin care to prevent stomatitis and skin breakdown

▶ Promote activity and position changes to prevent prolonged pressure and tissue necrosis

■ Nursing interventions for a patient receiving intraperitoneal chemotherapy

◆ Intervene as appropriate for systemic chemotherapy (see Nursing implications in oncology care, page 351), and perform interventions specific to intraperitoneal chemotherapy

◆ Warm the drug, which typically is given in 2 L of normal saline solution, to body temperature, and infuse it by gravity as rapidly as tolerated; to improve flow, check for kinks in the tubing or catheter obstruction, and encourage the patient to gently turn from side to side

◆ Gently irrigate the catheter with normal saline solution; use an I.V. infusion to promote flow as long as the catheter is patent

◆ After instillation, clamp the tubing and let the solution remain in the peritoneal cavity for 4 hours (the dwell time)

◆ Unclamp the drainage tubing after the dwell time to let fluid drain out of the peritoneum; facilitate drainage by aspiration, frequent changes in patient position, Valsalva's maneuver, and application of mild pressure to the abdomen

◆ After drainage is completed, flush the catheter first with preservative-free saline solution and then with heparinized saline, and remove the needle from the port; the drainage may be sent to the laboratory for analysis

◆ Monitor the patient for fluid and electrolyte imbalances related to chemotherapy-induced nephrotoxicity and intraperitoneal fluid infusion

  ❱ Administer I.V. fluid supplemented with potassium and magnesium on the evening before treatment, as prescribed

  ❱ Measure fluid intake and output, and notify the practitioner if the 4-hour urine output falls below 240 ml

  ❱ Monitor electrolyte levels daily

◆ Monitor the patient for infection, and take steps to prevent it by using strict aseptic technique when handling the peritoneal access device and checking for local erythema, fever, and other signs of sepsis or peritonitis

◆ Check for alterations in respiratory status; keep the head of the bed elevated, and make sure that oxygen is nearby

◆ Watch for complications resulting from a detached or obstructed catheter; if severe pain occurs, stop the infusion, and obtain X-rays to confirm catheter migration into the peritoneal cavity

◆ Promote comfort by administering antiemetics, pain medications, and sedatives as needed; also provide extra blankets because the patient may feel chilled during the procedure as a result of the instilled fluids

◆ Prepare the patient for discharge by providing verbal and written instructions about pain medications, adverse effects of chemotherapy, catheter care, activity restrictions, and follow-up treatment

■ Nursing interventions for a patient undergoing other treatments

◆ Provide care related to abdominal hysterectomy and bilateral salpingo-oophorectomy and pelvic radiation therapy (see "Cervical cancer," page 279)

◆ Provide care related to systemic chemotherapy (see Nursing implications in oncology care, page 351)

❖ Prostate cancer

■ Description

◆ Prostate cancer is the second leading cause of cancer death in men in the United States and the most common type of cancer overall, the most common type in black men, and the second most common type in American men older than age 55

◆ Risk factors for prostate cancer include advancing age; North American, African, and Northwestern European descent; a high-fat diet; physical inactivity; and a family history

◆ Adenocarcinoma is the type of tumor found in prostate cancer

◆ Common metastatic sites are the brain, lungs, bone, and lymph nodes

■ Signs and symptoms

◆ Early prostate cancer is asymptomatic; in about 50% of patients, the disease is in the advanced stages or has metastasized by the time it's discovered

◆ As the disease progresses and the size of the neoplasm increases, urinary obstruction occurs, thereby producing dysuria, urinary frequency, blood in the ejaculate, urine retention, decreased size and force of the urinary stream, and hematuria

◆ Signs and symptoms of metastasis include hip pain, backache, rectal or perineal discomfort, anemia, nausea, weight loss, weakness, shortness of breath, and edema

■ Diagnosis and treatment

◆ A firm nodule felt on digital rectal examination suggests prostate cancer; a biopsy of surgically removed tissue can confirm the diagnosis

◆ Other helpful diagnostic tests include serum acid phosphatase, PSA, and testosterone levels; bone scans to detect metastasis; and kidney function tests

◆ Treatment is based on the patient's age, overall health, symptoms, stage of the disease, and survival prognosis

◆ Radical perineal prostatectomy is the standard surgical procedure for patients with potentially curable disease; bilateral orchiectomy is commonly performed along with prostatectomy

◆ Curative radiation therapy may be indicated if the patient is in the early stages of prostate cancer; this treatment may preserve sexual functioning

◆ Palliative measures are indicated for patients with advanced tumors or signs of metastasis (see *Palliative treatments for prostate cancer,* page 290)

■ Nursing interventions

◆ Assess the patient's and family's understanding of the disease, diagnostic tests, and treatments, and intervene accordingly

◆ Encourage the patient to discuss his fears and concerns

◆ Evaluate the patient's support systems, and refer him to clergy members, home health care services, hospices, or support groups as needed

◆ Evaluate the patient's response to pain control; notify the practitioner if pain-control measures are ineffective

◆ Promote comfort by applying heat or ice, massaging painful areas, providing pillows and a firm mattress, and teaching the patient to use relaxation techniques and guided imagery

◆ Monitor the patient for complications of radiation therapy, such as systemic adverse reactions (including nausea, vomiting, headache, skin reactions, fatigue, and malaise) and transitory proctitis and cystitis

---

Palliative treatments for prostate cancer

Several palliative treatments may be used for a patient with advanced or metastatic prostate cancer.

● Radiation therapy may be used for patients with late-stage disease. Because it alters cell growth and reproduction through ionization, it affects cancerous — and healthy — cells.
● Suppressive hormone therapy may be used to decrease tumor size and relieve pain because prostatic adenocarcinomas are hormone-dependent. Suppression may be achieved by orchiectomy or administration of drugs, such as luteinizing hormone-releasing hormone analogs, antiandrogens, and other androgen-suppressing drugs (such as diethylstilbestrol).

● Chemotherapy may slow the disease process and provide palliative relief. It directly interferes with the biochemistry of the cancer cells, altering their growth, metabolism, and reproduction.
● Cryosurgery, which freezes the target tissue, is another palliative measure used for locally recurrent disease.
● Repeated transurethral resections of the prostate may be needed to maintain urine flow. Eventually, permanent urinary or suprapubic catheterization may be needed.
● Corticosteroids and neurosurgery may relieve pain by interrupting pain receptors in the spinal cord.

◆ Monitor the patient for complications of chemotherapy (see Nursing implications in oncology care, page 351); handle chemotherapeutic agents according to federal safety guidelines
◆ Promote adequate nutritional intake by collaborating with the dietitian to determine what types of food the patient should eat, how much, and how often; assessing the need for supplements; administering antiemetics as prescribed; and providing meticulous oral hygiene to improve the patient's ability and desire to eat
◆ Prevent alterations in skin integrity by observing the patient's skin and mucous membranes for signs of impaired skin integrity; radiation therapy, chemotherapy, inadequate nutrition, and impaired mobility can predispose him to skin breakdown and mucous membrane irritation
▶ Provide oral hygiene and skin care to prevent stomatitis and skin breakdown
▶ Promote activity and position changes to prevent prolonged pressure and tissue necrosis
◆ Maintain adequate urinary elimination
▶ Determine the patient's urinary elimination pattern
▶ Monitor him for urine retention; record the frequency and amount of urine output, and assess him for urinary urgency, dysuria, and suprapubic distention
▶ Facilitate bladder emptying
● Ensure adequate fluid intake, and encourage the patient to urinate when he feels the need
● Help the patient to a normal position for voiding when possible, and unless contraindicated, use the Valsalva maneuver to initiate urine flow
● Administer cholinergics, as prescribed, to stimulate bladder contraction
● Determine whether the patient needs intermittent or indwelling urinary catheterization

◆ Assess the patient's potential for injury, and take safety precautions; bone metastasis, pain, weakness, and peripheral neuropathy may predispose the patient to falls or other injuries

◆ Prepare the patient for discharge

❱ Provide sexual counseling, emotional support related to alopecia, and self-catheterization and catheter care instructions as needed

❱ Teach the patient exercises to strengthen the perineal muscles

❱ Caution the patient to avoid taking rectal temperatures and to allow suppositories to reach room temperature before inserting them into the rectum

❱ Provide referrals for home health care and other services as needed

❱ Provide verbal and written instructions about prescribed medications, activity restrictions, diet, and follow-up care

❖ Sexually transmitted diseases

■ Description

◆ STDs are the most common infections in the United States; acquired immunodeficiency syndrome (AIDS), herpes, gonorrhea, and hepatitis are considered epidemic (see chapter 17, Immune system disorders, for details on AIDS)

◆ These contagious diseases are usually transmitted through intimate sexual contact with an infected person; some are transmitted to an infant during pregnancy or childbirth

◆ People younger than age 25, those with multiple sex partners, and those with a history of STDs are at higher risk for infection; the incidence of STDs is higher among prostitutes and people having sexual contact with prostitutes, drug abusers, or prison inmates

◆ Morbidity and mortality depend on the type and stage of STD; many STDs are easy to treat when detected early

◆ STDs can be prevented by educating the public, identifying and treating partners and contacts of infected people, and identifying and treating symptomatic or asymptomatic infected patients; barrier methods of contraception, such as a condom and a diaphragm with spermicide, reduce the risk of certain infections

◆ More than 21 diseases are classified as STDs; they're caused by bacteria, viruses, protozoans, fungi, and ectoparasites

■ Signs and symptoms

◆ The chief signs of STDs are vaginitis, recurrent vaginitis, epididymitis, lower abdominal pain, pharyngitis, proctitis, and skin or mucous membrane lesions

◆ Many STDs are asymptomatic, especially in women; by the time the STD is detected, the woman may have severe complications, such as pelvic inflammatory disease (PID), infertility, ectopic pregnancy, or chronic pelvic pain

■ Diagnosis and treatment

◆ The diagnosis of a specific STD is made by physical examination, patient history, and laboratory tests to determine the causative organism

◆ Treatment is based on the specific causative organism; treatment guidelines for each STD are available from the Centers for Disease Control and Prevention (CDC) (see *Sexually transmitted diseases*)

◆ The CDC recommends that specific resources be available for patients with STDs: medical evaluation and treatment facilities for patients with HIV infection; hospitalization facilities for patients with complicated STDs, such as PID and disseminated gonococcal infection; referrals for medical, pediatric, infectious disease, dermatologic, and gynecologic-obstetric services; family-planning services; and substance abuse treatment programs

■ Nursing interventions

◆ Develop a therapeutic relationship with the patient that fosters trust and preserves the patient's dignity; ensure privacy and confidentiality, and avoid judging the patient's lifestyle and making assumptions about his sexual preference

◆ Provide emotional support, and encourage the patient to discuss feelings; he may be anxious and fearful and may experience altered self-esteem and self-image

◆ Teach the patient about the STD and its treatment

  ▶ Discuss disease transmission, signs and symptoms, the length of the infectious period, infection prevention, and cure (if the STD can be cured)

  ▶ Discuss the health consequences of improper treatment, and emphasize that the patient's partner is also at risk

  ▶ Clarify common misconceptions and promote understanding of healthful sexual practices

    • Inform the patient that washing his hands and genital area before and after sexual contact doesn't prevent STDs

    • Encourage the patient to urinate after intercourse

    • Advise women to avoid douching because it can alter the normal vaginal flora

    • Tell the patient that condoms and a diaphragm with spermicide may provide some protection against certain STDs, but intrauterine devices and birth control pills don't

  ▶ Encourage a sexually active patient who has multiple partners and no STD symptoms to have an STD examination twice a year

  ▶ Tell the patient to seek immediate treatment if STD symptoms develop

  ▶ Inform the patient that treatment doesn't provide immunity from the same or a different STD

  ▶ Advise the patient to abstain from sexual activity until the posttreatment follow-up verifies a cure

  ▶ Discuss modifications of sexual activity to prevent recurrence: reducing the number of sex partners, avoiding partners who have multiple partners, and questioning partners about their STD history

◆ Teach the patient about the prescribed medication and its dosing schedule and adverse effects; stress the importance of completing the medication regimen, even if symptoms disappear; advise the patient to

Sexually transmitted diseases

Name and organism	Possible signs and symptoms	Treatment	Special considerations
Chlamydia Chlamydia trachomatis	• Purulent discharge • *Males:* burning on urination and symptoms of epididymitis • *Females:* usually asymptomatic	Doxycycline or azithromycin	• All sexual contacts must be treated. • Potential complications in females are pelvic inflammatory disease (PID), infertility, and spontaneous abortion; in males, urethritis, epididymitis, and prostatitis. • Patient should take medication as prescribed, follow up in 7 to 10 days, and abstain from sexual activity until treatment is completed.
Genital herpes, herpes simplex Type 2	• *Females:* purulent vaginal discharge • Multiple vesicles on genital area, buttocks, or thighs • Painful dysuria • Fever • Headache • Malaise	Famciclovir; valacyclovir, acyclovir, topical anesthetic ointment	• Warm baths and mild analgesics may relieve pain. • Patient should avoid sexual activity during the prodromal stage and during outbreaks until all lesions have dried up. • Many patients have recurrences every 2 to 3 months; local hyperesthesias may occur 24 hours before outbreak of lesions.
Gonorrhea Neisseria gonorrhoeae	• Purulent discharge • Dysuria • Urinary frequency	Ceftriaxone plus azithromycin or doxycycline	• All sexual contacts must be treated. • Potential complications in females are PID, sterility, and ectopic pregnancy; in males, prostatitis, urethritis, epididymitis, and sterility. • Patient should take medication as prescribed, follow up in 7 to 10 days, and abstain from sexual activity until treatment is completed.
Human papillomavirus (HPV)	• Pink-gray soft lesions, singularly or in clusters	Podophyllin 10% to 25% or Imiquimod to lesions, cryosurgery	• Patient should receive frequent Papanicolaou tests. • HPV has an 80% chance of recurrence. • HPV is the most common cause of cervical cancer.
Syphilis Treponema pallidum	• Chancre on genitalia, mouth, lips, or rectum • Fever • Lymphadenopathy • Positive results for Venereal Disease Research Laboratories test, fluorescent treponemal antibodies test, and rapid plasma reagin test	Penicillin	• Syphilis may be characterized as primary, secondary, or tertiary. • All sexual contacts must be treated. • Patient should take medication as prescribed, follow up in 7 to 10 days, and abstain from sexual activity until treatment is completed.
Trichomoniasis Trichomonas vaginalis	• *Males:* urethritis or penile lesions; usually asymptomatic • *Females:* frothy vaginal discharge with erythema and pruritus; may be asymptomatic	Metronidazole	• All sexual contacts must be treated. • Complications in females include recurrent infections and salpingitis. • Patient should take medication as prescribed, follow up in 7 to 10 days, and abstain from sexual activity until treatment is completed. • Patients should avoid alcohol during treatment and for at least 3 days after its completion

return if he develops any adverse reactions so that another drug can be prescribed

◆ Teach the patient about lesion care, including soaking in a tub two to three times a day, keeping lesions clean and dry between baths, wearing cotton underwear, avoiding panty hose and restrictive clothing, and avoiding creams, lotions, and ointments except those specifically prescribed

◆ Refer the patient to other social and health services as needed

◆ Report the STD according to local health department or state health board requirements

❖ Testicular cancer

■ Description

◆ Testicular cancer is the most common type of cancer in men between ages 15 and 35; it's the third leading cause of death in these men but has an overall cure rate of 95% when detected early

◆ Although the cause of testicular cancer is unknown, incidence is higher in men with cryptorchidism; the disease is also associated with scrotal trauma, heredity, infection, hormonal abnormalities, and orchiopexy (surgical repair of undescended testis)

◆ Testicular tumors are histologically classified as seminomas or non-seminomas

❭ Seminomas typically are localized and highly sensitive to radiation therapy; the prognosis is good with early treatment

❭ Nonseminomas are faster growing and more diffuse; they require more aggressive treatment with surgery and chemotherapy

◆ Educating men to perform testicular self-examination facilitates earlier detection and intervention; however, many patients don't seek treatment for 3 to 6 months after detecting a tumor

■ Signs and symptoms

◆ Most patients with testicular cancer report unilateral testicular enlargement, a "dragging" sensation in the lower abdomen, and heaviness in the scrotum; 70% to 90% of patients don't report pain as an early symptom

◆ A patient with a palpable tumor that doesn't transluminate may have testicular cancer

◆ A patient with metastasis to retroperitoneal lymph nodes may report lower back pain, lymphadenopathy, fatigue, weight loss, and anorexia; the next most common site of metastasis is the lungs

◆ The patient also may experience breast enlargement and tenderness

■ Diagnosis and treatment

◆ Diagnosis of suspected testicular cancer is based on the patient's symptoms and history, testicular examination, urine estrogen and testosterone levels, scrotal illumination, and scrotal ultrasonography; radioimmunoassay studies, which measure antigens produced by malignant cells, aid in diagnosis

◆ Excretory urography may be used to evaluate renal function and structure; chest X-ray, CT, and MRI are used to evaluate metastasis

---

Treatments for testicular cancer

Testicular cancer may be treated with radiation therapy, chemotherapy, surgery, or any combination of these.

Radiation therapy

Radiation therapy is primarily used to treat pure semi-nomas after surgery because these tumors are highly sensitive to radiation. It also may be indicated for patients who are poor candidates for surgery or who don't respond to chemotherapy. To preserve fertility, the unaffected testis is shielded to prevent irradiation.

Chemotherapy

When used with surgery, chemotherapy has provided the most effective treatment of nonseminoma tumors. Cisplatin commonly is used to treat testicular cancer in combination with bleomycin, etoposide, vinblastine, ifosfamide, and cyclophosphamide.

Surgery

Unilateral radical orchiectomy is performed through an inguinal incision. It typically is a 1-day surgical procedure performed under local or spinal anesthesia, depending on the patient's health status. It may be the only surgery needed for patients with stage I and II seminomas who also undergo postoperative radiation therapy.

Orchiectomy and *retroperitoneal lymph node dissection* (RPLND) are used to treat stage II and III disease. Because RPLND is major abdominal surgery, it poses all the associated risks and potential complications. Therefore, the patient is monitored in the intensive care unit for the first 24 hours after surgery, and the expected postoperative hospital stay is 7 to 8 days. RPLND typically is performed after the staging orchiectomy and intensive chemotherapy. A unilateral (modified) RPLND is performed, unless regional metastasis is present. After full RPLND, orgasm and libido remain intact, but the patient is sterile.

◆ The histologic diagnosis is made by inguinal orchiectomy; testicular biopsy isn't done because it can promote the spread of tumor cells
◆ Testicular cancer is treated with radiation therapy, chemotherapy, and surgery; one, two, or all three of these treatments may be used, depending on the stage of the disease and the type of tumor (see *Treatments for testicular cancer*)
■ Nursing interventions for a patient in the early stages of testicular cancer
◆ Assess the patient's and family's understanding of the disease, diagnostic tests, and treatments, and intervene accordingly
◆ Encourage the patient to discuss his fears and concerns; clarify misconceptions, and be aware that orchiectomy can change the patient's body image and self-concept; discuss the possibility of joining a sperm bank if sterility is a concern
■ Nursing interventions for a patient undergoing orchiectomy
◆ Monitor the patient for complications of anesthesia and hemorrhage immediately after surgery
◆ Prepare the patient for discharge
❯ Teach the patient and family about wound care at home
❯ Provide verbal and written instructions about pain medications, activity restrictions (including sexual activity), and follow-up care
■ Nursing interventions for a patient undergoing retroperitoneal lymph node dissection

◆ Observe the patient for postoperative complications, such as hemorrhage, fluid and electrolyte imbalances, atelectasis, paralytic ileus, DVT, and wound infection

◆ Monitor hemodynamics and fluid and electrolyte status

◆ Initiate leg and breathing exercises and early ambulation to prevent circulatory, respiratory, and GI complications

◆ Assess the patient's pain and response to analgesia; patient-controlled analgesia is an effective way of administering opioids

◆ Prepare the patient for discharge

▶ Provide verbal and written instructions about pain medications, activity restrictions, and follow-up care

▶ Tell the patient to avoid lifting and straining until after he returns to the practitioner for his 6-week postoperative visit

▶ Inform the patient that sexual activity generally can be resumed in 4 to 6 weeks

■ Nursing interventions for a patient receiving chemotherapy

◆ Be fully knowledgeable about the prescribed chemotherapeutic agents, including their administration protocols, therapeutic and adverse effects, and specific nursing considerations; handle chemotherapeutic agents according to federal safety guidelines

◆ Monitor and treat the patient for complications of chemotherapy (see Nursing implications in oncology care, page 351)

◆ Prepare the patient for discharge

▶ Provide verbal and written instructions about pain medications, wound care, activity restrictions (including sexual activity), and follow-up care

▶ Make sure the patient understands how to manage the adverse effects of chemotherapy

▶ Teach the patient how to perform testicular self-examination; patients who have had testicular cancer are at higher risk for developing another tumor than those who haven't had the disease

▶ Tell the patient about the need for follow-up visits; recurrence is most common in the first year after treatment

■ Nursing interventions for a patient receiving radiation therapy

◆ Observe the patient for complications of treatment; common systemic adverse reactions include nausea, vomiting, headache, skin reactions, fatigue, and malaise

◆ Check for alterations in skin integrity

Review questions

1. Which patient has the highest risk of ovarian cancer?

○ **A.** 30-year-old woman taking an oral contraceptive

○ **B.** 45-year-old woman who has never been pregnant

○ **C.** 40-year-old woman with three children

○ **D.** 36-year-old woman who had her first child at age 22

Correct answer: B The incidence of ovarian cancer increases in women who have never been pregnant, are older than age 40, are infertile, or have menstrual irregularities. Other risk factors include a family history of breast, bowel, or endometrial cancer. The risk of ovarian cancer is reduced in women who have taken oral contraceptives (option A), who have had multiple births (option C), or who had their first child at a young age (option D).

2. A patient with a small, well-defined breast nodule asks the nurse about her treatment options. Which treatments would be considered for this patient?

○ **A.** Lumpectomy and radiation

○ **B.** Partial mastectomy and radiation

○ **C.** Partial mastectomy and chemotherapy

○ **D.** Total mastectomy and chemotherapy

Correct answer: A Treatment for breast cancer depends on the disease stage and type, the patient's age and menopausal status, and the disfiguring effects of the surgery. For this patient, lumpectomy is the most likely option. Lumpectomy involves a small incision with removal of the surrounding tissue and, possibly, the nearby lymph nodes. The patient usually undergoes radiation therapy afterward. With partial mastectomy (options B and C), the tumor is removed along with a wedge of normal tissue, skin, and possibly axillary lymph nodes. With a total (simple) mastectomy (option D), the entire breast is removed.

3. The nurse is assessing a male patient with gonorrhea. Which symptom most likely prompted him to seek medical attention?

○ **A.** Rashes on the palms of the hands and soles of the feet

○ **B.** Cauliflower-like warts on the penis

○ **C.** Painful red papules on the shaft of the penis

○ **D.** Foul-smelling discharge from the penis

Correct answer: D Signs and symptoms of gonorrhea in men include purulent, foul-smelling drainage from the penis and painful urination. Rash on the palms of the hands and soles of the feet (option A) is a sign of the secondary stage of syphilis. Cauliflower-like warts on the penis (option B) are a sign of human papillomavirus. Painful red papules on the shaft of the penis (option C) may be a sign of the first stage of genital herpes.

4. The nurse is speaking to a group of women about early detection of breast cancer. The average age of the women in the group is 47. Following the American Cancer Society guidelines, the nurse should recommend that the women:

○ **A.** perform breast self-examination (BSE) annually.

○ **B.** have a mammogram annually.

○ **C.** have a hormonal receptor assay annually.

○ **D.** have a practitioner conduct a clinical examination every 2 years.

Correct answer: B The American Cancer Society guidelines state "Women older than age 40 should have a mammogram annually and a clinical examination at least annually; all women should perform breast self-examination monthly." Option A is incorrect because women should perform BSE monthly. The hormonal receptor assay (option C) is done on a known breast tumor to determine whether the tumor is estrogen- or progesterone-dependent. Option D is incorrect because women older than age 40 should have an annual clinical examination.

5. The nurse is teaching a male patient to perform monthly testicular self-examinations. What is the appropriate point to make?

○ **A.** Testicular cancer is highly curable.

○ **B.** Testicular cancer is difficult to diagnose.

○ **C.** Testicular cancer is the number one cause of cancer deaths in men.

○ **D.** Testicular cancer is more common in older men.

Correct answer: A Testicular cancer is highly curable, particularly when it's treated in its early stage. Option B is incorrect because self-examination allows early detection and facilitates the early initiation of treatment. Option C is incorrect because the highest mortality rates from cancer among men are in men with lung cancer. Option D is incorrect because testicular cancer is found more commonly in younger men.

Immune system disorders

❖ **Introduction**

■ The immune system is a complex organization of highly specialized cells and tissue that protect the body from various foreign organisms

■ The bone marrow and thymus manufacture the immune cells, which work together with lymphoid tissue to destroy foreign organisms that enter the body; B lymphocytes and T lymphocytes are the primary cells of the immune system

■ Nursing history

   ◆ The nurse asks the patient about his *chief complaint*

   ▶ The patient with an immunologic disorder reports vague signs and symptoms, such as lack of energy, light-headedness, frequent infections or bruising, and slow wound healing

   ◆ The nurse then questions the patient about his *present illness*

   ▶ Ask the patient about his symptom, including when it started, associated symptoms, location, radiation, intensity, duration, frequency, and precipitating and alleviating factors

   ▶ Ask about the use of prescription and over-the-counter drugs, herbal remedies, vitamin and nutritional supplements, and alternative therapies

   ◆ The nurse asks about the *medical history*

   ▶ Question the patient about changes in overall health, allergies, childhood diseases, recurrent infections, and immunizations

   ▶ Ask about unexplained rashes, visual disturbances, fever, and changes in elimination patterns

   ▶ Question the patient about a history of immune disorders

   ▶ Ask the female patient about changes in menstrual patterns

   ◆ The nurse then assesses the *family history*

   ▶ Ask about a family history of immune disorders

   ▶ Also ask about a family history of recurrent infections, allergies, and cancer

   ◆ The nurse obtains a *social history*

   ▶ Ask about work, exercise, diet, use of recreational drugs and alcohol, and hobbies

   ▶ Also ask about stress, support systems, and coping mechanisms

   ▶ Question the patient about exposure to chemicals and pathogens

■ Physical assessment

   ◆ The nurse begins with *inspection*

▶ Inspect the patient's appearance, and note signs of acute and chronic illness, pain, fatigue, and malnutrition

▶ Observe the patient's movements, posture, gait, coordination, balance, range of motion, and strength

▶ Inspect the skin, noting color, rashes, and lesions; evaluate skin integrity

▶ Note hair growth, including texture, distribution, color, and amount

▶ Check the nose for evidence of chronic allergies; observe mucous membranes for ulcers, patches, and plaques; and observe the eyes for redness, infection, and hydration

▶ Inspect the extremities for blanching, cyanosis, pallor, edema, and reddening

▶ Assess level of consciousness and mental status, noting behavior, emotional stability, and cognition

◆ Next, the nurse performs *palpation* and *percussion*

▶ Take the patient's vital signs

▶ Feel the lymph nodes, noting any enlargement or tenderness

▶ Palpate and percuss various organs, noting enlargement, inflammation, masses, or tenderness

▶ Assess musculoskeletal integrity and range of motion, particularly in the hands, wrists, and knees

▶ Palpate the joints to detect nodules, swelling, tenderness, and pain

◆ Then the nurse performs *auscultation*

▶ Listen to the lungs, noting abnormal breath sounds

▶ Auscultate the heart, listening for abnormal sounds, rhythm, and rate

▶ Listen for bowel sounds in all abdominal quadrants

❖ The immune response

■ General information

◆ The primary function of the immune system is to protect the body against pathogenic microorganisms and malignant cells

◆ The immune response is a complex sequence of events triggered by a stimulus (antigen) and culminating in the elimination of the foreign substance; the process requires the differentiation of intrinsic organisms from foreign organisms

▶ Antigens (immunogens) are any substances recognized as foreign that stimulate an immune response; viruses, bacteria, fungi, and parasites are antigens

▶ Antibodies (immunoglobulins) are proteins that are formed in response to exposure to an antigen

◆ The following factors can decrease the immune response: genetics, age extremes, protein-calorie malnutrition, vitamin or mineral deficiency, certain drugs, radiation, and stress

■ Natural immunity

◆ Natural, innate immunity is the body's first line of defense against invading pathogens; this nonspecific mechanism can differentiate intrinsic from foreign organisms but can't identify the specific pathogen

Types of hypersensitivity

The following chart summarizes the four major types of hypersensitivity.

Type and description	Effects	Common causes
Type I (immediate type) Humoral hypersensitivity mediated by immunoglobulin (Ig) E antibodies	• Local reactions, such as allergic rhinitis and urticaria • Systemic, life-threatening (anaphylactic) reactions that can lead to respiratory distress and shock	• Hay fever, drugs, and foods (local reactions) • Penicillin allergy and insect stings (systemic reactions) • Diagnostic agents
Type II (tissue specific) Humoral hypersensitivity (cytotoxic or cytolytic reaction) mediated by IgG or IgM antibodies; cell-specific	• Inflammation, phagocytosis, and cell breakdown through complement system activation	• Blood transfusion reaction • Hemolytic disease of the newborn
Type III (immune complex-mediated) Humoral hypersensitivity (immune complex reaction) mediated by IgG or IgM antibodies; tissue versus cell-specific	• Itching and discomfort at the injection site (early) • Lymphadenopathy, fever, urticaria, and joint pain (late)	• Drugs such as penicillin • Serum sickness, caused by injection of bovine or equine serum antitoxin, renal damage, and vasculitis
Type IV (delayed type; cell mediated) Cell-mediated hypersensitivity (T cell-mediated reaction)	• Delayed response caused by direct or indirect antigen destruction	• Poison ivy • Graft rejection • Tuberculin reaction • Latex allergy

◆ Types of natural immunity include *physical barriers,* such as intact skin and mucous membranes; *chemical barriers,* such as gastric acidity and enzymes in the saliva; and *inflammation,* which is the sequence of vascular and cellular responses to tissue injury and immunologic stimuli (see chapter 6, Disruptions in homeostasis, for details)
■ Acquired immunity
◆ Adaptive, acquired immunity is the body's second line of defense; it's gained through exposure to pathogens, distinguishes intrinsic from foreign organisms, identifies the specific pathogen, and responds to previously encountered pathogens
◆ Four types of acquired immunity exist
▶ *Passive immunity* occurs when antibodies, such as immunoglobulin, of an infectious agent are supplied to the host's body, providing temporary immunity; antibodies may be obtained by injection, or they may be transferred from mother to neonate
▶ *Active immunity* results from direct exposure to an antigen by immunization (such as by tetanus toxoid) or exposure to disease
▶ *Humoral immunity,* primarily mediated by B cells, is the body's ability to respond to antigens by forming specific antibodies; the term *humoral* indicates that immunity is transferable by serum

> ▶ *Cell-mediated immunity* is primarily mediated by T cells and macrophages, which are responsible for antigen destruction and delayed hypersensitivity; unlike humoral immunity, cell-mediated immunity isn't readily transferred to another person by serum

■ Hypersensitivity and allergic reactions
  ◆ Hypersensitivity and allergic reactions are destructive immune responses that occur after reexposure to an antigen; they can produce various symptoms within minutes to several days
  ◆ Hypersensitivity reactions may be humoral or cell mediated (see *Types of hypersensitivity*, page 301)

❖ Acquired immunodeficiency syndrome

■ Description
  ◆ Acquired immunodeficiency syndrome (AIDS) compromises the competency of the immune system
  ◆ To provide statistical data for public health purposes, the Centers for Disease Control and Prevention (CDC) has developed a case definition for AIDS, based on laboratory evidence of human immunodeficiency virus (HIV) infection and indicator diseases (a seropositive HIV test and laboratory confirmation of one of the indicator diseases supports a diagnosis of AIDS)
  ◆ The CDC also has developed a classification method that covers the spectrum of the progression of HIV infection (see *Classification system for HIV infection and expanded AIDS surveillance case definition for adolescents and adults*)
  ◆ AIDS is caused by infection with HIV type 1 (HIV-1) or HIV type 2 (HIV-2); HIV is a retrovirus that selectively infects cells with a CD4+ surface marker, usually T_4 lymphocytes
  ◆ HIV is transmitted primarily through sexual intercourse, during which blood, semen, and vaginal secretions are shared
  ◆ HIV is also transmitted through contaminated blood that enters the body by way of parenteral or percutaneous routes or by way of mucous membranes or open wounds; such transmission can result from sharing or accidental injection with a contaminated needle, transfusion of contaminated blood, or perinatal transfer in the womb, during birth, or through breast milk
  ◆ HIV infection reduces cell-mediated immunity by destroying T_4 lymphocytes
    ▶ This decreases the ratio of helper T cells to suppressor T cells, which normally is 2:1 (CD4+ – CD8+ ratio)
    ▶ It also increases the patient's susceptibility to opportunistic infections and cancers
  ◆ HIV infection also affects humoral immunity by producing more nonspecific antibodies that are ineffective and by altering the function of monocytes and macrophages; these cells may be responsible for transporting the virus to other organs, such as the brain and lungs
■ Signs and symptoms

Classification system for HIV infection and expanded AIDS surveillance case definition for adolescents and adults

Diagnostic categories

As of January 1, 1993, people with acquired immunodeficiency syndrome (AIDS) indicator conditions (clinical category C) and those in categories A3 or B3 were considered to have AIDS.

CD4+ T-cell and clinical categories	Clinical category A: Asymptomatic, acute (primary) HIV or PGL	Clinical category B: Symptomatic not (A) or (C) conditions	Clinical category C: AIDS-indicator conditions
(1) 500/μl	A1	B1	C1
(2) 200 to 499/μl	A2	B2	C2
(3) < 200/μl AIDS indicator T-cell count	A3	B3	C3

Clinical category A
Includes one or more of the following in an adult or adolescent with confirmed human immunodeficiency virus (HIV) infection and without conditions in clinical categories B and C:
- Asymptomatic HIV infection
- Persistent generalized lymphadenopathy
- Acute (primary) HIV infection with accompanying illness or history of acute HIV infection

Clinical category B
Examples of conditions in clinical category B include, but aren't limited to:
- Bacillary angiomatosis
- Candidiasis, oropharyngeal (thrush) or vulvovaginal (persistent, frequent, or poorly responsive to therapy)
- Cervical dysplasia (moderate or severe) or cervical carcinoma in situ
- Constitutional symptoms, such as fever (101.3° F [38.5° C]) or diarrhea exceeding 1 month in duration
- Hairy leukoplakia, oral
- Herpes zoster (shingles), involving at least two distinct episodes or more than one dermatome
- Idiopathic thrombocytopenic purpura
- Listeriosis
- Pelvic inflammatory disease, particularly if complicated by tubo-ovarian abscess
- Peripheral neuropathy

Clinical category C
Examples of conditions in adults and adolescents include:
- Candidiasis of bronchi, trachea, lungs, or esophagus
- Cervical cancer, invasive
- Coccidioidomyocosis, disseminated or extrapulmonary
- Cryptococcosis, extrapulmonary
- Cryptosporidiosis, chronic intestinal (exceeding 1 month's duration)
- Cytomegalovirus disease (other than liver, spleen, or lymph nodes)
- Cytomegalovirus retinitis (with loss of vision)
- Encephalopathy, HIV-related
- Herpes simplex: chronic ulcers (exceeding 1 month's duration); or bronchitis, pneumonitis, or esophagitis
- Histoplasmosis, disseminated or extrapulmonary
- Isosporiasis, chronic intestinal (exceeding 1 month's duration)
- Kaposi's sarcoma
- Lymphoma, Burkitt's (or equivalent term); immunoblastic (or equivalent term); primary, of brain
- *Mycobacterium avium complex* or *M. kansasii*, disseminated or extrapulmonary
- *M. tuberculosis,* any site (pulmonary or extrapulmonary)
- *Mycobacterium,* other species or unidentified species, disseminated or extrapulmonary
- *Pneumocystis carinii* pneumonia
- Pneumonia, recurrent
- Progressive multifocal leukoencephalopathy
- *Salmonella* septicemia, recurrent
- Toxoplasmosis of brain
- Wasting syndrome due to HIV

Adapted from Centers for Disease Control and Prevention, U.S. Department of Health and Human Services, 1993 revised classification system for HIV infection and expanded AIDS surveillance case definition for AIDS among adolescents and adults. MMWR CDC Recommendations and Reports 41 (RR-17), 1-19.

◆ HIV infection may be asymptomatic or cause a mononucleosis-like syndrome associated with seroconversion; symptoms include headache, malaise, and swollen lymph nodes and last about 2 weeks (see *AIDS indicator diseases*)

▶ Persistent generalized lymphadenopathy at two or more extrainguinal sites may persist for more than 3 months in the absence of concurrent illness

▶ The infected patient also may display signs of opportunistic infections and other diseases

◆ HIV can produce central nervous system effects

▶ AIDS dementia complex, also called HIV encephalopathy, causes cognitive changes, such as confusion, impaired concentration, and memory loss; motor disturbances, such as ataxia, leg weakness, and diminished fine motor movements; and behavioral changes, such as apathy, depression, reduced spontaneity, social withdrawal, anxiety, agitation, and personality changes

▶ Atypical aseptic meningitis causes headache, fever, and signs of meningeal infection

▶ Vacuolar myelopathy (spinal cord degeneration) may produce leg weakness, incontinence, and ataxia

◆ HIV wasting syndrome may occur as a complication of advanced HIV infection; it causes involuntary weight loss of more than 10% of body weight and diarrhea, recurrent or sustained fevers, and chronic weakness for more than 1 month in the absence of a causative illness, such as cancer or tuberculosis

■ Diagnosis and treatment

◆ The enzyme-linked immunosorbent assay (ELISA) detects the presence of HIV-1 antibodies; if a patient's blood has a positive reaction on two ELISA tests, the Western blot test is used to confirm the results

◆ The Western blot test detects the presence of HIV antibodies and determines their type; two positive ELISA tests and a positive Western blot test indicate infection and a high probability of developing AIDS over months to years

◆ CD_4 + T-cell count is less than 200 cells/μl

◆ Polymerase chain reaction may detect viral genetic material in patients in whom antibodies haven't yet developed

◆ Other laboratory tests may include hematocrit (below 30%, indicating anemia), white blood cell count (below 2,500/cm^3, indicating leukopenia), the ratio of helper T cells to suppressor T cells (decreased to 1:2), and platelet count (below 100,000/mm^3)

◆ Because many opportunistic infections are reactivations of previous infections, the patient may also be tested for syphilis, hepatitis B, tuberculosis, and toxoplasmosis

◆ Drug therapy for HIV infection includes four types of antiretrovirals

▶ Protease inhibitors, such as ritonavir, indinavir, nelfinavir, amprenavir, and saquinavir

▶ Nucleoside reverse transcriptase inhibitors, such as zidovudine, didanosine, zalcitabine, lamivudine, abacavir, and stavudine

AIDS indicator diseases

The following chart summarizes the clinical signs and symptoms and treatments of major indicator diseases of acquired immunodeficiency syndrome (AIDS).

Disease	Clinical signs and symptoms	Treatments
Viral infections *Cytomegalovirus retinitis*	• Floaters • Blurred vision • Decreased vision that may lead to blindness	• I.V. ganciclovir (DHPG, Cytogene) • I.V. foscarnet (Foscavir)
Herpes simplex virus (HSV) infection	• Vesicular lesions around mucosal orifices of the face and genitals • Debilitation	• I.V. acyclovir (Zovirax) for HSV encephalitis • Oral acyclovir to suppress HSV • Topical acyclovir for a small outbreak of local lesions
Protozoal infections Pneumocystis carinii *pneumonia*	• Fever • Nonproductive cough • Progressive shortness of breath	• I.V. co-trimoxazole (TMP-SMX, Bactrim) for treatment and prevention • I.V. or inhalation pentamidine for patients who can't tolerate or don't respond to TMP-SMX
Toxoplasmosis	• Focal neurologic defects, such as seizures and hemiparesis • Encephalitis manifestations, such as headache, confusion, and lethargy	• Oral pyrimethamine (Daraprim) and sulfadiazine
Cryptosporidiosis	• Protracted watery stoool • Severe vomiting • Fluid and electrolyte imbalances	• Oral antidiarrheals • Fluid replacement • Nutritional support
Bacterial infections Myobacterium avium-intracellulare *infection*	• Fever • Weight loss • Weakness • Abdominal pain • Frequent watery stools • Anorexia	• Oral clarithromycin
M. tuberulosis *infection*	• Fever • Fatigue • Weight loss • Productive, purulent cough	• Combination oral therapy with isoniazid and rifampin plus either pyrazinamide or ethambutol

(continued)

AIDS indicator diseases *(continued)*

Disease	Clinical signs and symptoms	Treatments
Fungal infections *Candidiasis*	• Painless mouth lesions • Pain with swallowing • Retrosternal chest pain • Nausea and vomiting	• Nystatin suspension for oral candidiasis • Topical antifungal creams, such as clotrimazole (Mycelex) or ketoconazole (Nizoral), for cutaneous candidiasis • Oral ketoconazole for esophageal candidiasis • Clotrimazole or miconazole creams, vaginal tablets, or suppositories for vaginal candidiasis • Ketoconazole, itraconazole, or fluconazole for systemic candidiasis
Cryptococcosis	• High fever, headache, and malaise (early) • Photophobia, stiff neck, nausea, vomiting, and mental changes (late)	• Systemic therapy with amphotericin B or fluconazole
Neoplasms *Kaposi's sarcoma*	• Pigmented, raised, nonblanching skin lesions • Pain when lesion impinges on organs or nerves	• Intralesional and systemic chemotherapy • Cryotherapy • Radiation therapy • Biological response modifiers and antiretrovirals
Non-Hodgkin's lymphoma	• Painless, enlarged lymph node, usually in the neck (early) • Fever, night sweats, and weight loss (late)	• Chemotherapy

❱ Nonnucleoside reverse transcriptase inhibitors, such as nevirapine, efavirenz, and delavirdine

❱ Fusion inhibitors, such as enfuviritide, which interfere with the virus' ability to fuse with the cellular membrane, thereby blocking entry into the host cell

❱ These antiretrovirals are used in various combinations to inhibit HIV viral replication; this is called highly active antiretroviral therapy

❱ Treatment protocols combine two or more drugs in an effort to gain the maximum benefit with the fewest adverse reactions

❱ Combination therapy helps to inhibit the production of resistant, mutant strains

❱ Combination agents that combine two or three drugs in one dose are available and help improve compliance

◆ Different treatments are required for AIDS indicator diseases (see *AIDS indicator diseases)*

■ Nursing interventions

◆ Provide respiratory care

◆ Encourage activity as tolerated to prevent fatigue and dyspnea

▶ Administer medications, as prescribed, to relieve symptoms and prevent or treat infection

▶ Monitor vital signs and laboratory values (arterial blood gas levels, oxygen saturation by pulse oximetry, sputum cultures, CD4$^+$ count, and complete blood count [CBC]) to determine the effectiveness of treatment

▶ Provide pulmonary hygiene (including coughing and deep breathing every 2 hours), splinting while coughing, and suctioning to prevent atelectasis and clear airway secretions; maintain adequate hydration to thin mucus secretions

▶ Provide throat lozenges and warm saline gargles to soothe an irritated throat

▶ Administer antitussives and expectorants, as prescribed, for cough

▶ If appropriate, help the patient to decrease or stop smoking

◆ Perform GI care

▶ Monitor fluid intake and output, weight, urine specific gravity, serum electrolyte levels, and skin turgor to evaluate hydration

▶ Obtain stool cultures to identify enteric pathogens

▶ Encourage the patient to drink at least 3 qt (3 L) of fluid daily; administer I.V. therapy, as prescribed, to maintain hydration

▶ Administer antibiotics and antivirals to treat infectious diarrhea and antidiarrheals to lessen the severity of diarrhea

◆ Promote good nutrition

▶ Offer small, frequent meals to reduce fatigue

▶ Engage the patient in menu planning, and invite the patient's family and friends to meals to encourage eating

• Allowing the patient to include personal food preferences gives him some control over the diet

• Eating with others may improve appetite

▶ Encourage the patient to eat meals sitting up and out of bed; sitting up aids digestion and decreases the risk of aspiration

▶ Provide a low-residue, high-protein, high-potassium, high-calorie, lactose-free diet to minimize diarrhea and maximize caloric, electrolyte, and fluid intake

▶ Use oral dietary supplements, such as Vivonex T.E.N.; initiate and monitor tube feedings or total parenteral nutrition as prescribed

▶ Avoid serving rare meats and raw vegetables, which may harbor living microbes

▶ Monitor daily weight and laboratory values—including serum protein, albumin, blood urea nitrogen, hemoglobin, and serum electrolyte levels and hematocrit—to evaluate nutrition

▶ Provide mouth care, using viscous oral lidocaine (Xylocaine) before meals to relieve mouth, pharyngeal, and esophageal pain; use saline rinses after meals to prevent exacerbation of infection

◆ Perform skin care

▶ Use pressure-relieving devices (convoluted foam mattress, pressure mattress, or pressure pads), and turn the patient every 2 hours to prevent skin deterioration caused by pressure and inadequate circulation
▶ Apply A + D Original Ointment or other skin barrier to the perianal area to prevent further maceration of the anal mucosa
▶ Maintain wound and skin precautions to prevent further spread of infection

◆ Prevent and control infection
▶ Restrict the patient's contact with visitors, staff members, and other patients who have infections, such as colds or flu
▶ Make sure that staff members and visitors adhere to hand-washing procedures before approaching the patient
▶ Use reverse isolation if the patient is immunocompromised
▶ Consider moving the patient to a private room and leaving equipment—such as a thermometer, blood pressure cuff, and stethoscope—in the room to minimize pathogen exposure
▶ Follow standard precautions to reduce pathogen transfer
▶ Inspect the skin, I.V. sites, vascular access devices, and invasive cardiovascular monitoring lines; loss of skin integrity is a potential source of infection
▶ Monitor antimicrobial therapies; antibiotics can increase the likelihood of superinfection and the development of resistant organisms
▶ Encourage and maintain adequate nutritional intake, which promotes healing and prevents infection

◆ Provide neuropsychiatric care
▶ Encourage the patient to discuss emotional issues; mood swings may be related to an inability to cope with a terminal illness
▶ Identify resources for patient and family support
▶ Use reminder devices, such as pictures and appointment books, to help orient the patient
▶ Arrange for continuity of caregivers, and avoid frequent room changes to prevent patient confusion
▶ Consult occupational and physical therapists; the patient may need special devices, such as a cane or walker, and physical therapy to maintain or prevent further loss of function

◆ Promote health maintenance
▶ Teach the patient, family, significant others, and caregivers about the diagnosis, treatments, modes of transmission, and symptoms to report
▶ Explain medications to the patient, including dose, frequency, and adverse effects; reinforce the importance of compliance to help suppress the virus and to prevent the development of drug-resistant strains
▶ Discuss the importance of avoiding high-risk behaviors and reducing the risk of transmission to others
▶ Make appropriate referrals—for example, for home care, pain management, legal services, support groups, financial support, and hospice care

❖ Latex allergy
- ■ Description
  - ◆ Latex allergy is a type 1, immunoglobulin E (IgE)-mediated hypersensitivity reaction or type IV cell-mediated response to products that contain natural rubber latex
  - ◆ It can cause reactions that range from local dermatitis to life-threatening anaphylaxis
- ■ Signs and symptoms
  - ◆ Hypotension due to vasodilation and increased vascular permeability, tachycardia, urticaria and pruritis may occur
  - ◆ Other signs or symptoms include difficulty breathing and bronchospasm, wheezing, stridor, and angioedema
- ■ Diagnosis and treatment
  - ◆ Diagnosis is based primarily on history and physical assessment of the patient
  - ◆ Radioallergosorbent test shows IgE antibodies specific to latex
  - ◆ Patch test causes hives along with itching and redness
  - ◆ The best treatment is prevention by avoiding exposure to airborne particles and use of latex-free products
  - ◆ Drug therapy may include corticosteroids, antihistamines, and histamine-2-receptor antagonists before and after latex exposure
  - ◆ For acute emergency, perform cardiopulmonary resuscitation, administer epinephrine, assist with tracheostomy, oxygen therapy, volume expanders, I.V. vasopressors, and other drugs to reverse broncospasm
- ■ Nursing interventions
  - ◆ Make sure that products that aren't available free of latex are wrapped in cloth before they come in contact with the skin of a hypersensitive patient
  - ◆ Use powder-free, vinyl gloves
  - ◆ When adding medication to an I.V. bag, inject the drug through the spike port, and not the rubber latex port
  - ◆ Urge the patient to wear a tag identifying his latex allergy
  - ◆ Instruct the patient to avoid tomatoes, bananas, avocados, chestnuts, and kiwifruits because they contain proteins similar to those present in rubber
  - ◆ Teach the patient to be aware of all latex-containing products and to use vinyl or silicone products instead

❖ Rheumatoid arthritis
- ■ Description
  - ◆ Rheumatoid arthritis is a chronic, systemic inflammatory disease that affects the small joints of the hands and wrists and the surrounding muscles, tendons, ligaments, and blood vessels; it may progress to other joints and body tissues, including the heart, lungs, kidneys, and skin
  - ◆ This autoimmune disease has no known cause; it affects three times as many women as men between ages 30 and 50 and becomes more evident during the winter
- ■ Signs and symptoms

◆ Edema and stiffness may affect one or more joints, symmetrically and bilaterally, especially on arising and in the morning

◆ Other signs and symptoms may include malaise; fever; anemia; rheumatoid nodules near joints; dull, aching joint pain; and joint deformity

◆ Rheumatoid arthritis may be associated with pericarditis and pneumonitis

■ Diagnosis and treatment

◆ Diagnosis is based on patient history, physical examination, and serologic blood tests, including rheumatoid factor, CBC, erythrocyte sedimentation rate (ESR), serum complement, and C-reactive protein; 75% to 80% of patients with a positive rheumatoid factors test have the disease

◆ Other diagnostic tests may include immunologic studies, synovial biopsy, X-rays, and magnetic resonance imaging

◆ Treatment aims to reduce inflammation and maintain or increase joint mobility

◆ Affected joints are rested, and splints may be used to help maintain functional positions

◆ Physical therapy exercises are recommended to maintain joint motion

◆ A paraffin "glove" may be applied to the affected joints; the patient dips his hands into melted paraffin to form a ⅛"-thick glove, which draws blood to the areas to resolve the inflammation

◆ Use of ice or cold compresses alternating with the paraffin glove reduces edema and inflammation

◆ Various anti-inflammatories are prescribed: salicylates (primarily aspirin), low-dose steroids (primarily prednisone), and nonsteroidal anti-inflammatory drugs (NSAIDs), including ibuprofen, naproxen, flurbiprofen, indomethacin, sulindac, tolmetin, piroxicam, diclofenac; misoprostol may be given to prevent NSAID-induced gastric ulcers

◆ Gold compounds also may be prescribed to reduce inflammation; opioid analgesics may be used to relieve pain; antimalarials (primarily chloroquine and hydroxychloroquine), immunosuppressants (such as azathioprine), and cytotoxic agents (such as methotrexate) may be used to decrease synovial inflammation; and sulfasalazine may be used to reduce inflammation in patients who have responded inadequately to salicylates or NSAIDS

◆ Surgical interventions include joint repair or prosthetic replacement and synovectomy (removal of the synovium)

◆ Lymphapheresis or plasmapheresis may be used for some patients

■ Nursing interventions

◆ Explain the treatment regimen and the involvement of each member of the health care team

◆ Administer drugs as prescribed, and monitor for therapeutic and adverse reactions; drug therapy may need to be changed if adverse reactions are intolerable, or therapeutic effects don't occur

◆ Monitor the patient for relief of pain, stiffness, and soreness; patients have periods of remission and "flare" when symptoms increase

◆ Help the patient with self-care, including range-of-motion exercises, splint application, and ambulatory aid use

◆ Provide modified utensils and equipment suggested by the occupational therapist to help conserve small-joint and muscle function

◆ Provide rest periods in the morning and evening, with the patient lying supine in bed to maintain strength while preventing flexion contractures; teach him not to overexert himself

◆ Provide a quiet environment for nighttime sleep; patients with acute rheumatoid arthritis require 8 to 10 hours of sleep

◆ Discuss home maintenance activities recommended by the occupational therapist to ensure that the patient understands needed changes

◆ Prepare the patient for surgery if indicated

◆ Provide postoperative care appropriate for the surgery

◆ Encourage compliance with treatments to achieve optimal results

◆ Teach the patient about medications and adverse effects, activity prescription, rest periods, and relaxation techniques

◆ Encourage the patient to verbalize concerns about body image and changes in quality of life

❖ Systemic lupus erythematosus
■ Description
◆ Systemic lupus erythematosus (SLE) is a chronic, systemic autoimmune disease that causes skin, heart, lung, and kidney inflammation

◆ It varies in severity from mild to rapidly progressing with multiple organ involvement

◆ Although its cause is unknown, SLE affects nine times as many women as men, primarily between ages 15 and 45; it's more common in Blacks and Asians than in Whites

◆ Discoid lupus is a less-severe form of SLE that chiefly affects the skin, producing raised, red, scaly lesions on the face, shoulders, and upper back as well as hair loss

■ Signs and symptoms
◆ Primary features include arthritis with synovitis, a characteristic butterfly rash over the nose and cheeks (develops in 50% of patients), and photosensitivity

◆ Constitutional signs and symptoms of SLE include fever, malaise, weight loss, and extreme fatigue

◆ Other effects may include diffuse and patchy hair loss, seizures, psychosis, pleuritis, endocarditis, myocarditis, Raynaud's phenomenon, anemia, abdominal pain, menstrual irregularities, and lymph node enlargement throughout the body

■ Diagnosis and treatment
◆ Diagnosis may be based on patient history; physical examination; serologic studies, such as CBC, ESR, antinuclear antibody tests, and lupus erythematosus cell test; electrocardiography; chest X-ray; and kidney function studies

◆ Treatment typically calls for NSAIDs and corticosteroids to decrease inflammation

◆ Other drugs — such as immunosuppressants, cardiotonics, and anti-malarials — are prescribed based on the severity of the disease

■ Nursing interventions

◆ Monitor vital signs to evaluate the extent of inflammation

◆ Observe the patient for rash to help differentiate SLE from discoid lupus

◆ Monitor the patient for reports of arthritis, joint or chest pain, respiratory difficulties, and other symptoms; SLE symptoms vary among patients

◆ Monitor the patient for seizures, headaches, and vision disturbances; neurologic problems may accompany the disease

◆ Monitor the patient for numbness and tingling of the hands and feet; peripheral neuropathy may occur

◆ Monitor the degree of fatigue, color of skin and conjunctivae, and color of stools; anemia is common in patients with SLE

◆ Test urine and stool for occult bleeding, a possible adverse effect of prescribed medications

◆ Provide for rest periods to avoid fatigue; promote independence in activities of daily living to improve self-esteem

◆ Encourage the patient to express feelings about changes in body image and the chronic nature of the disease

◆ Teach the patient about family planning, genetic counseling, medications, his treatment plan, avoidance of sun exposure, and wearing protective clothing and sunscreen when outdoors.

Review questions

1. The nurse is preparing a patient with SLE for discharge. Which instructions should the nurse include in the teaching plan?

○ **A.** Exposure to sunlight will help control skin rashes.

○ **B.** No activity limitations are necessary between flare-ups.

○ **C.** Monitor body temperature.

○ **D.** Corticosteroids may be stopped when symptoms are relieved.

Correct answer: C The patient should monitor his body temperature because fever can signal an exacerbation and should be reported to the practitioner. Option A is incorrect because sunlight and other sources of ultraviolet light may exacerbate the disease. Option B is incorrect because fatigue can cause a flare-up of SLE, and patients should be encouraged to pace activities and plan for rest periods. Corticosteroids, option D, must be gradually tapered because they can suppress the function of the adrenal gland. Abruptly stopping corticosteroids can cause adrenal insufficiency, a potentially life-threatening situation.

2. A patient with rheumatoid arthritis has a history of long-term NSAID use and, consequently, has developed peptic ulcer disease. To treat this condition, the nurse should expect to administer:

○ **A.** cyanocobalamin (vitamin B$_{12}$).

○ **B.** ticlopidine (Ticlid).

○ **C.** prednisone (Deltasone).

○ **D.** misoprostol (Cytotec).

Correct answer: D   NSAIDs decrease prostaglandin synthesis. Misoprostol (Cytotec), a synthetic analog of prostaglandin, is used to treat and prevent NSAID-induced gastric ulcers. Cyanocobalamin, option A, is used to treat vitamin B$_{12}$ deficiency. Ticlopidine, option B, is an antiplatelet drug used to reduce the risk of stroke. Prednisone, option C, is a glucocorticosteroid used to treat several inflammatory disorders and may promote gastric ulcer development.

3. The nurse is providing care for a patient with AIDS and *Pneumocystis carinii* pneumonia. The patient is receiving aerosolized pentamidine isethionate (Nebu-Pent). What's the best evidence that the therapy is working?

○ **A.** A sudden gain in lost body weight

○ **B.** Whitening of lung fields on the chest X-ray

○ **C.** Improved patient vitality and activity tolerance

○ **D.** A febrile body temperature and development of leukocytosis

Correct answer: C   *P. carinii* pneumonia is a protozoal infection of the lungs. Pentamidine isethionate is one drug used to treat this infection. Because a common manifestation of the infection is activity intolerance and loss of vitality, improvements in these areas suggest success of the therapy. Sudden weight gain (option A), whitening of the lung fields on chest X-ray (option B), and development of leukocytosis (option D) aren't evidence of therapeutic success.

4. A patient with SLE who receives immunosuppressants develops a fever. The nurse should:

○ **A.** administer prescribed antipyretics.

○ **B.** place the patient in isolation.

○ **C.** apply cooling measures immediately.

○ **D.** help identify the cause.

Correct answer: D Immunosuppressants impair the patient's immuno-competence and predispose him to infection. Fever is a sign of infection; therefore, it's important to discover the cause of the fever as soon as possible. Antipyretics (option A) should be withheld until cultures have been obtained. Isolation (option B) isn't indicated unless the absolute neutrophil count is less than 1,000/µl. Cooling measures (option C) may be indicated, but they don't have priority over organism identification.

5. Which finding distinguishes rheumatoid arthritis from osteoarthritis and gouty arthritis?

○ **A.** Crepitus with range of motion

○ **B.** Symmetry of joint involvement

○ **C.** Elevated serum uric acid levels

○ **D.** Dominance in weight-bearing joints

Correct answer: B Rheumatoid arthritis is bilateral and symmetrical; by contrast, osteoarthritis and gouty arthritis are unilateral. Crepitus (option A) is usually associated with osteoarthritis. Elevated serum uric acid levels (option C) are common in patients with gouty arthritis; weight-bearing joint dominance (option D), in those with osteoarthritis.

Eye, ear, and nose disorders

❖ Introduction

■ Disorders of the eye, ear, and nose can be particularly disruptive to activities of daily living

■ Full visual function requires normal brain function, an intact retina, a clear lens, and normal intraocular pressure

■ Common vision disorders result from alterations in acuity, trauma, and high intraocular pressure; patients with impaired vision are frightened and anxious and require special nursing care

■ Hearing loss is a common disability that affects millions of people and causes significant alterations in daily activities; sclerotic disorders and vestibular dysfunction can be especially upsetting

■ Although the nose is the primary organ of smell, nasal disorders can affect taste and the smooth passage of air during respirations

■ Nursing history

◆ The nurse asks the patient about his *chief complaint*

▶ A patient with an eye disorder usually reports having diplopia, visual floaters, iridescent vision, vision loss, or eye pain

▶ The patient may also report decreased visual acuity or clarity, defects in color vision, and difficulty seeing at night

▶ A patient with an ear disorder may experience hearing loss, tinnitus, pain, discharge, or dizziness

▶ A patient with a nose disorder may experience nasal stuffiness, nasal discharge, or epistaxis

◆ The nurse then questions the patient about his *present illness*

▶ Ask the patient about his symptom, including when it started, associated symptoms, location, radiation, intensity, duration, frequency, and precipitating and alleviating factors

▶ Ask about the use of glasses or contact lenses

▶ Ask about the use of prescription and over-the-counter drugs, herbal remedies, and vitamin and nutritional supplements

◆ The nurse asks about the *medical history*

▶ Question the patient about a history of allergies, hypertension, diabetes, cerebrovascular accident, multiple sclerosis, syphilis, or human immunodeficiency virus

▶ Ask about corrective eye surgery

▶ Ask the patient about previous ear problems or injuries, frequent colds, hay fever, headaches, nose or head trauma, and sinus trouble

◆ The nurse then assesses the *family history*

▶ Ask about a family history of eye disorders, such as cataracts, glaucoma, or blindness

▶ Question the patient about a family history of diabetes and hypertension

▶ Question the patient about a family history of eye, ear, and nose problems

◆ The nurse obtains a *social history*

▶ Ask about work, exercise, diet, use of recreational drugs and alcohol, and hobbies

▶ Also ask about stress, support systems, and coping mechanisms

▶ Question the patient about exposure to chemicals, flying debris, noise, fumes, or infectious agents; ask about the use of protective eyewear

▶ Ask the visually impaired patient how well he can manage activities of daily living

■ Physical assessment

◆ Nurse begins with *inspection*

▶ Observe the patient's eye movements and ability to focus

▶ Note the appearance of the eyelids, eyeballs, and lacrimal apparatus

▶ Examine the conjunctiva, sclera, iris, anterior chamber, and cornea

▶ Check both pupils for equality of size and shape, pupillary reaction to light, and accommodation

▶ Test visual acuity using a Snellen chart and near-vision chart

▶ Test extraocular muscles by assessing the corneal light reflex and cardinal positions of gaze

▶ Examine intraocular structures using an ophthalmoscope

▶ Observe the ears for position and symmetry; inspect the auricles for lesions, nodules, or redness; check the ear canal for hair, foreign bodies, and cerumen

▶ Examine the auditory canal, tympanic membrane, and malleus with an otoscope

▶ Assess hearing using Weber's and Rinne's tests and pure tone audiometry

▶ Observe the nose for position, symmetry, swelling, deformity, and color; note any nasal discharge or flaring

▶ Inspect the nasal cavity for septal deviation or perforation; examine the vestibule and turbinates for redness, softness, and discharge

▶ Assess the patient's sense of smell

▶ Examine the nostrils using a nasal speculum

• Note color, patency, and the presence of exudate

◆ Next, the nurse uses *palpation*

▶ Gently palpate the eyelids, noting any swelling or complaints of tenderness; eyeballs should feel equally firm, but not hard or rigid

▶ Palpate the lacrimal sac while observing the punctum for excessive tearing or drainage

▶ Palpate the mastoid area and ear for tenderness, redness, or warmth

▶ Palpate the nose for pain, tenderness, swelling, and deformity

▶ Palpate the sinuses for tenderness

Types of cataracts	

There are several forms of cataracts. They occur at various points in the life cycle, however the treatment for each is the same.

Type of cataract	Description
Complicated	Develop as secondary effects in patients with uvetitis, glaucoma, retinitis pigmentosa, or retinal detachment or with systemic disease, such as diabetes, hypoparathyroidism, or atopic dermatitis; also develop after exposure to ionizing radiation or infrared rays
Congenital	Develop in utero at the anterior or posterior ocular pole; associated with heredity or maternal rubella infection in the first trimester
Senile	Occur after age 50 as part of aging; the nuclear portion of the lens becomes increasingly dense, transparency decreases, and light rays strike the opaque lens and scatter
Toxic	Result from drug or chemical toxicity with dinitrophenol, ergot, naphthalene, or phenothiazines
Traumatic	Can occur at any age and are caused by mechanical trauma or exposure to chemicals, radiation, or toxic substances; the capsule ruptures, swelling occurs, and opacity increases; usually unilateral

❖ Cataracts
- ■ Description
  - ◆ Cataracts, which come in several forms, cause a loss of transparency of the lens of the eye or its capsule (See *Types of cataracts*)
  - ◆ It is a common cause of gradual vision loss that usually affects both eyes
- ■ Signs and symptoms
  - ◆ Gradual painless blurring eventually leads to poor reading vision, reduced vision at night and in bright sunlight, and vision loss
  - ◆ Other effects may include halos around lights, milky pupils, and unpleasant glares
- ■ Diagnosis and treatment
  - ◆ Indirect ophthalmoscopy or slit-lamp examination confirms the diagnosis
  - ◆ Cataracts are treated surgically by extracapsular extraction, which removes the anterior capsule and its contents; intracapsular extraction, which removes the entire lens in the capsule; or phacoemulsification, which uses ultrasonic vibration to fragment the lens
    - ◆ Corrective lenses may be prescribed to improve vision
      - ▶ A plastic intraocular lens implant may be inserted in the eye as part of the surgical procedure
      - ▶ Cataract glasses (glasses with magnifying lenses) or contact lenses may be prescribed 6 to 8 weeks after surgery
- ■ Preoperative nursing interventions
  - ◆ Explain the importance of compliance in a preadmission interview

◆ Make sure that someone can drive the patient to and from the day surgery center

◆ Tell the patient to tilt his head backward when shampooing, to prevent jarring the eye and increasing intraocular pressure

◆ Administer a preoperative laxative to prevent straining during defecation, which increases intraocular pressure

◆ Explain preoperative and postoperative care to decrease the patient's anxiety

◆ Answer questions and encourage the patient to discuss concerns

■ Postoperative nursing interventions

◆ Review postoperative instructions to improve compliance and prevent complications; the patient may have difficulty reading instructions because of impaired vision

◆ Tell the patient not to bend, strain, lift, cough, sneeze, or rub the eye postoperatively; these actions can increase intraocular pressure, which can lead to complications, such as bleeding, vitreous herniation, vision loss, pain, and wound dehiscence; rubbing also increases the chance of infection

◆ Tell the patient not to make quick movements or read, which could irritate the patched eye or dislodge an implanted lens

◆ Teach the patient or family member how to administer eye medications properly

◆ Teach the patient how to clean the eye to prevent infection

◆ Have the patient wear an eye shield and patch to protect the eye from injury; tell him to keep the eye patch dry and to wear an eye shield while sleeping

◆ Tell the patient to call the practitioner if any of these signs or symptoms occur: eye pain that isn't relieved with analgesics, yellow or green discharge, temperature above 100°F (37.8°C), blurred vision, nausea and vomiting, and seeing halos around lights

◆ Explain postoperative activity restrictions

▶ The patient may walk, climb stairs, watch television, and perform daily activities but should avoid engaging in strenuous physical activity and lifting more than 10 lb (4.5 kg)

▶ The patient may bathe or shower but should avoid getting water on the eye patch by tilting his head back when shampooing

▶ The patient should avoid bending from the waist and hanging the head forward; a long-handled grabber may be used to pick up objects

◆ Make sure the patient is cared for by a family member or friend after surgery

◆ Advise the patient to refrain from sexual activity until he receives his practitioner's approval

❖ Deviated nasal septum

■ Description

◆ The nasal septum, which bisects the nasal cavity, is made up of cartilage and bone; deviations are common

◆ Although septal deviation typically is asymptomatic, it can cause nasal obstruction and increase the risk of sinusitis and epistaxis

◆ Deviated nasal septum may be congenital or caused by trauma

■ Signs and symptoms

◆ Signs and symptoms of deviated septum include drying, crusting, nasal discharge and other mucosal changes as well as bleeding that can block the sinus opening

◆ The patient may report shortness of breath and difficulty breathing through the nose; he may also report sinusitis and headache

◆ Upper respiratory tract infection, a blow to the nose, or nasal trauma can exacerbate symptoms

■ Diagnosis and treatment

◆ Diagnosis is based on visual inspection of the nasal mucosa with a bright light and nasal speculum

◆ Short-term treatment consists of decongestants, antihistamines, and nasal saline douches to open the nasal airway and analgesics to relieve headache

◆ Long-term treatment may require septoplasty or submucous resection of the septum; in these procedures, the septum is surgically straightened and then stabilized with sutures and packing (consisting of petroleum jelly, iodoform, and soft gauze) for 24 to 48 hours

◆ Indications for surgery include nasal hemorrhage and an inability to pack the nose adequately because of deformity, recurrent sinusitis resulting from blocked sinus openings, and such signs and symptoms as snoring, breathing through the mouth, dry mouth, and shortness of breath

◆ Surgery is performed under local or general anesthesia and may require overnight hospitalization; its complications include septal hematoma, infection, hemorrhage, septal perforation, anosmia, and cosmetic deformity

■ Preoperative nursing interventions

◆ Determine the severity of the nasal airway obstruction; a patient with a blocked nasal airway needs humidification, oral hygiene, and other comfort measures

◆ Teach the patient about postoperative care to reduce anxiety and promote compliance

■ Postoperative nursing interventions

◆ Keep the patient's head elevated 30 degrees to promote drainage, reduce edema, and maintain a patent airway

◆ Check his vital signs and airway frequently to ensure that the packing hasn't slipped posteriorly, which could block the oral airway; take rectal temperatures while the packing is in place because the patient's only airway is his oral airway

◆ Watch for nasal bleeding and frequent swallowing; inspect the pharynx with a penlight if bleeding is suspected

◆ Encourage the patient to expectorate oral secretions, and measure and record the amount

◆ Change the 2″ × 3″ gauze dressing or drip pad as needed, and record the frequency and amount of drainage

◆ Urge the patient to avoid swallowing blood, which can lead to nausea and vomiting

◆ Provide comfort measures, and administer analgesics, as needed, to decrease pain and promote participation in care

◆ Use a face tent to provide humidified air, and frequently perform oral hygiene measures; because air breathed in through the mouth isn't humidified like air breathed in through the nose, the oral mucous membranes can become dry

◆ Inform the patient of limitations and safety measures, such as not blowing his nose, to prevent injury to the surgical site; if sneezing is necessary, the patient should open the mouth to release the pressure of the sneeze

◆ Tell the patient to notify the practitioner if signs or symptoms of infection, hemorrhage, or hematoma occur, including bleeding, pain, swelling, redness, fever, or foul-smelling drainage

❖ Glaucoma

■ Description

◆ This group of disorders is characterized by high intraocular pressure (IOP) and optic nerve damage that affects peripheral vision

◆ There are two main forms of glaucoma:

▶ *Open-angle* (also known as *chronic, simple,* or *wide angle*) glaucoma, which begins insidiously and progresses slowly

▶ *Angle-closure* (also known as *acute* or *narrow angle*) glaucoma, which occurs suddenly and can cause permanent vision loss in 48 to 72 hours

■ Signs and symptoms

◆ Open-angle glaucoma—possibly no symptoms, dull, morning headache; mild aching in the eyes, loss of peripheral vision; halos around lights; and reduced visual acuity (especially at night) that's uncorrected by glasses

◆ Angle-closure—rapid onset with pain and pressure over the eye, blurred vision, decreased visual acuity, halos around lights, and nausea and vomiting

■ Diagnosis and treatments

◆ Tonometry measurements reveal increased IOP; perimetry or visual field tests measure loss of peripheral vision

◆ Ophthalmoscopy shows effects of glaucoma on the optic disk (called cupping) whereas gonioscopy measures the angle of the anterior chamber of the eye

◆ Other diagnostic tests may include slit-lamp examination and fundus photography

◆ Drugs that may be used to treat glaucoma include topical adrenergic agonists, cholinergic agonists, beta-adrenergic blockers, and topical or oral carbonic anhydrase inhibitors that reduce IOP by decreasing the production of aqueous humor

◆ Surgery or laser treatments may be peformed for patients who're unresponsive to drug therapy (see *Procedures for glaucoma*)

Procedures for glaucoma

Argon laser trabeculoplasty (ALT) is a first-line therapy for different types of glaucoma. It's used either instead of drug therapy or if drug therapy can't control the increased intraocular pressure (IOP). Performed as an outpatient procedure, ALT directs 40 to 80 laser beams into the trabecular network, creating holes through which the aqueous humor can return to the venous circulation.

For patients who're unresponsive to drug therapy or ALT, or aren't suitable candidates for these treatments, a trabeculectomy may be performed. In this glaucoma filtration procedure, a flap of sclera is dissected free to expose the trabecular meshwork. This discrete tissue block is then removed, and a surgical hole is made in the periphery of the iris. The opening allows aqueous humor to flow out under the conjunctiva by creating a filtering bleb. Often, drugs such as 5-fluorouracil are applied during or after the procedure to control scarring and reclosure of the hole.

Patients whose trabeculectomy have failed to maintain lower IOPs or who're at high risk for failure may need a tube shunt implanted to keep the drainage pathway artificially open. These shunts are surgically kept closed with an absorbable suture to allow healing time. Because of the time required before the shunt is operational, and the difficulty of medically controlling the IOP after surgery, the patient may undergo a trabeculectomy at the same time. Usually, this site fails about the same time as the shunt is healed, providing for continuous pressure reduction.

When other treatments have failed to control IOP, transscleral cyclophotocoagulation may be performed. Twenty to 40 laser beams are directed into the ciliary body of the eye to decrease its production of aqueous fluid.

Laser peripheral iridotomy is used to correct the narrow angle between the iris and the trabecular meshwork that blocks appropriate drainage of aqueous humor in patients with angle-closure glaucoma. A laser beam creates a small hole in the peripheral iris, allowing the fluid to flow to the anterior chamber of the eye, which also results in opening of the angle of the eye.

◆ Bed rest is recommended for patients with acute angle-closure glaucoma
■ Nursing interventions
  ◆ Encourage patient compliance by teaching the patient about medications
  ◆ Postoperatively, give medications, as ordered, to dilate the pupil and topical corticosteroids to rest the pupil and protect the affected eye
  ◆ Administer pain medication as ordered
  ◆ Encourage the patient to be ambulatory immediately after surgery

❖ Otosclerosis
■ Description
  ◆ Otosclerosis (or hardening of the ear) is an overgrowth of bone that impedes normal ossicular motion and can fix the stapes to the oval window
  ◆ It's the most common cause of progressive conductive hearing loss in adults with normal tympanic membranes
  ◆ The disease has a familial tendency and usually occurs between ages 15 and 50; twice as many women are affected as men
  ◆ Pregnancy may trigger the onset in women

■ Signs and symptoms
◆ Progressive hearing loss, which may be unilateral at first and may become bilateral, typically begins at an early age
◆ Vertigo also can occur
◆ The patient may report hearing his own voice better than the voices of others
■ Diagnosis and treatment
◆ Diagnostic tests may include audiometry; electronystagmography; caloric testing; Weber's, Rinne, and Romberg's tests; and facial nerve testing
◆ Hearing aids are recommended to improve hearing
◆ Stapedectomy (surgical removal of the stapes) may be done, and the stapes may be replaced by a prosthesis; complications of this procedure, which is typically performed under local anesthesia, include continued hearing loss, granuloma, oval window rupture that causes perilymph fistula, inflammation, infection, prosthesis displacement, and temporary taste changes
■ Preoperative nursing interventions
◆ Use alternative communication methods as needed; a patient with severe hearing loss may need written instructions or a signing oral interpreter
◆ Discuss preoperative tests and postoperative care to reduce anxiety and promote compliance
◆ Encourage the patient to discuss anxieties and expectations; clarify misconceptions, and inform him that his hearing won't improve until 6 weeks after surgery because of edema and packing
■ Postoperative nursing interventions
◆ Elevate the head of the patient's bed 30 degrees; position him according to the practitioner's orders — on the unaffected side to prevent graft displacement or on the affected side to facilitate drainage
◆ Monitor vital signs, and check dressings for bleeding; attempt to quantify bleeding
◆ Check for headache, stiff neck, fever, and vertigo, which are signs and symptoms of complications
◆ Observe the patient for edema, meningitis, labyrinthitis, and infection
◆ Keep dressings intact; when removed, observe the site for bleeding, redness, drainage, and edema
◆ Clean the suture line as directed; use aseptic technique to prevent infection, and watch for signs of infection
◆ Keep packing intact; it's absorbable, and it shouldn't be removed
◆ Assess facial nerve functioning twice daily to detect nerve compromise
◆ Administer pain medications, as needed, to allow the patient to participate in care
◆ Help the patient get out of bed to prevent falls
◆ Remind the patient to avoid rapid head movements, which can cause the dizziness that commonly occurs after surgery
◆ Tell the patient not to blow his nose and to keep his mouth wide open when coughing or sneezing; the Valsalva maneuver can displace the graft

over the oval window and could introduce bacteria to the middle ear by way of the eustachian tube
- Discharge nursing interventions
  - ◆ Provide written instructions to increase compliance
  - ◆ Tell the patient to avoid strenuous activity for 1 to 3 weeks but to return to work after 1 week as prescribed; strenuous activity can result in perilymph fistula and may dislodge the prosthesis
  - ◆ Instruct the patient to keep the ear dry for 6 weeks; he can shampoo his hair after 1 week; to avoid getting water in the affected ear while bathing, he should plug the ear with a cotton ball coated with petroleum jelly
  - ◆ Tell the patient not to travel by air for 2 to 3 weeks to prevent barotrauma
  - ◆ Tell the patient to avoid people with colds or upper respiratory tract infections for 4 to 6 weeks; these infections can spread to the middle ear by way of the eustachian tube
  - ◆ Instruct the patient to report drainage, fever, otalgia, vertigo, redness, and tenderness of the incision site
  - ◆ Tell the patient to change the cotton ball covering the ear canal daily and as needed but not to disturb the packing in the ear canal
  - ◆ Show the patient how to perform daily incision care

❖ Retinal detachment
- Description
  - ◆ Retinal detachment is the separation of the sensory layers of the retina from the underlying retinal pigment epithelium; without treatment, the entire retina may detach, causing severe vision impairment and possible blindness
  - ◆ It may be caused by degenerative changes in the retina or vitreous gel, intraocular inflammation, or mechanical trauma
  - ◆ In this disorder, vitreous body traction causes retinal tears or holes, which allow vitreous fluid to leak behind the retina and cause it to separate
  - ◆ Retinal detachment may be primary or secondary; a primary detachment occurs spontaneously due to a change in the retina or vitreous; a secondary detachment results from another problem, such as inflammation or trauma
- Signs and symptoms
  - ◆ Signs and symptoms may occur slowly or suddenly
  - ◆ They may include dark or irregular vitreous floaters, flashes of light, and progressive loss of vision in one area (as though a curtain is being pulled before the eye)
- Diagnosis and treatment
  - ◆ Diagnosis depends on ophthalmoscopy (both direct and indirect) after full pupil dilation
  - ◆ Treatment requires bed rest with the affected eye patched and the patient's head positioned so that the retinal hole is at the lowest point of the eye

◆ One of several types of surgery may be performed to find and seal retinal holes or tears

▶ *Diathermy* uses extreme heat to seal the hole

▶ *Laser photocoagulation* uses laser-generated heat to injure the tissue and cause scars, which create a fibrous adhesion to seal the hole

▶ *Cryotherapy* uses nitrous oxide (also known as laughing gas) or carbon dioxide to injure the tissue by freezing it; the injury leaves a scar, which seals the retinal hole

▶ *Scleral buckling* places a band around the globe of the eye to bring the choroid into contact with the retina and hold it in place until adhesion occurs

■ Preoperative nursing interventions

◆ Place the patient on bed rest, patch the eye as prescribed, and position the patient's head so that the retinal tear or hole is at the lowest point of the eye (if the detachment is toward the outer side of the head, have the patient lie on the affected side with the bed flat); these interventions help prevent further detachment

◆ Provide emotional support to the patient who may be distraught at the potential loss of vision

◆ Prepare the patient for surgery by cleaning his face and giving him antibiotics and eyedrops, as ordered

◆ Teach the patient about the role of the retina and why floaters, flashes of light, and decreased vision occur

◆ Allow the patient and family to discuss their concerns

◆ Explain the preoperative routines and the surgical procedure

■ Postoperative nursing interventions

◆ Position the patient as directed; the position varies according to the surgical procedure

◆ Tell the patient to avoid activities that increase intraocular pressure, such as sneezing, coughing, vomiting, lifting, straining during defecation, bending from the waist, and rapidly moving the head; increased intraocular pressure may cause more fluid to flow behind the retina before healing is complete

◆ Administer eyedrops, antiemetics, analgesics, and antibiotics, as ordered; to reduce corneal edema and discomfort, apply ice packs as ordered

◆ Tell the patient to notify the practitioner if he experiences floaters, flashes of light, blurred vision, or pain that isn't relieved with analgesics; these symptoms indicate recurrence of detachment

◆ Teach the patient to recognize and report the signs and symptoms of infection, such as temperature above 100° F (37.8° C), yellow or green discharge, increased redness or pulling of the eye or lid, and vision loss

◆ Show the patient how to administer eye medications and change dressings using sterile technique to decrease the risk of infection

◆ Tell the patient to wear the eye shield at night or when napping to prevent accidental injury to the eye

◆ Discuss when the patient can return to work, resume activities of daily living, and drive or perform strenuous activities

Review questions

1. The nurse is caring for a patient who underwent stapedectomy. To prevent postoperative complications, the nurse should instruct the patient to:

○ **A.** sneeze with her mouth open.

○ **B.** frequently blow her nose.

○ **C.** clean her operated ear with a cotton-tipped applicator twice a day.

○ **D.** resume bending and straining when she's no longer experiencing ear pain.

Correct answer: A   If sneezing can't be avoided, the patient should sneeze with her mouth open. This will prevent changes of air pressure in the middle ear, which can dislodge the prosthesis and graft. Option B is incorrect because blowing the nose and coughing should be avoided. Option C is incorrect because small objects, such as cotton-tipped applicators, shouldn't be inserted into the ear. Option D is incorrect because straining during a bowel movement and bending should be avoided for at least 2 to 3 weeks, or as instructed by the practitioner.

2. The nurse is assessing a 32-year-old patient with otosclerosis. The nurse should be aware that the patient's hearing loss:

○ **A.** affects only one ear.

○ **B.** affects both ears.

○ **C.** occurred suddenly.

○ **D.** is associated with ear pain.

Correct answer: B   The hearing loss associated with otosclerosis is bilateral, although one ear may show a greater impairment. Option A is incorrect because otosclerosis is bilateral. Option C isn't correct because otosclerosis develops slowly over time. Because otosclerosis doesn't cause ear pain, option D is incorrect.

3. The nurse is teaching a patient with a detached retina who underwent scleral buckling on the left eye. The procedure included gas injection into the vitreous. Which of the following statements indicates that the patient understands the nurse's instructions?

○ **A.** "I should lie on my abdomen with my head turned to the right."

○ **B.** "I'll lie face down with my head turned to the left."

○ **C.** "I'll lie face up with my head turned to the right."

○ **D.** "I should lie on my back with my head turned to the left."

Correct answer: B In a scleral buckling, the sclera is flattened against the retina. A piece of silicone is attached to the sclera with a band that encircles the eye to keep the retina in contact with the choroid and sclera. Air or other gases may be injected into the vitreous to float up against the retina and promote retinal reattachment. When a gas is used, the patient is positioned on his abdomen with the head turned to the affected eye (in this situation, the left side) so that the gas will float up against the retina and aid in reattachment. The positions in options A, C, and D don't allow the gas to float up against the retina.

4. The nurse is providing care for a patient following right cataract removal surgery. In which position should the nurse place the patient?

○ **A.** Right-side lying

○ **B.** Prone

○ **C.** Supine

○ **D.** Trendelenburg's

Correct answer: C Positioning the patient on his back or inoperative side prevents pressure on the operative eye. Right side-lying (option A) or prone position (option B) may put external pressure on the affected eye. Trendelenburg's position (option D) may increase intraocular pressure.

CHAPTER 19

Perioperative nursing

❖ Introduction

■ Perioperative nursing includes three phases of the surgical experience: the preoperative, intraoperative, and postoperative phases

■ It's a specialty that provides multidisciplinary continuity of care of the surgical patient

■ It occurs in various inpatient and outpatient settings

❖ Preoperative phase

■ Description

◆ The preoperative period begins when the decision for surgery is made

◆ It ends when the patient is transferred to the operating room table, but functionally ends when the patient is transferred to the holding area

■ Psychosocial assessment

◆ The preoperative psychosocial assessment aims to identify sources of the patient's anxiety; it includes assessing the patient's understanding of the surgery, previous surgical experiences, specific concerns or feelings about the surgery, and religious beliefs that may affect anxiety

◆ Determine the patient's language and communication patterns and arrange for assistance as needed

■ Health history

◆ Obtain a history of allergies, such as to drugs, adhesive tape, latex, betadine, or soap

◆ Ask about preexisting illness, such as liver, respiratory, renal, cardiac, bowel, endocrine, and blood disease

◆ Inquire about use of medications, herbal or over the counter remedies, tobacco, or alcohol that could interfere with anesthesia or contribute to postoperative complications

◆ Ask about the patient's level of pain or discomfort and expectations about postoperative pain relief; perform a baseline pain assessment

■ Physical assessment

◆ Assess the cardiovascular, pulmonary, gastrointestinal, and neurologic systems for baseline functioning

◆ See that a chest X-ray is done, if ordered, to detect lung disease

◆ If the patient is age 40 or older, obtain an electrocardiogram to provide a baseline and detect arrhythmias

◆ Obtain a blood sample for a complete blood count and electrolyte levels as a baseline; if the patient is undergoing major surgery that may involve considerable blood loss, draw blood for typing and crossmatching

◆ Review the results of liver function tests, blood urea nitrogen and serum creatinine, and urinalysis to determine postoperative risk factors

◆ Obtain baseline objective data, beginning with vital signs, height, and weight, then check for skin lesions and presence of dentures or caps

■ Preoperative teaching

◆ Provide a description of and reasons for preoperative tests, description of preoperative routines, time of surgery, probable length of surgery, and estimated amount of time in the postanesthesia care unit (PACU)

◆ Explain the recovery process, including the place where the patient will awaken, nursing care provided, monitoring of vital signs, equipment used, and the time he'll return to the room

◆ Cover the probable postoperative course, anticipated treatments, need to increase activity as soon as possible, need to cough and deep-breathe despite discomfort, pain medication administration, and anticipated discharge needs

◆ Tell family members what time the patient will leave for surgery, where they can wait during surgery, when the practitioner will contact them about surgery results, and when they can visit with the patient

■ Preanesthesia medication

◆ Preanesthesia medication is usually given while the patient is in the holding area, to decrease anxiety, provide sedation, induce amnesia, prevent infection, decrease pharyngeal secretions, slow hydrochloric acid production, and prevent allergic reactions to anesthetics

■ Informed consent

◆ Informed consent must be obtained by the practitioner before the patient receives his preanesthesia medication and be placed in the chart

◆ The informed consent document indicates the specific procedure to be performed; includes a list of possible complications, disfigurement, disability, and removal of body parts; is clearly worded in simple terms; and contains the patient's or guardian's signature

■ Preoperative checklist

◆ On the preoperative checklist, the nurse documents actions, such as removing jewelry and dentures; checking patient identification; surgical site verification; asking the patient to void; ensuring that all needed documents are available; and administering medications as prescribed

❖ Intraoperative phase

■ Description

◆ The intraoperative phase begins when the patient is transferred to the operating table and ends when he's transferred to the PACU or recovery room

◆ Various types of anesthesia and anesthetics may be used (see *Types of anesthesia*)

❖ Postoperative phase

■ Description

◆ The postoperative phase begins when the surgery is complete and ends with a follow-up evaluation in the clinical setting or at home

◆ PACU nurses provide initial assessment, care, and treatments while the patient recovers from the anesthesia; when the patient's activity level,

Types of anesthesia

A patient may receive general, regional, or local anesthesia.

Type of anesthesia	Description
General	<ul><li>Blocks awareness centers in the brain</li><li>Produces unconsciousness, body relaxation, and loss of sensation</li><li>Is administered by inhalation or I.V. infusion</li></ul>
Regional	<ul><li>Inhibits excitatory processes in nerve endings or fibers</li><li>Provides analgesia over a specific body area</li><li>Doesn't produce unconsciousness</li><li>Is administered by nerve block, I.V. regional block with tourniquet, spinal (intrathecal) block, or epidural block</li></ul>
Local	<ul><li>Blocks nerve impulse transmission at the site of action</li><li>Provides analgesia over a limited area</li><li>Doesn't produce unconsciousness</li><li>Is administered topically or by infiltration</li></ul>

respirations, blood pressure, level of consciousness (LOC), and oxygen saturation are stable, per PACU discharge criteria, he's returned to the regular unit.

■ Basic nursing actions
   ◆ Verify the patient's identity, position him properly in bed, and obtain report from the PACU nurse
   ◆ Assess the patient's airway, respirations, and lung sounds; administer oxygen if ordered
   ◆ Obtain baseline vital signs and blood pressure, and assess apical and peripheral pulsations, skin temperature and color, and capillary refill
   ◆ Assess the patient's LOC and neuromotor function
   ◆ Inspect surgical site dressings for drainage and bleeding; reinforce dressings as required
   ◆ Check I.V. fluids, medications being given, and new orders; assess I.V. site for patency; and start new record
   ◆ Check the patency of drainage tubes and urinary catheters; note character of drainage; and start output record
   ◆ Assess postoperative pain, and provide comfort measures and prescribed drug therapies
   ◆ Assess bowel sounds and maintain NG suction, if present; continue nothing-by-mouth status until active peristasis is present
   ◆ Relieve other postoperative discomforts, such as vomiting, abdominal distention, hiccups, and constipation (see *Managing postoperative discomforts,* page 330)
■ Promoting recovery
   ◆ Monitor fluid balance, including elctrolyte levels
   ◆ Maintain nutrition by gradually increasing diet, as tolerated, and encouraging foods high in protein and vitamin C
   ◆ Increase activity daily; consult with physical therapy staff as needed
   ◆ Care for surgical wounds and drains, and urinary catheter aseptically

Managing postoperative discomforts

The following chart summarizes the causes of postoperative discomforts and related nursing interventions.

Discomfort	Cause	Nursing interventions
Vomiting	• Fluid or air accumulation in the stomach • Stomach inflation • Food and fluid ingestion before peristalsis returns • Psychological factors • Adverse drug reactions • Pain • Electrolyte imbalances	• Encourage the patient to lie quietly in bed. • Administer antiemetics, as prescribed. • Prevent aspiration of vomitus. • Maintain an accurate record of fluid intake and output.
Abdominal distention	• Loss of normal peristalsis for 24 to 48 hours after surgery • Swallowing air during recovery from anesthesia	• Have the patient turn in bed, ambulate as tolerated, and perform leg exercises if able • Have the patient avoid hot or cold liquids when peristalsis is sluggish. • Insert a rectal tube to stimulate lower colonic peristalsis and gas passage. • Apply heat to the abdomen to expand the gas and stimulate peristalsis. • Insert a nasogastric tube to aspirate fluid or gas. • Administer an enema as prescribed.
Hiccups	• Intermittent spasms of the diaphragm that may result from direct, indirect, or reflexive irritation of the phrenic nerve	• Have the patient rebreathe carbon dioxide at 5-minute intervals by inhaling and exhaling into a paper bag. • Aspirate the patient's stomach if the hiccups are caused by gastric dilation. • Request blockage of the phrenic nerve by using local infiltration. • Administer a phenothiazine as prescribed.
Constipation	• Local inflammation, peritonitis, or abscess • Weakness resulting from surgery	• Administer an enema as prescribed. • Administer a stool softener, as prescribed, in the early postoperative phase. • Encourage early ambulation. • Increase fluids and dietary intake as prescribed.

◆ Monitor for signs and symptoms of infection and other complications
◆ Teach the patient about the care being provided and how to continue postoperative recovery after discharge; obtain home health referral if needed
◆ Provide psychosocial support; refer for inpatient pastoral or social services assistance as needed; refer to outpatient support groups or services

❖ **Postoperative complications**
  ■ Femoral phlebitis or thrombosis
    ◆ Description
      ▶ Femoral phlebitis or thrombosis usually occurs in patients who have undergone lower abdominal surgery and in those with peritonitis or a ruptured ulcer

◗ It may result from injury to the vein by tight straps on leg holders at the time of surgery, pressure from a blanket roll under the knees, or concentration of blood caused by loss of fluid or dehydration (see chapter 7, Cardiovascular disorders, for details)

■ Hemorrhage

◆ Description

◗ Hemorrhage after an operation may be caused by anesthetic interventions or internal bleeding due to surgical manipulation

◗ It's classified as primary, intermediary, or secondary

• Primary hemorrhage occurs at the time of the operation

• Intermediary hemorrhage occurs within the first few hours after the operation as a result of the return of normal blood pressure and its effect on clots in untied vessels

• Secondary hemorrhage occurs some time after the operation as a result of insecure taping or erosion of a vessel by a drainage tube

◆ Signs and symptoms

◗ A patient with hemorrhage may experience apprehensiveness, restlessness, agitation, thirst, tinnitus, and progressive weakness followed by cold, moist, pale skin and pallid lips and conjunctivae; increased pulse rate; reduced blood pressure; decreased temperature; rapid, deep respirations; and rapid decrease in hemoglobin level

◆ Nursing interventions

◗ Apply pressure to the area of bleeding, if accessible

◗ Provide supplemental oxygen, and maintain a patent airway

◗ Monitor the patient's vital signs frequently

◗ Give blood transfusions, I.V. fluids, and drugs to hemodynamically stabilize the patient's condition

◗ Prepare the patient for surgery, if necessary

■ Paralytic ileus

◆ Description

◗ Paralytic ileus is a physiologic form of intestinal obstruction that can develop after abdominal surgery, after anesthesia, after manipulation of the GI tract, or because of the stress response; it usually resolves spontaneously in 2 to 3 days

◆ Signs and symptoms

◗ A patient with paralytic ileus may have severe abdominal distention, extreme distress and, possibly, vomiting with diminished or absent bowel sounds

◗ The patient may be severely constipated or may pass flatus and small, liquid stools

◆ Nursing interventions

◗ Maintain nothing-by-mouth status until bowel sounds return

◗ Provide I.V. fluids as ordered

◗ Encourage frequent position changes and ambulation

◗ If paralytic ileus doesn't resolve, insert an NG tube

■ Pulmonary embolism

◆ Description

◗ An embolus is a foreign body, gas bubble, blood clot, or piece of tissue that travels in the bloodstream

❱ A pulmonary embolism occurs when an embolus is dislodged from its original site and carried in the blood to the main pulmonary artery or one of the pulmonary branches (see chapter 9, Respiratory disorders, for details)

❱ It's common in patients who have experienced trauma as well as in immobilized patients and elderly patients and is a serious complication

■ Respiratory complications
◆ Description
❱ Respiratory complications are serious, and they're the most common postoperative problems; their incidence is higher in patients undergoing abdominal surgery
❱ The most common respiratory complications are atelectasis, bronchitis, bronchopneumonia, lobar pneumonia, and pleurisy
◆ Signs and symptoms
❱ Signs and symptoms vary according to the cause of the respiratory complication but may include adventitious breath sounds, chest pain, cough, sputum production, hemoptysis, cyanosis, nasal flaring, shortness of breath, dyspnea, tachypnea, orthopnea, retractions, accessory muscle use, and decreased respiratory excursion
❱ Other findings include changes in mentation, anxiety, diaphoresis, fatigue, and tachycardia
◆ Nursing interventions
❱ Monitor respiratory status, including breath sounds, pulse oximetry, respiratory rate and depth, skin color, use of accessory muscles, vital signs, and LOC
❱ Provide supplemental oxygen, and initiate continuous monitoring of oxygen saturation levels by pulse oximetry
❱ Obtain a chest X-ray, as ordered
❱ Provide chest physiotherapy, and encourage coughing, deep breathing, and use of incentive spirometry to mobilize and facilitate removal of secretions
❱ Reposition the patient frequently, and assist with ambulation
❱ Administer drugs, such as antibiotics and bronchodilators, as prescribed
■ Shock
◆ Shock is the most serious postoperative complication
◆ Shock may be hypovolemic, cardiogenic, neurogenic, or septic (see chapter 6, Disruptions in homeostasis, for details)
■ Wound dehiscence and evisceration
◆ Description
❱ Wound dehiscence may occur when the edges of the wound fail to join or separate after they seem to be healing normally
❱ Evisceration may occur if a portion of the viscera protrudes through the incision
❱ Dehiscence and evisceration are most likely to occur 6 to 7 days after surgery
❱ Factors that may contribute to dehiscence and evisceration include poor nutrition, diabetes, chronic pulmonary or cardiac disease, localized wound infection, and stress on the incision

❯ Stress on the incision from coughing or vomiting may cause abdominal distention or severe stretching, leading to dehiscence

◆ Nursing interventions

❯ Place sterile dressings soaked in normal saline over exposed viscera

❯ Monitor vital signs and report any signs of shock

❯ Place the patient on bed rest, and notify the surgeon immediately

❯ Don't allow the patient to have anything by mouth; he may need to have surgery

■ Wound infection

◆ Description

❯ Infections of the surgical wound account for 38% of postoperative infections (see chapter 5, Principles of wound care)

Review questions

1. A patient undergoes a surgical procedure that requires the use of general anesthesia. Following general anesthesia, the patient is most at risk for:

○ **A.** atelectasis.

○ **B.** anemia.

○ **C.** dehydration.

○ **D.** peripheral edema.

Correct answer: A   Atelectasis occurs when the postoperative patient fails to move, cough, and breath deeply. With good nursing care, this is an avoidable complication. Anemia (option B) is a rare complication that usually occurs in patients who lose a significant amount of blood or continue bleeding postoperatively. Fluid shifts that occur postoperatively may result in dehydration (option C) and peripheral edema (option D), but the patient is most at risk for atelectasis.

2. The nurse is administering preoperative medication to a patient going to the operating room for an aortobifemoral bypass. After administering preoperative medication to the patient, the nurse should:

○ **A.** allow him to walk to the bathroom unassisted.

○ **B.** place the bed in low position with the side rails up.

○ **C.** tell him that he'll be asleep before he leaves for surgery.

○ **D.** take his vital signs.

Correct answer: B   When the preoperative medication is given, the bed should be placed in low position, with the side rails raised. The patient should void before the preoperative medication is given—not after. Option A is incorrect because the patient shouldn't get up without assistance. The patient may not be asleep (option C), but he may be drowsy. Vital signs (option D) should be taken before the preoperative medication is given.

3. The nurse is caring for a patient who was given pain medication before leaving the recovery room. Upon returning to her room, the patient states that she's experiencing pain and requests more pain medication. Which is the best action for the nurse to take?

○ **A.** Tell the patient that she must wait 4 hours for more pain medication.

○ **B.** Give one-half of the ordered as-needed dose.

○ **C.** Document the patient's pain.

○ **D.** Notify the practitioner that the patient is continuing to experience pain.

Correct answer: D   The practitioner should be notified of the patient's complaint so that new medication orders can be established. A patient who's experiencing pain after surgery shouldn't have to wait 4 hours for pain relief (option A). A nurse can't alter a dose without first consulting the practitioner (option B); if she does, she could be charged with practicing medicine without a license. The patient's pain should be documented (option C); however, the nurse also needs to follow up with the patient about it.

4. The nurse is evaluating a patient postoperatively for infection. Which of the following would be most indicative of infection?

○ **A.** The presence of an indwelling urinary catheter

○ **B.** A rectal temperature of 100°F (37.8°C)

○ **C.** Redness, warmth, and tenderness in the incision area

○ **D.** A white blood cell (WBC) count of 8,000/µl

Correct answer: C   Redness, warmth, and tenderness in the incision area would lead the nurse to suspect a postoperative infection. The presence of any invasive device (option A) predisposes a patient to infection but alone doesn't indicate infection. A rectal temperature of 100°F (option B) is normal in a postoperative patient because of the inflammatory process. Because a normal WBC count ranges from 4,000 to 10,000/µl, option D is incorrect.

5. The nurse is caring for a patient with a postoperative wound evisceration. Which action should the nurse perform first?

○ **A.** Explain to the patient what is happening, and provide support.

○ **B.** Cover the protruding organs with sterile gauze moistened with sterile saline solution.

○ **C.** Push the protruding organs back into the abdominal cavity.

○ **D.** Ask the patient to drink as much fluid as possible.

Correct answer: B   Immediately covering the wound with moistened gauze prevents the organs from drying. Both the gauze and the saline solution must be sterile to reduce the risk of infection. Explaining what is happening and providing support (option A) may reduce the patient's anxiety, but it isn't the first priority. Option C is incorrect because pushing the organs back into the abdomen may tear or damage them; therefore, the nurse should avoid doing this. Option D is incorrect because evisceration requires emergency surgery, so the nurse should immediately place the patient on nothing-by-mouth status.

Appendices and index

NANDA *nursing diagnoses*

The following is a list of the NANDA International 2005-2006 nursing diagnosis classification according to their domain (area of activity, investigation, or interest).

Domain: Health promotion

- Effective therapeutic regimen management
- Health-seeking behaviors (specify)
- Impaired home maintenance
- Ineffective community therapeutic regimen management
- Ineffective family therapeutic regimen management
- Ineffective health maintenance
- Ineffective therapeutic regimen management
- Readiness for enhanced management of therapeutic regimen
- Readiness for enhanced nutrition

Domain: Nutrition

- Deficient fluid volume
- Excess fluid volume
- Imbalanced nutrition: Less than body requirements
- Imbalanced nutrition: More than body requirements
- Impaired swallowing
- Ineffective infant feeding pattern
- Readiness for enhanced fluid balance
- Risk for deficient fluid volume
- Risk for imbalanced fluid volume
- Risk for imbalanced nutrition: More than body requirements

Domain: Elimination/Exchange

- Bowel incontinence
- Constipation
- Diarrhea
- Functional urinary incontinence
- Impaired gas exchange
- Impaired urinary elimination
- Perceived constipation
- Readiness for enhanced urinary elimination
- Reflex urinary incontinence
- Risk for constipation
- Risk for urge urinary incontinence
- Stress urinary incontinence
- Total urinary incontinence
- Urge urinary incontinence
- Urinary retention

Domain: Activity/Rest

- Activity intolerance
- Bathing or hygiene self-care deficit
- Decreased cardiac output
- Deficient diversional activity
- Delayed surgical recovery
- Disturbed energy field
- Disturbed sleep pattern
- Dressing or grooming self-care deficit
- Dysfunctional ventilatory weaning response
- Fatigue
- Feeding self-care deficit
- Impaired bed mobility
- Impaired physical mobility
- Impaired spontaneous ventilation
- Impaired transfer ability
- Impaired walking
- Impaired wheelchair mobility
- Ineffective breathing pattern
- Ineffective tissue perfusion (specify type: renal, cerebral, cardiopulmonary, gastrointestinal, peripheral)

- Readiness for enhanced sleep
- Risk for activity intolerance
- Risk for disuse syndrome
- Sedentary lifestyle
- Sleep deprivation
- Toileting self-care deficit

Domain: Perception/Cognition

- Acute confusion
- Chronic confusion
- Deficient knowledge (specify)
- Disturbed sensory perception (specify: visual, auditory, kinesthetic, gustatory, tactile, olfactory)
- Disturbed thought processes
- Impaired environmental interpretation syndrome
- Impaired memory
- Impaired verbal communication
- Readiness for enhanced communication
- Readiness for enhanced knowledge (specify)
- Unilateral neglect
- Wandering

Domain: Self-perception

- Chronic low self-esteem
- Disturbed body image
- Disturbed personal identity
- Hopelessness
- Powerlessness
- Readiness for enhanced self-concept
- Risk for loneliness
- Risk for powerlessness
- Risk for situational low self-esteem
- Situational low self-esteem

Domain: Role relationships

- Caregiver role strain
- Dysfunctional family processes: Alcoholism
- Effective breast-feeding
- Impaired parenting
- Impaired social interaction
- Ineffective breast-feeding
- Ineffective role performance
- Interrupted breast-feeding
- Interrupted family processes
- Parental role conflict
- Readiness for enhanced family processes
- Readiness for enhanced parenting

- Risk for caregiver role strain
- Risk for impaired parent/infant/child attachment
- Risk for impaired parenting

Domain: Sexuality

- Ineffective sexuality patterns
- Sexual dysfunction

Domain: Coping/Stress tolerance

- Anticipatory grieving
- Anxiety
- Autonomic dysreflexia
- Chronic sorrow
- Compromised family coping
- Death anxiety
- Decreased intracranial adaptive capacity
- Defensive coping
- Disabled family coping
- Disorganized infant behavior
- Dysfunctional grieving
- Fear
- Impaired adjustment
- Ineffective community coping
- Ineffective coping
- Ineffective denial
- Posttrauma syndrome
- Rape-trauma syndrome
- Rape-trauma syndrome: Compound reaction
- Rape-trauma syndrome: Silent reaction
- Readiness for enhanced community coping
- Readiness for enhanced coping
- Readiness for enhanced family coping
- Readiness for enhanced organized infant behavior
- Relocation stress syndrome
- Risk for autonomic dysreflexia
- Risk for disorganized infant behavior
- Risk for dysfunctional grieving
- Risk for posttrauma syndrome
- Risk for relocation stress syndrome

Domain: Life principles

- Decisional conflict (specify)
- Impaired religiosity
- Noncompliance (specify)
- Readiness for enhanced religiosity
- Readiness for enhanced spiritual well-being

- Risk for impaired religiosity
- Risk for spiritual distress
- Spiritual distress

Domain: Safety/Protection

- Hyperthermia
- Hypothermia
- Impaired dentition
- Impaired oral mucous membrane
- Impaired skin integrity
- Impaired tissue integrity
- Ineffective airway clearance
- Ineffective protection
- Ineffective thermoregulation
- Latex allergy response
- Risk for aspiration
- Risk for falls
- Risk for imbalanced body temperature
- Risk for impaired skin integrity
- Risk for infection
- Risk for injury
- Risk for latex allergy response
- Risk for other-directed violence
- Risk for perioperative-positioning injury
- Risk for peripheral neurovascular dysfunction
- Risk for poisoning
- Risk for self-directed violence
- Risk for self-mutilation
- Risk for sudden infant death syndrome
- Risk for suffocation
- Risk for suicide
- Risk for trauma
- Self-mutilation

Domain: Comfort

- Acute pain
- Chronic pain
- Nausea
- Social isolation

Domain: Growth/Development

- Adult failure to thrive
- Delayed growth and development
- Risk for delayed development
- Risk for disproportionate growth

Nursing implications of diagnostic tests

To provide appropriate care for a patient undergoing a diagnostic test, the nurse must understand the test and its uses, prepare the patient properly (including verifying that informed consent has been obtained and explaining the procedure), and monitor the patient carefully before and after the test.

Test and description	Uses of test	Patient preparation	Nursing implications
Radiologic (X-ray) tests			
Abdominal flat plate of abdomen or kidneys, ureters, and bladder			
X-ray of the abdomen or kidneys, ureters, and bladder	● Detecting abdominal masses, bowel obstructions, ileus or perforation ● Detecting renal and bladder masses and some renal calculi	● Have the patient remove clothing and metal objects. ● Instruct the patient to take a deep breath and hold it while the X-ray is taken.	● Cover a male patient's testes with a lead shield. ● Don't perform this test on a pregnant patient.
Angiography X-ray of arterial blood vessels using contrast media (dye)	● Identifying femoral artery occlusion ● Detecting arterial peripheral vascular disease ● Checking for aneurysms, tumors, vascular anomalies ● Determining status of cerebral circulation ● Determining condition of coronary arteries ● Identifying blood flow dynamics	● Give nothing by mouth (NPO) after midnight. ● Mark peripheral pulses with a pen. ● Tell the patient to expect a warm, flushing sensation when the dye is injected.	● Check for allergies to shellfish or iodine and for a prior reaction to dye before the X-ray. ● Observe the patient for signs of hemorrhage or hematoma at the insertion site. ● Monitor vital signs. ● Document the type of vascular closure device used and status of the dressing. ● Ambulate the patient per the standards for the type of closure device used. ● Check the peripheral pulses bilaterally. ● Compare color and temperature in extremities. ● Monitor the patient for allergic reactions to the dye, such as diaphoresis, hypotension, wheezing, angioedema, and laryngospasm. ● Monitor the patient for signs of cerebral emboli, such as slurred speech, confusion, and hemiparesis (one-sided weakness). ● Encourage the patient to drink plenty of fluids.

Test and description	Uses of test	Patient preparation	Nursing implications
Radiologic (X-ray) tests *(continued)*			
Arthrography Visualization of the shape and integrity of a joint capsule following the injection of contrast media, air, or both	● Determining the cause of joint pain and swelling ● Diagnosing joint disorders and synovial cysts	● Tell the patient that crackling noises may be heard in the joint after the procedure due to the injection of air during the procedure. ● Explain that a local anesthetic will be used.	● Assess the patient for allergies to contrast media or local anesthesia. ● After the test, assess the joint for swelling, and apply ice if needed. ● Administer an analgesic for pain and discomfort.
Bone densitometry Measures bone mineral density	● Diagnosing osteoporosis and monitoring its progression	● Tell the patient to wear clothing that's easily removed from the hip area and without zippers or metal fasteners. ● Make sure the patient avoids calcium products for 24 hours before the test.	● Tell patient to remain still during the test.
Cardiac catheterization and coronary angiography X-ray examination of coronary vessels using dye injected through a catheter in the femoral or antecubital vein (for right-sided cardiac catheterization) or in the femoral or brachial artery (for left-sided cardiac catheterization)	● Determining size and structure of cardiac chambers ● Measuring pressures and volumes in cardiac chambers ● Determining valve structure and function ● Determining pressure in pulmonary vessels ● Determining extent of damage from heart disease ● Determining condition of coronary vessels ● Facilitate infusion of thrombolytic agents into occluded coronary arteries ● Performing angioplasty, atherectomy, and stent insertion	● Have the patient fast for 3 to 8 hours before the test. ● Prepare the patient for a warm, flushing sensation when the dye is injected. ● Scrub and shave the catheter insertion site. ● If prescribed, administer pretest medications, such as an antihistamine, a steroid, a sedative, or a tranquilizer. ● Have the patient void before receiving the pretest medication or before going to the cardiac catheterization laboratory.	● Check for allergies to shellfish or iodine and for a prior reaction to dye before the test. ● Have the patient remove dentures and jewelry before the test. ● Start an I.V. infusion before the test and maintain it during and after the test. ● Obtain baseline vital signs, and monitor them continuously during the test and frequently after the test. ● Monitor peripheral pulses below the insertion site each time vital signs are taken. ● Maintain bed rest for 4 to 6 hours then ambulate the patient. ● Tell the patient to avoid heavy lifting and vigorous activity for several days unless the practitioner orders further restrictions. ● Check the catheter insertion site for hemorrhage or hematoma; apply ice if needed. ● Document the type of vascular closure device used and status of the dressing. ● Maintain pressure to the insertion site, and keep the extremity flat and immobilized with a sandbag. ● Have emergency equipment available to treat complications, such as arrhythmias, anaphylaxis, pneumothorax, and hemopericardium. ● Encourage the patient to drink fluids after thet test.

Test and description	Uses of test	Patient preparation	Nursing implications
Radiologic (X-ray) tests *(continued)*			
Chest X-ray Visualization of the lungs, heart, and bony structures	● Detecting lung diseases or tumors ● Diagnosing chronic obstructive pulmonary disease ● Identifying infections ● Diagnosing abnormal rib conditions ● Detecting cardiomegaly ● Identifying location of central lines ● Identifying fluid or air accumulation	● Have the patient remove metal objects. ● Instruct the patient to take a deep breath and hold it while the X-ray is taken.	● Cover the patient's reproductive organs with a lead shield. ● Don't perform this test on a pregnant patient.
Computed tomography (CT) scan, or computed axial tomography scan, and spiral CT scan			
Multi-dimensional visualization of a body part using a computer-controlled, focused X-ray beam of various speeds; contrast media may be used to enhance visualization	● Visualizing brain lesions, tumors, edema, and other conditions (cerebral CT scan) ● Identifying herniated disks, tumors, and other abnormalities (spinal CT scan) ● Visualizing tumors and chest lesions (thoracic CT scan) ● Visualizing liver, pancreas, spleen, gallbladder, reproductive tract, and abdominal cavity for abnormalities (abdominal CT scan) ● Detecting kidney abnormalities, such as tumors and calculi (renal CT scan)	● If dye is used, maintain NPO status 3 to 8 hours before the test. ● If the patient is undergoing a cerebral CT scan, remove hair pins and jewelry, and administer a sedative, as prescribed. ● Explain that flushing or nausea may occur after injection of contrast media. ● Patients taking metformin (Glucophage) should be instructed to withhold medication for 48 hours prior to the test.	● Check for allergies to shellfish or iodine and for a prior reaction to dye before the test. ● Tell the patient to remain still during the test and breathe steadily. ● Prepare the patient for the large and confining machinery; assess him for claustrophobia. ● If dye was used, check for signs of iodine reaction and acute renal failure after the test. If an allergic reaction occurs, administer an antihistamine as prescribed. ● Monitor for hypoglycemia or acidosis in patients who withheld Glucophage prior to the test. ● Encourage the patient to drink fluids after the test.
Excretory urography X-ray visualization of the urinary tract using I.V. injected, iodine-based contrast media that concentrates in the urinary tract; also known as intravenous pyelography (IVP)	● Determining the size, shape, and function of the kidneys, ureters, and bladder ● Detecting tumors, cysts, or renal calculi ● Detecting other renal diseases ● Detecting urinary outlet obstruction	● Maintain NPO status 8 to 12 hours before the test. ● Administer a laxative the evening before the test.	● Check for allergies to shellfish or iodine and for a prior reaction to dye. ● Check urine output and blood urea nitrogen (BUN) level; the test usually isn't performed on oliguric patients or on those with a BUN level greater than 40 mg/dl. ● Observe for an allergic reaction to the dye. If an allergic reaction occurs, administer a steroid or antihistamine as prescribed. ● Monitor urine output. ● Encourage the patient to drink fluids after the test.
GI series *Upper:* X-ray examination of the esophagus, stomach, and small bowel after the patient swallows contrast media, such as barium or diatrizoate meglumine (Gastrografin)	● Examining the stomach for ulcerations, cancer, or other diseases ● Diagnosing hiatal hernia ● Detecting esophageal varices, pyloric stenosis, or foreign bodies	● Maintain NPO status after midnight. ● Tell the patient that the test may take 1 to 6 hours.	● Don't allow the patient to eat until the test is completed. ● Give a laxative, such as magnesium salts (milk of magnesia), as prescribed, after an X-ray series using barium. ● Note stool color and consistency to ensure that the barium has been passed. ● Advise the patient who has received diatrizoate meglumine that diarrhea may occur.

Test and description	Uses of test	Patient preparation	Nursing implications
Radiologic (X-ray) tests *(continued)*			
GI series *(continued)* *Lower:* X-ray examination of the large intestine by inserting barium by way of an enema	● Detecting diverticula ● Checking for tumors or obstructions ● Detecting inflammatory bowel disease	● Make sure the patient receives a clear liquid diet the day before the test. ● Instruct the patient on the bowel cleansing preparation ordered. ● Maintain NPO status after midnight.	● Administer enemas, bisacodyl suppositories, or saline enemas at 6 a.m. the morning of the test; make sure the drainage is clear. ● Encourage increased fluid intake on the day before the test. ● Administer a laxative, such as magnesium citrate (milk of magnesia), or an enema, as prescribed, to expel the barium. ● Advise the patient that the barium may make his stools appear a light color for several days after the test. ● Tell the patient to report lack of bowel movements to the physician; retained barium can cause bowel obstruction and fecal impaction.
Hysterosalpingography X-ray that visualizes the uterine cavity, fallopian tubes, and peritubal area; fluoroscopic radiographs obtained as contrast medium flows through the uterus and fallopian tubes	● Detecting tubal abnormalities ● Detecting uterine abnormalities such as congenital malformations ● Confirming the presence of fistulas or peritubal adhesions ● Evaluating the cause of repeated miscarriage ● Diagnosing infertility	● Check the patient's history for recent pelvic infection and notify practitioner. ● Tell the patient that antibiotics may be given before or after the test. ● Explain that the test should take place 2 to 5 days after menstruation ends. ● Warn the patient that she might experience moderate cramping during the test. ● Tell the patient to perform bowel preparation the night before the test, as ordered.	● Teach the patient that she can return to pretest activities gradually. ● Monitor the patient for signs and symptoms of infection, uterine perforation, bleeding, and adverse reaction to the contrast medium. ● Premedicate the patient for cramping as ordered.
Mammography X-ray examination of the breast's soft tissue structures	● Detecting benign breast cysts, mastitis or abscess ● Screening for malignant breast tumors	● Have the patient remove clothing and jewelry from the waist up and put on a gown. ● Prepare the patient for pinching and discomfort as the breast tissue is compressed. ● Tell the patient not to use powder or deodorant the day of the test because both may leave residue that could be mistaken for areas of calcification.	● Tell the patient to remain still during the test. ● Tell the patient that breast augmentation may be an interfering factor.

Test and description	Uses of test	Patient preparation	Nursing implications
Radiologic (X-ray) tests *(continued)*			
Myelography X-ray examination of the spinal column using contrast media	● Detecting tumors or other obstructions of the spinal tract ● Locating herniated intervertebral disks	● Tell the patient to increase fluid intake the day before the test; fasting for 2 to 6 hours before the test may be required. ● Tell the patient to remain still on the X-ray table, which will be tilted downward. ● Inform the patient that a lumbar puncture is performed to instill the dye. ● Notify the radiologist if there is history of seizures or asthma, or use of an antidepressant, phenothiazine, blood thinner, or diabetic drugs like metformin, as these drugs may be stopped 1 to 2 days before the test.	● Check for allergies to shellfish or iodine and for a prior reaction to dye. ● Maintain the patient's position, as prescribed, after the test; maintain bed rest for 3 to 4 hours, then tell the patient to avoid bending over or strenuous activities for 1 to 2 days. ● Keep the patient's head elevated at 30 to 45 degrees to prevent seizures. ● Encourage fluid intake to eliminate the contrast media and prevent headache. ● Observe the patient for signs of dye reactions. ● Observe the patient for signs of meningeal irritation. ● Monitor the patient's ability to void after the test. ● Monitor vital signs after the test.
Percutaneous transhepatic cholangiography Visualization of the biliary system using contrast media injected I.V. or through a T tube	● Identifying calculi or obstructions in the biliary system ● Detecting calculi or other obstructions in the common bile duct after surgery (T-tube cholangiography)	● There are no special preparations. ● An I.V. antibiotic may be administered prior to the test via a T tube. ● Tell the patient that an anesthesia will be injected into the abdominal skin site, and will sting.	● Check for allergies to shellfish or iodine and for a prior reaction to dye before the test. ● Observe the patient for allergic reactions, inflammation, and sepsis. ● Watch for nausea and vomiting after the test.
Venography X-ray examination of the peripheral venous system using contrast media	● Detecting deep vein thrombosis ● Evaluating varicose veins	● Explain the test to the patient.	● Check for allergies to shellfish or iodine and for a prior reaction to dye before the test. ● Check the examination site for signs of inflammation or infection. ● Observe the patient for systemic signs of infection. ● Monitor vital signs and pulses in the affected area.
Endoscopic tests			
Arthroscopy Visualization of the internal joint structures, usually in the knee	● Detecting torn cartilage or ligaments ● Assessing arthritic changes ● Performing corrective surgery through arthroscope	● Perform standard preoperative preparations. ● If the patient will receive general anesthesia, maintain NPO status after midnight. ● Shave and scrub the affected area.	● Check the incision site for infection. ● Assess neurovascular status of the affected extremity. ● Keep the joint elevated and extended. ● Apply ice to decrease edema and administer an analgesic, as prescribed, to relieve pain. ● Instruct the patient to avoid using the joint for several days and, if necessary, teach crutch walking. ● Tell the patient that sutures are usually removed in 7 days.

Test and description	Uses of test	Patient preparation	Nursing implications
Endoscopic tests (continued)			
Bronchoscopy Visualization of the trachea and bronchi	• Detecting tumors or inflammation • Obtaining sputum culture • Biopsying accessible lesions • Removing foreign bodies and excessive secretions • Locating bleeding sites in the tracheobronchial tree	• Maintain NPO status for 6 to 12 hours before the test. • Have the patient remove dentures and contact lenses. • Administer pretest medications, such as atropine to decrease secretions and a sedative or tranquilizer to relax the patient.	• Maintain NPO status until the gag reflex returns. • Monitor vital signs. • Monitor respiratory status; this test poses a risk of laryngospasm. • Note any hemoptysis. • Provide gargling solutions or lozenges to relieve sore throat.
Colonoscopy Visualization of the colon using a flexible endoscope	• Detecting tumors • Detecting and removing polyps • Identifying sites of bleeding • Detecting ulceration and bowel inflammation	• Confirm that the patient hasn't undergone a barium test in the past 14 days. • Have the patient maintain a clear fluid diet for up to 3 days before the test. • Make sure the patient performs the bowel cleansing preparation ordered. • Maintain NPO status after midnight. • Administer an analgesic and a sedative, as prescribed.	• Maintain NPO status after the test until the patient is alert. • Observe the patient for bleeding and abdominal pain; the patient is at risk for bowel perforation and hemorrhage, especially if a biopsy was performed or polyps were removed. • Monitor vital signs until the patient is stable. • Explain that flatus and gas pains are common after the test. • Encourage fluid intake.
Cystoscopy Visualization of the urethra and bladder cavity; may include retrograde pyelography (X-ray visualization of the ureters after dye is injected)	• Detecting tumors and calculi • Establishing cause of hematuria • Determining cause of infection • Biopsying prostate (bladder), or urethra • Resecting bladder tumors	• If the patient will receive general anesthesia, maintain NPO status after midnight. • Encourage fluid intake before the test. • Administer a pretest analgesic, if prescribed, 1 hour before the test. • Prepare the patient for the lithotomy position and the use of an irrigation system. • Tell the patient that an anesthetic gel may be inserted into the urethra before the test.	• Monitor urine output and vital signs. • Remember that urine may be pink and contain clots. • Report any hemorrhage or difficulty voiding. • Monitor the patient for signs of gram-negative sepsis, such as chills, fever, tachycardia, and hypotension; administer a prophylactic antibiotic if prescribed. • Encourage fluid intake. • If bladder spasms occur, give warm sitz baths and an antispasmodic, as prescribed.
Endoscopic retrograde cholangiopancreatography Visualization of the bile and pancreatic ducts using an endoscope and contrast media	• Detecting obstructions, such as tumors, cysts, and calculi • Detecting cirrhosis and pancreatic disease	• Maintain NPO status after midnight. • Administer a pretest medication, such as an opioid analgesic or sedative, as prescribed.	• Check for allergies to shellfish or iodine and for a reaction to previous tests using dye. • Maintain NPO status until the gag reflex returns. • Check vital signs, and observe the patient for signs of inflammation and sepsis. • Monitor the patient for signs of pancreatitis, such as abdominal pain, nausea, and vomiting. • Monitor the patient for signs of respiratory distress. • Provide gargling solutions or lozenges to relieve sore throat.

Test and description	Uses of test	Patient preparation	Nursing implications

Endoscopic tests *(continued)*

Test and description	Uses of test	Patient preparation	Nursing implications
Esophagogastroduodenoscopy Direct visualization of the esophagus, stomach, and duodenum	• Detecting gastric ulcers or esophagitis • Detecting tumors • Determining site of bleeding • Detecting hiatal hernia	• Maintain NPO status for 8 to 12 hours before the test. • Have the patient remove dentures. • Administer medications, such as atropine, a sedative or tranquilizer, or an opioid analgesic, 1 hour before the test, as prescribed.	• Maintain NPO status until the gag reflex returns. • Place the patient on his side to prevent aspiration. • Monitor vital signs. • Check for complications, such as fever, hemorrhage, abdominal pain, and dyspnea. • Inform the patient that retained air may cause bloating, belching, and flatus, and he may have a sore throat or hoarseness.
Sigmoidoscopy Visualization of the rectum and sigmoid colon using a flexible endoscope	• Screening for polyps and colorectal cancer • Inspecting for inflammatory disease • Detecting hemorrhoids and other perirectal conditions	• Administer two saline enemas the morning of the test. • Let the patient eat a light breakfast the morning of the test. • Confirm that the patient hasn't undergone a barium test in the past 14 days.	• Observe the patient for signs of bleeding or perforation. • Explain that the test may cause gas pain and flatus and may cause slight rectal bleeding if biopsies were obtained.

Nuclear (radioisotope) scans

Test and description	Uses of test	Patient preparation	Nursing implications
Bone scan I.V. administration of a radioisotope followed by a bone scan 2 to 3 hours later	• Determining condition of bone • Detecting bone disease and degeneration • Detecting metastasis	• Don't limit oral intake. • Force fluids (four to six glasses of water between isotope administration and scanning). • Have the patient void before the scan.	• Tell the patient to remain still during the test. • Remember that no radiation precautions are needed after the test. • Encourage fluid intake to hasten isotope elimination, which occurs in 6 to 24 hours.
Brain scan I.V. administration of a radioisotope followed by a brain scan 30 minutes to 3 hours later	• Detecting intracranial lesions • Evaluating cerebral perfusion	• Don't limit oral intake. • Explain the test to the patient.	• Tell the patient to remain still during the test with his hands at his sides. • Remember that no radiation precautions are needed after the test. • Encourage fluid intake.
Cardiac perfusion scan I.V. administration of a radioisotope followed by imaging in 10 to 60 minutes; if part of a stress test, thallium is given before exercise, then re-imaging is done at peak exercise	• Screening for ischemic heart disease • Determining coronary perfusion after a myocardial infarction (MI) • Assessing cardiac chambers	• Have the patient fast per facility procedure. • Restrict smoking before a thallium stress test. • Tell the patient to avoid drugs for erectile dysfunction (ED) for 48 hours before the test	• Remember that no special radiation precautions are needed for this test. • If a stress test is performed, monitor vital signs after the test. • Encourage the patient to drink fluids after the test. • ED drugs can cause severe hypotension when mixed with nitroglycerin, which may be required during the test.

Test and description	Uses of test	Patient preparation	Nursing implications
Nuclear (radioisotope) scans *(continued)*			
Gallbladder scan I.V. administration of a radioisotope followed by imaging	● Determining gallbladder function ● Identifying gallstones or other obstruction ● Detecting infection of the gallbaldder	● Tell the patient not to eat for 4 hours before the scan. ● Explain that images will be taken at 10- to 15-minute intervals over 1 to 2 hours. ● Tell the patient with acute pain that a positive test may result in further medical treatment or surgery.	● Don't perform the test on a pregnant or nursing patient. ● Encourage fluid intake to hasten radio-isotope elimination over 1 to 2 days.
Leukocyte scan Injection of indium-tagged leukocytes to detect infection location	● Locating sources of infec-tion that are difficult to de-tect such as those in bone, the abdomen, or the kidneys	● Make sure the patient's blood is drawn, tagged with indium, and reinjected be-fore imaging.	● No special follow-up care is required.
Liver and spleen scan I.V. administration of a radioisotope followed by imag-ing within 30 min-utes	● Determining size, shape, and position of liver and spleen ● Identifying liver path-ology ● Assess condition of liver after abdominal trauma	● Check with the radiology department about oral in-take limitations. ● Explain the test to the pa-tient, especially the positions used.	● Tell the patient to remain still during the test. ● Remember that no radiation precau-tions are needed after the test. ● Encourage fluids posttest ● Watch the patient for analphylactoid or pyrogenic reaction
Lung scan I.V., inhalation, or ventilation adminis-tration of a radio-isotope followed by imaging; time varies with route of ad-ministration	● Determining lung func-tion ● Assessing pulmonary vas-cular perfusion ● Determining presence of pulmonary embolism ($\dot{V}/\dot{Q}$ scan)	● Don't limit oral intake. ● Explain the test to the patient.	● Tell the patient to remain still during the test. ● Inform the patient undergoing a xenon ventilation scan that he must hold his breath on request during the test. ● Remember that no radiation precau-tions are needed after the test.
Lymphoscintigraphy Following subcuta-neous administra-tion of a radioiso-tope, a scanner de-tects the gamma rays emitted by affected lymph nodes	● Diagnosing lymphedema ● Locating sentinal lymph nodes in breast cancer and malignant melanoma	● Explain that the skin around the tumor site or in the distal extremity will be injected with a very tiny nee-dle.	● Don't perform the test on a pregnant patient. ● Tell the patient that the length of time after injection until scanning varies and may include post exercise testing in pa-tients with lymphedema. ● Remember that no radiation precau-tions are needed after the test.
Positron emission tomography (PET) scan Inhalation or infu-sion of high-energy radioactive tracers (attached to glu-cose, water, or am-monia) and use of computer-based nuclear imaging to measure blood flow, tissue compo-sition, and meta-bolism	● Detecting coronary artery disease (CAD) and assessing ischemic tissue and myocar-dial viability with or without exercise testing ● Detecting tumor, stroke , and epilepsy ● Charting progress of CAD, collateral coronary artery cir-culation, head injury, stroke, Alzheimer's disease, Parkin-son's disease, and certain biochemical abnormalities associated with psychiatric disorders	● Tell the patient not to eat for 4 hours before the scan, but to drink plenty of water. ● If the patient is diabetic, tell him to follow the practi-tioner's instructions on which diabetic drugs to take before the test. ● Patients who are confused or agitated may require se-dation. ● Urinary catheterization may be necessary for colon or kidney studies.	● Check blood glucose level; the test usu-ally isn't performed on patients with a blood glucose level greater than 150 g/dl. ● Prepare patient for the length of the test and any sensations the patient may hear or feel. (Light-headedness, dizziness, and headache are common.) ● Don't perform this test on a pregnant patient. ● Document the patient's weight for use in determining dose of radioactive material. ● Encourage the patient to drink fluids after the test.

Test and description	Uses of test	Patient preparation	Nursing implications
Nuclear (radioisotope) scans *(continued)*			
Positron emission tomography (PET) scan *(continued)*	• Providing measurements of V̇/Q̇ relationship and lung perfusion	• Tell the patient to abstain from caffeine, alcohol, tobacco 24 hours prior to the test.	
Renal scan I.V. administration of a radioisotope followed immediately or within 30 minutes by imaging	• Determining renal function • Identifying kidney position, size, and shape	• Don't limit oral intake. • Encourage fluid intake (two to three glasses of water about 30 minutes before the test). • Have the patient void before the scan.	• Make sure the test isn't scheduled within 24 hours of excretory urography because the patient should be well hydrated. • Remember that no radiation precautions are needed after the test. • Encourage fluid intake to hasten radioisotope elimination.
Single-photon emission computed tomography (SPECT) Following injection of radionuclide, the scanner detects the radiation emitted as it rotates around to obtain a 3D image of the target	• Detecting specific types of cancer such as neuroendocrine tumors • Detecting cancer that has metastasized to the bone • Confirming diagnosis of Alzheimer's disease • Detecting location of an infection, stress fractures, spondylosis, brain abnormalities, cardiac dysfunction, thyroid tumors, plus flow of blood	• Maintain NPO status 4 hours before the scan • Tell the patient the test takes about 1 hour	• Prepare patient for the length of the test and any sensations the patient may hear or feel (lightheadedness, dizziness, and headache are common). • Encourage the patient to drink fluids after the test.
Thyroid scan Oral administration of radioactive iodine followed by scanning within 2 to 24 hours	• Determining thyroid size, shape, and function • Identifying pathologic conditions, especially adenomas	• Check on drug restrictions; thyroid drugs, cough syrup, multiple vitamins, and some oral contraceptives may be restricted from 1 to several weeks before the test.	• Check for iodine allergies. • Make sure the test isn't administered to a pregnant patient because it can damage the fetus. • Remember that no radiation precautions are needed after the test.
Magnetic and ultrasound studies			
Endoscopic ultrasonography Combines ultrasonography and endoscopy to visualize the GI wall and adjacent structures and allows ultrasound imaging with high resolution	• Evaluating or staging lesions of the esophagus, stomach, duodenum, pancreas, ampulla, biliary ducts, and rectum • Evaluating submucosal tumors	• Instruct the patient to fast for 6 to 8 hours before the test. • Administer an I.V. sedative to help the patient relax before the test. • Some procedures may require prior bowel cleansing.	• Make sure the patient is scheduled for abdominal ultrasonography before a barium test is done; retained barium interferes with ultrasound readings. • Obesity and excess gas in the bowel can interfere with the accuracy of the results.
Magnetic resonance imaging (MRI) Visualization of body parts by exposing body cells to small magnets and tracking the cells' reaction	• Detecting abnormalities in all body parts, including bones and joints • Studying bone structure	• Have the patient remove metal objects, such as jewelry and hairpins. • Identify surgeries or wounds with metal implants, rods or pacemakers which would be contraindication to MRI. • Have the patient take preprocedure anxiolytic for claustrophobia, if ordered.	• Prepare the patient for being placed inside the large, doughnut-shaped electromagnet. (Open MRIs are available in some areas.) • Tell the patient to remain still during the test; assess him for claustrophobia. • Tell the patient to expect loud clicking sounds during the test. • Encourage the patient to relax during the test.

Test and description	Uses of test	Patient preparation	Nursing implications
Magnetic and ultrasound studies *(continued)*			
Transesophageal echocardiography Invasive procedure using an esophageal scope to place a probe behind the heart to better visualize the heart and its structures	• Assessing left atrial anatomy and function and prosthetic valve function • Diagnosing cardiac masses and aneurysms • Assessing cardiac tamponade, endocarditis and intracardiac thrombi	• Maintain NPO status for six hours before the test. • Attach electrocardiogram (ECG) leads and blood pressure cuff. • Position the patient on the table to allow for esophageal intubation. • Administer sedatives as ordered. • Remove the patient's dentures.	• Prepare the patient for the procedure and use of sedation and local anesthetic. • Closely monitor ECG, blood pressure, and oxygen saturation during and after the test. • Have suctioning equipment readily available in case of vomiting. • Keep the patient NPO until he's fully awake and his gag reflex has returned.
Ultrasonography Visualization of underlying soft tissues and body structures using high-frequency sound waves that echo from the underlying body parts, producing scans, waveforms, or sounds	• Identifying gallstones • Differentiating between liver masses and other causes of jaundice • Diagnosing renal masses • Determining fetal presence and growth; visualizing uterus, ovaries, and fallopian tubes • Assessing blood flow (Doppler) and detecting occlusion or aneurysm • Assessing heart valve movement and heart size, position, and shape (echogram) • Evaluating thyroid gland size and structure • Detecting abdominal aneurysms	• Explain the test to the patient based on the body site being evaluated. • For a transabdominal scan, which requires a full bladder, instruct the patient to drink several glasses of water and not to void. For a kidney, gallbladder, spleen, or abdominal scan, instruct the patient to fast for 8 to 12 hours before the test.	• Tell the patient he can resume activity and diet as ordered. • Monitor the patient for signs and symptoms of perforation or bleeding. • Tell the patient to avoid alcohol and driving for 24 hours after the test if I.V. sedation was used.
Biopsies			
Liver biopsy Removal of hepatic tissue by way of needle aspiration for microscopic examination	• Detecting tumors • Diagnosing hepatocellular disease, especially cirrhosis	• Check the patient's platelet count and coagulation studies; this test is contraindicated in a patient with a platelet count less than 100,000/µl. • Maintain NPO status for 6 to 8 hours before the test. • Give vitamin K, if prescribed, before and after the test. • Administer a sedative as prescribed. • Tell the patient to report use of aspirin, NSAIDs, or anticoagulants to the practitioner before the test.	• Report abnormal prothrombin times to the practitioner. • Tell the patient that the test requires supine positioning and placement of the right hand under the head. • Have the patient practice exhaling and holding his breath in that position. • Place the patient on his right side for 2 hours after the test to apply pressure on the liver and prevent hemorrhage. • Monitor vital signs and assess for pain in the chest or shoulder; give an analgesic as prescribed. • Observe the patient for signs of hemorrhage. • Monitor respirations to detect pneumothorax.

Test and description	Uses of test	Patient preparation	Nursing implications
Biopsies *(continued)*			
Other tissue biopsies Removal of organ tissue for microscopic examination	• Detecting malignant tumors • Identifying pathologic cellular changes	• Preparation for a patient undergoing other tissue biopsy is similar to that for a liver biopsy.	• Nursing care for the patient undergoing other tissue biopsy is similar to that for a liver biopsy.
Electrodiagnostic tests			
Electrocardiography Noninvasive test that gives a graphic representation of the heart's electrical activity; ambulatory or Holter monitoring records the ECG over a 24-hour period; stress testing records the ECG during increasing levels of exercise	• Detecting ischemia, injury, and necrosis • Identifying conduction delays, bundle blocks, fascicular blocks, and arrhythmias • Identifying chamber enlargement • Determining cardiac status after MI • Assessing the effectiveness of cardiac drugs and treatments • Determining pacemaker activity • Determining safe limits of exercise	• Tell the patient that his skin may be prepared with alcohol, sandpaper, or shaved so the electrodes hold. • Withhold food and fluids for 2 to 4 hours before the test. • Instruct the patient to wear loose-fitting clothing and supportive shoes. • Tell the patient to immediately report chest discomfort, shortness of breath, fatigue, leg cramps, or dizziness. • Show the patient how to record activity and symptoms in a diary for Holter monitor. • Tell the patient that there's no risk of electrical shock.	• Withhold medications, as ordered, before the stress test. • Have emergency equipment available during stress testing. • Obtain a resting ECG and baseline vital signs before the stress test. • Monitor vital signs, and assess the patient for signs and symptoms of cardiovascular instability during and after the stress test. • Help the patient remove electrodes after the test.
Electroencephalography Noninvasive test that records the electrical activity of the brain via scalp electrodes	• Identifying seizure activity • Assessing and locating cerebral lesions and injury • Evaluating trauma and drug intoxication • Determining brain death • Evaluating sleep disorders	• Explain to the patient that he'll be subjected to stimuli, such as lights and sounds. • Tell the patient he must lie still during the test. • Reassure the patient that electrical shock won't occur. • Tell the patient to wash his hair the night before the test but not to apply any conditioners, sprays, or gels. • Tell the patient he may need to avoid sleep the night before the test if his study requires sleep testing.	• Withhold caffeine-containing beverages and chocolate and refrain from smoking 8 hours before the test. • Withhold medications, as indicated, for 24 to 48 hours before the test. • Help the patient remove any electrode gel from his hair and scalp after the test.
Electromyography Needle insertion into selected muscles at rest and during voluntary contraction picks up nerve impulses and measures nerve conduction time	• Determining the severity and location of nerve entrapment to diagnose conditions, such as carpal tunnel syndrome or herniated disk • Diagnosing peripheral nervous system disorders such as polyneuropathies • Evaluating disorders of the muscles and motor neurons, such as amyotrophic lateral sclerosis and myasthenia gravis	• Explain to the patient that he'll experience discomfort during needle insertion. • Tell the patient that he'll be asked to flex and relax muscles during the procedure.	• Withhold medications, such as nonsteroidal anti-inflammatory drugs or pyridostigmine bromide before the test, as ordered. • Administer analgesics, as prescribed, after the test. • Check the needle insertion sites for bleeding and inflammation.

Test and description	Uses of test	Patient preparation	Nursing implications
Electrodiagnostic tests (continued)			
Evoked potential studies Electrodes on the skin and scalp to record electrical activity in the brain in response to sensory (visual, auditory, or somatosensory) stimulation	● Diagnosing multiple sclerosis ● Assessing hearing and vision, optic nerve disorders, and acoustic neuromas ● Detecting abnormalities affecting the brain and spinal cord such as neuropathies ● Determining brain death	● Have the patient wash his hair the night before the test but not to apply any conditioners, sprays, or gels. ● Tell the patient what to expect, based on the type of stimulus being used.	● Help the patient remove any electrode gel from his hair after the test.

Nursing implications in oncology care

Cancer is a group of diseases characterized by uncontrolled growth and spread of abnormal cells. In the United States, it's the second leading health problem and the cause of one of every four deaths.

Various risk factors for cancer have been identified:

- Tobacco is associated with cancers of the lung, mouth, tongue, upper airway, bladder, kidney, pancreas, and esophagus.
- Alcohol is associated with cancers of the mouth, pharynx, larynx, esophagus, and liver.
- Occupational exposure to carcinogens is associated with leukemia and cancers of the lung, skin, liver, bladder, nose, kidney, esophagus, and pancreas.
- Viruses are associated with cancers of the liver and cervix, Burkitt's lymphoma, Kaposi's sarcoma, and lymphoma.
- Radiation exposure is associated with leukemia, melanoma, and cancers of the lip, thyroid, lungs, breast, and digestive organs.
- Hormones are associated with endometrial and breast cancer.
- High-fat, low-fiber diet is associated with cancers of the colon, prostate, breast, esophagus, and stomach.

In patients with cancer, normal cells go through a multistage process of change. During initiation, they're exposed to factors that damage them, causing mutation of their genetic codes. There are at least 4 types of genes which, when damaged, cause a normal cell to behave abnormally. These are oncogenes, tumor supressor genes, suicide genes, and DNA-repair genes. During promotion, the mutated cells respond to additional factors that promote their growth. During invasion, continuous cellular division causes pressure and destruction of surrounding tissues by enzymes released from the cancer cells to promote the spread of disease. During metastasis, the cancer cells spread to other sites in the body that are far from the primary tumor site.

Tumors are classified as benign or malignant. In benign tumors, cells grow abnormally but don't metastasize or invade surrounding tissue. In malignant tumors, abnormal cells can spread, resulting in death for the host cells.

Cancers are anatomically staged using the TNM (tumor, node, metastasis) classification, which stages disease based on the size, penetration, and invasion of the primary tumor; the presence, extent, and location of regional node involvement; and the presence or absence of metastasis. Cancer also can be histologically graded as grade 1 (highly differentiated cells that resemble the tissue of origin most closely), 2 (intermediate differentiation), 3 (essentially undifferentiated cells), and 4 (highly undifferentiated, anaplastic cells). Patients with grade 4 disease have the poorest prognosis.

Cancer treatment has four goals:
- Cure by eradicating the cancer to ensure long-term survival
- Control by arresting tumor growth
- Palliation by alleviating symptoms when the disease is beyond control
- Prophylaxis by providing treatment when the patient is at increased risk for tumor development, spread, or recurrence.

Treatment may include surgery, radiation therapy, chemotherapy, bone marrow transplantation, biotherapy, or any combination of these options.

Surgery

For a patient with cancer, different types of surgery may be performed for different reasons.

Diagnostic surgery is used to diagnose specific types of cancer. Examples include laparotomy and incisional, excisional, aspiration, or needle biopsies.

Staging surgery determines the extent of the disease and the need for additional therapy. Examples include exploratory surgery, tumor delineation, and multiple biopsies.

Definitive and curative surgery removes as much of the tumor as possible. Examples include local excision of cancer in situ, cryosurgery, laser surgery, electrosurgery, and en bloc (in one piece) dissection.

Preventive and prophylactic surgery is performed on tissues or organs at high risk for developing subsequent cancer because of family history, congenital disposition, or underlying conditions. Examples include colectomy, orchiopexy, and oophorectomy.

Reconstructive surgery is used to repair anatomic defects and improve function and appearance after cancer surgery. Examples include ostomies, breast reconstruction, and prosthesis placement.

Palliative surgery promotes patient comfort and quality of life by relieving the symptoms of advanced disease. Examples include neurosurgical management of pain, removal of obstructive metastasis, and treatment of oncologic emergencies.

Surgery to insert a mechanical device is performed to facilitate treatment or patient comfort. Devices may be inserted to facilitate drug administration, collect blood samples, or implant radioactive substances.

Preoperative and postoperative care related to these types of surgery is similar to that for other types of surgery.

Radiation therapy

Radiation therapy is the use of high-energy radiation in doses large enough to eradicate disease but small enough to miminize adverse effects. Radiation rays cause one or both strands of the deoxyribonucleic acid (DNA) molecule to break, thereby preventing cellular division or replication. Rapidly dividing, well oxygenated, poorly differentiated cancer cells are most sensitive to the effects of radiation.

Various types of radiation therapy may be used. With external beam therapy, the radiation source is outside the body. With internal therapy (brachytherapy), the radiation source is placed directly on the body surface or near the body area to be irradiated. With interstitial therapy, the radiation source is implanted into the involved tissues. With systemic therapy, the radiation source is absorbed into the circulation and travels throughout the body.

For internal, interstitial, or systemic radiation, safety guidelines include following safety procedures based on the type, dose, method, and half-life of the radioisotope and minimizing exposure to radiation by maintaining a safe distance and placing shields between people and radioisotope devices.

Follow additional safety guidelines for interstitial radiation therapy with sealed (contained in seals, wires, or ribbons) or unsealed sources:
- Assign the patient to a private room, and mark the door with a radiation therapy safety sign.
- Assess the patient's self-care ability.
- Protect staff and the patient's family members from exposure to radiation by implementing time and distance restrictions, using shielding devices, and safely handling body fluids, depending on the sealed or unsealed status of the radiation source. Keep a safety container in the patient's room.
- Prevent dislodgment of implanted radiation devices. Check linens, bedpans, and other equipment for signs of a dislodged implant.
- If the implant becomes dislodged, contact the radiation therapy department.
- Provide reassurance that when the radiation source is gone, the patient is no longer radioactive.

Also follow additional safety guidelines for systemic radiation therapy:
- Wear protective gloves when handling the patient's radioactive body fluids or items that come in contact with the patient's body fluids.
- Use disposable food trays and eating utensils.
- Keep nondisposable items, linens, and other equipment in plastic bags in the patient's room to be scanned for radioactivity before removal.

Chemotherapy

Chemotherapy is the use of antineoplastics to destroy or retard cancer cell growth. Chemotherapeutic drugs affect normal and cancer cells by interfering with DNA synthesis or cellular function during the cell cycle. They have the greatest effect on rapidly dividing cells, such as those found in bone marrow, mucous membranes, and hair follicles. The guiding principle of chemotherapy is to administer agents in doses large enough to eradicate disease but small enough to minimize adverse effects and the damage to the normal cells.

Chemotherapeutic drugs are used as adjuvant therapy with either surgery or radiotherapy. Many classes of antineoplastics are used for chemotherapy. Alkylating agents are cell-cycle nonspecific drugs that cross-link and break DNA strands, causing cell death. They're used to treat leukemias, lymphomas, and myelomas. Examples include cyclophosphamide (Cytoxan), thiotepa (Thioplex), nitrogen mustard (Mustargen), chlorambucil (Leukeran), lomustine (CeeNU), carmustine (Gliadel Wafer), and cisplatin (Platinol), which is also classified as a heavy metal with alkylating properties.

Antimetabolite agents are cell-cycle specific for the S phase. They block or interfere with normal DNA or ribonucleic acid synthesis by competing for placement as a metabolite needed by the cell. They're used to treat leukemias, testicular and ovarian tumors, lymphomas, sarcomas, and lung and breast cancers. Examples include methotrexate (Trexall), cytosine arabinoside (Cytosar-U), and 5-fluorouracil (Adrucil).

Antibiotics are cell-cycle nonspecific drugs that interfere with DNA synthesis by inserting a compound between the DNA helix strands. They're used to treat Wilms' tumor, neuroblastoma, lymphomas, ovarian and testicular cancers, and breast cancer. Examples include doxorubicin (Adriamycin), bleomycin (Blenoxane), plicamycin (Mithracin), and daunorubicin (Cerubidine).

Vinca or plant alkaloids are cell-cycle specific for the M phase. They block cell division by inhibiting spindle formation during mitosis. They're used to treat leukemia, Hodgkin's disease, non-Hodgkin's lymphoma, neuroblastoma, Wilms' tumor, and cancers of the lung, breast, and testes. Examples include vincristine (Oncovin), vinblastine (Velban), and etoposide (VePesid).

Topoisomerase I inhibitors cause DNA damage during DNA synthesis. They're used to treat colorectal cancer, metastatic ovarian cancer, and small cell lung cancer. Examples include irinotecan (Camptosar) and topotecan (Hyramtin).

Steroids and hormones, which are used in combination with other drugs, alter the environment that bathes the cell. They're used to treat leukemias, lymphomas, and reproductive organ tumors. Examples include prednisone (Deltasone), estrogen, progestin, and the anti-estrogen tamoxifen (Nolvadex).

Miscellaneous antineoplastics are also available; paclitaxel (Taxol), for example, inhibits microtubular function and is used to treat metastatic breast and ovarian cancer.

Follow these safety guidelines when preparing, administering, or disposing of chemotherapeutic drugs:

● Prepare drugs under a laminar hood to prevent air from flowing into your face (usually prepared by a pharmacist).

● Wear two pair of latex gloves and a cuffed gown when mixing drugs.

● Wash hands before putting gloves on and after removing gloves.

● Don't eat, drink, smoke, or chew gum in the drug preparation area.

● If a chemotherapeutic drug touches the skin, wash the area thoroughly with nonabrasive soap and water as soon as possible.

● If a chemotherapeutic drug touches the eye, flood the eye immediately with clear water or eyewash and seek medical attention.

● Use spill kits for large spills on work areas or the floor.

● Don't store food or drink with chemotherapeutic drugs.

● Wash hands before and after administering drugs and wear gloves.

● Don't dispose of materials by clipping needles, breaking syringes, or removing needles from syringes.

● Use needles, syringes, tubing, and connectors with luer-lock attachments.

● Use gauze pads when removing chemotherapy syringes and needles from injection ports or spikes from I.V. bags.

● Use an absorbent pad under the injection site to contain spillage.

● Avoid hand-to-eye and hand-to-mouth contact when handling chemotherapeutic drugs or contaminated body fluids.

● Dispose of equipment used to administer chemotherapeutic drugs in accordance with the regulations governing disposal of toxic and chemical wastes.

Bone marrow transplantation

Although bone marrow transplantation is a complex treatment with a high potential for severe complications, it has become a viable option for many patients with various malignant disorders. Bone marrow transplantation may be considered for patients with disorders, such as leukemia, lymphoma, multiple myeloma, neuroblastoma, metastatic breast cancer, ovarian cancer, and small cell lung cancer.

Before transplantation, the patient receives high and potentially lethal doses of radiation and chemotherapy that produce an immunosuppressed state and damage and destroy the patient's bone marrow, creating space for replacement with healthy donor marrow. There are three types of donor marrow:

1. Autologous donor marrow, the most commonly transplanted type, is harvested from the recipient during disease remission, processed, and kept in frozen storage to be reinfused at a later date. Peripheral blood stem cells can be similarly harvested by leukopheresis and are then processed and stored for later use.

2. Allogenic donor marrow is harvested from a relative or a person with similar human leukocyte antigen tissue type.

3. Synergic donor marrow is harvested from an identical twin.

The donor marrow is usually infused 48 to 72 hours after the last dose of radiation or chemotherapy. Potential immediate adverse reactions include allergic response (urticaria, chills, fever), fluid overload, and pulmonary system response to fat emboli. Potential complications include infection, hemorrhage, liver veno-occlusive disease, renal insufficiency, GI disturbances, multiple organ dysfunction syndrome, and graft-versus-host disease.

Nursing implications for care are based on the care plan for any severely immunosuppressed patient and include:

● prevention of exposure to nosocomial infections posttransplantation (strict aseptic techniques must be maintained.)

● recognition of early signs of posttransplantation complications and graft rejection (Early treatment may reverse the rejection process.)

● provision of extensive patient and family teaching before and after transplantation

● recognition of the critical patient's and his family's need for emotional support during the transplantation process.

Biotherapy

Biotherapy stimulates and enhances the body's immune response against tumor cells. Biotherapeutic drugs include bacillus Calmette-Guérin vaccine, human tumor antigens, monoclocal antibodies, interferon, and growth factors.

Many biological response modifiers (BRMs) have been approved by the FDA since the mid-1980's.

The following BRMs have experienced success in treating select cancers:

● Interferon is a protein that regulates the immune response and has antiviral and antiproliferative characteristics at the cellular level. Interferon alfa-Za (Roferon-A) is used to treat hairy cell leukemia and chronic myelogenous leukemia. Interferon alfa-2b (Intren A) also treats hairy cell leukemia plus malignant melanoma and follicular lymphoma

- Interleukins are produced by leukocytes to promote hematopoiesis. Interleukin-2 (Proleukin) treats metastatic melanomas and renal-cell cancers. Interleukin-II (Neumega) prevents or treats thrombocytopenia in non-myeloid cancers.
- Monoclonal antibodies may be tagged with radioisotopes for diagnostic testing or to kill target cancer cells; tositumomab (Bexxar) is used to treat B-cell lymphoma. Other monoclonal antibodies suppress autoimmune destruction of transplants or inhibit malignant cells (without radioactivity), such as ritoximab (Rituxan) for non-Hodgkin's lymphoma, cetuximab (Erbitux) for metastatic colorectal cancer, and trastuzumab (Herceptin) for breast cancer.
- Colony-stimulating factors occur naturally in the body and mediate hematopoiesis. Filgrastim (Neupogen) and Saragramostim (Leukine) are commonly used to stimulate white blood cell production; epoetin alfa (Epogen) is used to stimulate red blood cell production.

Many adverse effects are associated with these treatments. Nursing implications include:

- familiarity with potential adverse effects and complications of BRMs
- careful monitoring and documentation of patient response to treatment
- extensive patient and family teaching

Cancer-related problems

Various problems can result from cancer treatment or from the disease itself. To provide quality care, see the chart below for common cancer-related problems and their nursing implications.

Cancer-related problem	Nursing implications
Alopecia To the patient, alopecia may be the most distressing adverse reaction. If caused by chemotherapy, alopecia is temporary. Radiation-induced alopecia, however, may be permanent.	• Prepare the patient for alopecia. Inform the patient that hair loss is usually gradual and may be reversible after treatment ends. • Inform the patient that alopecia may be partial or complete and that it affects men and women. • Inform the patient that alopecia may affect the scalp, eyebrows, eyelashes, and body hair. • Discuss ways to improve self-image—for example, by using wigs, hats, cosmetics, and scarves.
Anemia Anemia can develop slowly over several courses of treatment or may be due to the disease.	• Assess the patient for dizziness, fatigue, pallor, and shortness of breath on minimal exertion. • Monitor the patient's hematocrit, hemoglobin level, and red blood cell count. Remember that a patient dehydrated from nausea, vomiting, or anorexia may exhibit a false-normal hematocrit. After this patient is rehydrated, the hematocrit will decrease. • Be prepared to administer a blood transfusion to a symptomatic patient, as prescribed. • Instruct the patient to rest frequently and to increase his dietary intake of iron-rich foods. Advise the patient to take a multivitamin with iron as prescribed.
Bone marrow suppression Bone marrow suppression is the most common and potentially serious adverse reaction to antineoplastics.	• Watch for the blood count nadir because that's when the patient is at greatest risk for the complications of leukopenia, thrombocytopenia, and anemia. • Plan a patient-teaching program about bone marrow suppression, including information about blood counts, potential infection sites, personal hygiene, and measures to take to prevent unnecessary exposure. • Place patient on neutropenic precautions per institution policy.

Cancer-related problem	Nursing implications
Constipation Constipation is common in patients with colon cancer; it may indicate neurotoxicity caused by chemotherapy, or it may be caused by narcotic pain control.	● Assess the patient for bowel sounds, abdominal distention or pain, and fecal impaction. ● Encourage fluid intake of 3 qt (2.8 L) daily unless contraindicated. ● Modify the diet to include more fiber. ● Administer a laxative, stool softener, enema, or suppository, as prescribed. ● Monitor amount and number of stools
Depression Depression is described as a persistent, sad, or dysphoric mood.	● Assess the patient's psychosocial status. ● Encourage the patient to verbalize his concerns and needs. ● Offer to refer the patient to a cancer care counselor. ● Administer antidepressants, as prescribed.
Diarrhea A common reaction to chemotherapy and radiation therapy, diarrhea can cause fluid and electrolyte imbalances if severe.	● Monitor fluid intake and output. ● Assess the patient for signs of dehydration and electrolyte imbalances. ● Assess the patient for bowel sounds, abdominal cramps, and rectal irritation. ● Obtain stool cultures as prescribed. ● Administer an antidiarrheal as prescribed. ● Provide good perianal hygiene. ● Encourage fluid intake, and modify the diet as needed.
Dyspnea Dyspnea may result from lung cancer and is typically described as shortness of breath but also refers to difficult or uncomfortable breathing.	● Assess the patient's breath sounds and pulse oximetry and for peripheral edema. ● Provide oxygen therapy if saturation levels fall below 92%, as ordered. ● Encourage the patient to pace activities with rest periods and assist with daily activities as needed. ● Administer respiratory therapy as prescribed.
Fatigue Fatigue is a general feeling of physical or emotional exhaustion and lack of energy that may result from anemia, decreased nutritional intake, or increased cell destruction by treatment.	● Assess the patient's inability to sleep or rest and level of fatigue. ● Assess the patient for signs of increased metabolic processes, such as fever and disease progression. ● Assist the patient with daily activities. ● Minimize physical fatigue by pacing activities and allowing adequate time for sleep and rest. ● Help the patient examine coping strategies.
Leukopenia Leukopenia increases the patient's risk of infection, especially if the granulocyte count is under 1,000/μl.	● Provide information about good hygiene, and assess the patient frequently for signs and symptoms of infection. ● Teach the patient to recognize and report the signs and symptoms of infection, such as fever, cough, sore throat, or a burning sensation on urination. ● Teach the patient how and when to take his temperature. ● Caution the patient to avoid crowds and people with colds or the flu during the nadir. ● Remember that the inflammatory response may be decreased and the complications of leukopenia more difficult to detect if the patient is receiving a corticosteroid. ● Administer colony-stimulating factors, as prescribed.
Nausea and vomiting Nausea and vomiting can result from gastric mucosal irritation, chemical irritation of the central nervous system, or psychogenic factors that may be activated by sensations, suggestions, or anxiety related to chemotherapy.	● Control the chemical irritation by administering combinations of antiemetics as prescribed. ● Monitor the patient for signs and symptoms of aspiration because most antiemetics sedate. ● Control psychogenic factors by helping the patient perform relaxation techniques before chemotherapy to minimize feelings of isolation and anxiety. ● Encourage the patient to express feelings of anxiety. ● Encourage the patient to listen to music or to engage in relaxation exercises, meditation, or hypnosis to promote feelings of control and well-being. ● Adjust the drug administration time to meet the patient's needs. Some patients prefer treatments in the evening when they find sedation comfortable. Patients who are employed may prefer their treatments on their days off.

Cancer-related problem	Nursing implications
Sexual dysfunction Sexual dysfunction is a physical or emotional inability to express oneself sexually that can result from treatment or the disease.	• Assess the patient for sexual concerns related to fatigue, anemia, nausea, vomiting, or body image. • If the patient is male, assess him for impotence; if the patient is female, menstrual problems. • Give the patient information about the disease's effects and treatment. • Discuss specific measures to help the patient adapt to sexuality changes, such as using different positions and lubrication. • Advise the patient that contraception is advisable during chemotherapy (or radiation therapy) to prevent birth defects from chromosomal damage. • Allow the partner to visit the patient in private. • Refer the patient to counselors or support groups, as needed.
Stomatitis Although epithelial tissue damage can affect any mucous membrane, the most common site is the oral mucosa. Stomatitis is temporary and can range from mild and barely noticeable to severe and debilitating. (Debilitation may result from poor nutrition during acute stomatitis.)	• Initiate preventive mouth care before chemotherapy to provide comfort and decrease the severity of the stomatitis. • Provide therapeutic mouth care, including topical antibiotics, if prescribed, and cessation of mouthwash use. • Encourage use of oral anesthetics before meals and/or pain medication, if prescribed. • Assess need for diet change or alternate form of nutrition (tube feedings, TPN).
Thrombocytopenia Thrombocytopenia may occur with leukopenia. When the platelet count is under 50,000/µl the patient is at risk for bleeding. When it's under 20,000/µl, the patient is at severe risk and may require a platelet transfusion.	• Assess the patient for bleeding gums, increased bruising or petechiae, hypermenorrhea, tarry stools, hematuria, and coffee-ground vomitus. • Advise the patient to avoid cuts and bruises and to use a soft toothbrush and an electric razor. • Instruct the patient to report sudden headaches, which could indicate potentially fatal intracranial bleeding. • Instruct the patient to use a stool softener, as prescribed, to prevent colonic irritation and bleeding. • Instruct the patient to avoid using a rectal thermometer and receiving I.M. injections to prevent bleeding.

Nursing implications in clinical pharmacology

The following chart identifies drugs by class and summarizes their indications, contraindications, adverse reactions, and nursing implications.

Common drugs	Indications	Contraindications	Adverse reactions	Nursing implications
Drugs that affect the autonomic nervous system				
Cholinergics (parasympathomimetics)				
ambenonium (Myte-lase); bethanechol (Urecholine), carbachol (Isopto Carbachol), edrophonium (Tensilon), neostigmine (Prostigmin), pilocarpine (Isopto Carpine), pyridostigmine (Mestinon, Regonol)	• Glaucoma (carbachol, pilocarpine) • Nonobstructive urine retention (bethanechol) • Neurogenic bladder (bethanechol) • Abdominal distention and ileus (bethanechol) • Myasthenia gravis (ambenonium, edrophonium, neostigmine, pyridostigmine)	• Potential GI or urinary obstruction • Enlarged prostate	• Nausea, vomiting, and diarrhea • Headache • Hypotension • Muscle weakness • Increased bronchial secretions, salivation, and sweating • Bradycardia • Abdominal cramping • Respiratory depression	• Monitor the patient's GI and urinary status. • Monitor vital signs. • Administer atropine as an antidote. • Determine what other drugs the patient is taking. Use of another cholinergic increases the risk of cholinergic crisis; use of an anticholinergic may inhibit the effects of the cholinergic.
Anticholinergics (parasympatholytics, cholinergic blockers)				
atropine, benztropine mesylate (Cogentin), dicyclomine (Bentyl), glycopyrrolate (Robinul), meclizine (Antivert) propantheline (Pro-Banthine), scopolamine (Transderm-Scōp), trihexyphenidyl (Artane)	• Bradycardia (atropine) • Decrease saliva and bronchial secretions preoperatively (atropine, scopolamine, glycopyrrolate) • Parkinsonism (benztropine, trihexyphenidyl) • Motion sickness (scopolamine) • Peptic ulcer or bowel spasm (propantheline, dicyclomine) • Produce mydriasis (atropine)	• Angle-closure glaucoma • Hemorrhage, tachycardia, and GI or urinary obstruction	• Dry mouth and difficulty swallowing • Photophobia, blurred vision, and dizziness • Constipation • Urinary retention	• Assess mucous membranes for dryness. • Tell the patient to report blurred vision and dizziness; if these symptoms are present, help the patient with daily activities to prevent injury. • Report sudden eye pain to the physician, and withhold next dose.

Common drugs	Indications	Contraindications	Adverse reactions	Nursing implications

Drugs that affect the autonomic nervous system *(continued)*

Adrenergics (sympathomimetics)

Common drugs	Indications	Contraindications	Adverse reactions	Nursing implications
albuterol (Proventil), dobutamine (Dobutrex), dopamine (Intropin), ephedrine (Pretz-D), epinephrine (Adrenalin, EpiPen Auto-Injector), isoetharine (Bronkosol), isoproterenol (Isuprel), metaproterenol (Alupent), norepinephrine (Levophed), phenylephrine (Neo-Synephrine), pseudoephedrine (Sudafed), salmeterol (Serevent)	• Bronchodilation (albuterol, isoproterenol) • Cardiac stimulation (epinephrine, dobutamine) • Hypotension (dopamine, norepinephrine) • Enhance renal perfusion (dopamine) • Allergic reactions (epinephrine) • Nasal congestion (ephedrine)	• Angle-closure glaucoma • Tachyarrhythmias	• Arrhythmias, tachycardia, and hypertension • Nervousness and restlessness • Hypotension	• Monitor vital signs, breath sounds, and electrocardiogram (ECG) results. • Measure output to detect adequate renal perfusion.

Adrenergic blockers (sympatholytics)

Common drugs	Indications	Contraindications	Adverse reactions	Nursing implications
Alpha-adrenergic blockers: ergotamine (Cafergot), phentolamine (Regitine) *Beta-adrenergic blockers:* atenolol (Tenormin), metoprolol (Lopressor), nadolol (Corgard), propranolol (Inderal), timolol (Blocadren)	• *Alpha-adrenergic blockers:* hypertension from pheochromocytoma (phentolamine), vascular headaches (ergotamine) • *Beta-adrenergic blockers:* hypertension (atenolol, propranolol, timolol), angina (atenolol, propranolol), arrhythmias (propranolol), vascular headache (propranolol), glaucoma (timolol)	• *Alpha-adrenergic blockers:* myocardial infarction (MI) and pregnancy • *Beta-adrenergic blockers:* heart failure (with caution), heart block, and bronchospasm	• *Alpha-adrenergic blockers:* cardiac arrhythmias, hypotension, and tachycardia • *Beta-adrenergic blockers:* bradycardia, dizziness, vertigo, and bronchospasm	• Monitor vital signs, especially blood pressure. • Monitor circulatory status.

Neuromuscular blockers

Common drugs	Indications	Contraindications	Adverse reactions	Nursing implications
atracurium (Tracrium), pancuronium (Pavulon), succinylcholine (Anectine), tubocurarine, vecuronium (Norcuron)	• Relax skeletal muscles during surgery (succinylcholine) • Reduce muscle spasm during induced seizures (tubocurarine) • Manage ventilator-dependent patients (pancuronium) • Facilitate intubation (atracurium)	• Hypersensitivity • Malignant hypertension	• Excessive bronchial secretions, respiratory depression, and bronchospasm • Malignant hyperthermia	• Protect the patient's airway. • Assess the patient's level of pain. • Monitor vital signs.

Common drugs	Indications	Contraindications	Adverse reactions	Nursing implications

Analgesics and opioids

Opioid analgesics

buprenorphine (Buprenex), codeine, fentanyl (Duragesic, Sublimaze), hydromorphone (Dilaudid), meperidine (Demerol), morphine (Duramorph, MS Contin), oxycodone (OxyContin, Percodan, Percocet), pentazocine (Talwin), propoxyphene (Darvon,Darvocet)	• Moderate to severe pain • Anesthesia adjunct (meperidine, morphine) • Acute pulmonary edema (morphine) • Cough (codeine) • Acute MI (morphine)	• Central nervous system (CNS) depression • Respiratory depression • Acute alcohol withdrawal • Liver disease, respiratory problems, and renal disease (use with caution)	• Respiratory depression • Orthostatic hypotension • Dizziness, ataxia, drowsiness, and euphoria • Tolerance • Physical and psychological dependence	• Assess the patient's level of pain and the effectiveness of pain relief measures. • Administer the drug before pain is severe. • Monitor respiratory status and blood pressure. • Assess bowel function; continued use of opioid agents can cause severe constipation.

Opioid antagonists

nalmefene (Revex), naloxone (Narcan), naltrexone (ReVia)	• CNS depression in opioid overdose • Respiratory depression in opioid overdose • Opioid detoxification in a former addict	• Opioid dependence (use with caution); acute withdrawal symptoms may develop • Cardiac irritability (use with caution)	• Hypotension and hypertension	• Monitor vital signs, respiratory status, and level of consciousness until the effects of the opioid have worn off. • Assess the patient's level of pain. • Protect the patient's airway.

Nonopioid analgesics and antipyretics

acetaminophen (Tylenol), acetylsalicylic acid (aspirin), phenazopyridine (Pyridium)	• Mild to moderate musculoskeletal or nerve pain (acetaminophen, aspirin) • Fever (acetaminophen, aspirin) • Inflammation (aspirin) • Arthritis (aspirin) • Urinary tract pain (phenazopyridine)	• Pregnancy (except acetaminophen) • Bleeding disorders and ulcers (aspirin) • Chickenpox (danger of Reye's syndrome with aspirin)	• GI upset and heartburn • Prolonged bleeding time (aspirin)	• Assess the patient's level of pain and the effectiveness of pain relief measures. • Administer the drug before meals for optimal effect or with meals to alleviate GI symptoms.

Nonsteroidal anti-inflammatory drugs (NSAIDs)

celecoxib (Celebrex), diclofenac (Voltaren), fenoprofen (Nalfon), ibuprofen (Advil, Motrin), ketorolac (Toradol), meclofenamate (Meclomen), naproxen (Aleve, Naprosyn), piroxicam (Feldene), sulindac (Clinoril), tolmetin (Tolectin)	• Inflammation associated with arthritis, gout, bursitis, and other inflammatory disorders • Pain associated with general aches • Fever	• Bleeding disorders (use with caution) • Ulcers and GI problems (use with caution) • Hypersensitivity to sulfonamides (celecoxib)	• GI bleeding, nausea, and vomiting • Prolonged bleeding time	• Assess the patient's level of pain and the effectiveness of pain relief measures. • Assess the patient for GI symptoms.

Common drugs	Indications	Contraindications	Adverse reactions	Nursing implications
Drugs that affect the central nervous system				
CNS stimulants				
amphetamine (Adderall, Biphetamine), caffeine (Vivarin), dextroamphetamine (Dexedrine), methamphetamine (Desoxyn), methylphenidate (Ritalin), pemoline (Cylert)	● Narcolepsy (amphetamine, methylphenidate, pemoline) ● Attention deficit hyperactivity disorder (methamphetamine, methylphenidate, pemoline) ● Appetite control (amphetamine, caffeine, dextroamphetamine, methamphetamine)	● Hypertension, angina, or cardiovascular disease ● Glaucoma ● Hyperthyroidism ● History of drug abuse	● Insomnia, restlessness, and irritability ● Hypotension and tachycardia ● Drug dependence and tolerance	● Tell the patient to avoid caffeine-containing drinks. ● Monitor blood pressure. ● Monitor weight.
Anticonvulsants				
Barbiturates: phenobarbital (Luminal), primidone (Mysoline) *Benzodiazepines:* clonazepam (Klonopin), diazepam (Valium), lorazepam (Ativan) *Hydantoins:* mephenytoin (Mesantoin), phenytoin (Dilantin), fosphenytoin (Cerebyx) *Succinimides:* ethosuximide (Zarontin), methsuximide (Celontin) *Other:* carbamazepine (Tegretol), lamotrigine (Lamictal), levetiracetam (Keppra), oxcarbazepine (Trileptal) valproic acid (Depakene)	● Generalized tonic-clonic seizures (barbiturates, hydantoins, carbamazepine) ● Partial seizures (barbiturates, hydantoins, carbamazepine, lamotrigine, levetiracetam, oxcarbazepine) ● Absence seizures (benzodiazepines, succinimides, valproic acid) ● Status epilepticus (benzodiazepines)	● Hypersensitivity ● Bone marrow suppression ● Blood dyscrasias	● Drowsiness, ataxia, sedation, and dizziness ● Leukopenia ● Gingival hyperplasia (hydantoins)	● Assess seizure activity. ● Administer the drug with food to decrease GI upset. ● Don't administer the drug with milk or antacids, which can interfere with absorption. ● Assess oral mucous membranes, particularly noting gum hyperplasia. ● Monitor serum levels.
Antiparkinsonians				
amantadine (Symmetrel), bromocriptine mesylate (Parlodel), carbidopa-levodopa (Sinemet), levodopa (Dopar, Larodopa), pergolide (Permax), ropinirole (Requip), selegiline (Carbex, Eldepryl)	● Parkinson's disease (increase levels of dopamine) ● Drug-induced extrapyramidal symptoms (amantadine) ● Antiviral (amantadine)	● Angle-closure glaucoma ● Cardiac disease and pyloric obstruction (use with caution)	● Nausea and vomiting ● Orthostatic hypotension ● Involuntary body movements	● Supervise the patient's activity when drug therapy is started. ● Tell the patient to get up slowly to prevent orthostatic hypotension. ● Be aware that some anticholinergics, such as trihexyphenidyl and benztropine, may also be used to treat Parkinson's disease.

Common drugs	Indications	Contraindications	Adverse reactions	Nursing implications

Drugs that affect the central nervous system *(continued)*

Sedatives, hypnotics, and anxiolytics

Common drugs	Indications	Contraindications	Adverse reactions	Nursing implications
Antihistamines: diphenhydramine (Benadryl), hydroxyzine (Atarax, Vistaril), promethazine (Phenergan) *Barbiturates:* pentobarbital (Nembutal), phenobarbital (Luminal), secobarbital (Seconal) *Other:* chloral hydrate (Aquachloral, Noctec), paraldehyde (Paral)	• Anxiety (hydroxyzine) • Insomnia (diphenhydramine, barbiturates, chloral hydrate) • Sedation (promethazine, barbiturates, chloral hydrate)	• Preexisting CNS depression • Respiratory depression • History of drug abuse	• Drowsiness, dizziness, and confusion • Decreased blood pressure and pulse rate	• Assess the patient's mental status. • Be aware that the effects of these drugs are potentiated by alcohol and other sedatives, hypnotics, or anxiolytics. • Keep in mind that barbiturates decrease the effectiveness of warfarin (Coumadin) and oral contraceptives.

Antidepressants

Common drugs	Indications	Contraindications	Adverse reactions	Nursing implications
Selective serotonin-reuptake inhibitors (SSRIs): citalopram (Celexa), escitalopram (Lexapro), fluoxetine (Prozac), paroxetine (Paxil), sertraline (Zoloft) *Tricyclics:* amitriptyline (Elavil), imipramine (Tofranil), nortriptyline (Pamelor) *Other:* venlafaxine (Effexor)	• Clinical depression • Obsessive-compulsive disorder (fluoxetine, paroxetine, sertraline) • Panic disorder (SSRIs, venlafaxine)	• Hypotension (tricyclics) • Cardiovascular disease (tricyclics) • Use of monoamine oxidase inhibitors (SSRIs) in combination or within 14 days of use	• Cardiac adverse effects (tricyclics) • Anticholinergic effects (tricyclics) • GI irritation (SSRIs) • Nervousness and insomnia (SSRIs) • Hypertension (venlafaxine)	• Monitor the patient carefully for adverse reactions, which may occur before therapeutic effect, which takes 2 to 4 weeks. • Monitor the patient taking SSRIs for nervousness and insomnia.

Drugs that affect the cardiovascular system

Antianginals

Common drugs	Indications	Contraindications	Adverse reactions	Nursing implications
Beta-adrenergic blockers (see page 360) *Calcium channel blockers:* amlodipine (Norvasc), diltiazem (Cardizem), nicardipine (Cardene), nifedipine (Procardia), verapamil (Isoptin) *Nitrates:* isosorbide dinitrate (Isordil), isosorbide mononitrate (IMDUR, ISMO), nitroglycerin (Nitro-Bid, Nitro-Dur, Transderm-Nitro)	• Chest pain caused by ischemia of the coronary arteries • Decrease the heart's workload and reduce the need for oxygen	• Uncontrolled hypotension or hypertension • Heart failure or heart block	• Headache • Hypotension • Flushing	• Assess anginal pain before, during, and after administration of nitroglycerin. • Be aware that the patient should avoid using these agents during the night to prevent drug tolerance. • Monitor pulse rate and blood pressure before administering antianginals. • Treat headache (a common adverse reaction) with mild analgesics.

Common drugs	Indications	Contraindications	Adverse reactions	Nursing implications

Drugs that affect the cardiovascular system *(continued)*

Antiarrhythmics

Class IA (sodium channel blockers): disopyramide (Norpace), moricizine (Ethmozine), procainamide (Procan SR), quinidine gluconate (Quinaglute) *Class IB (sodium channel blockers):* lidocaine (Xylocaine), mexiletine (Mexitil), phenytoin (Dilantin), tocainide (Tonocard) *Class IC (sodium channel blockers):* flecainide (Tambocor), propafenone (Rythmol) *Class II (beta-adrenergic blockers):* atenolol (Tenormin), metoprolol (Lopressor), propranolol (Inderal) *Class III:* amiodarone (Cordarone), bretylium (Bretylol) *Class IV (calcium channel blockers):* diltiazem (Cardizem), verapamil (Calan)	● Cardiac arrhythmias, specifically, atrial fibrillation, premature ventricular contractions, ventricular tachycardia and fibrillation, and supraventricular tachycardia ● Promote normal sinus rhythm with regular ventricular response	● Heart block ● Heart failure ● Sinus bradycardia	● Nausea ● Hypotension ● Dyspnea ● Heart failure, heart block, and new arrhythmias	● Monitor vital signs and ECG results. ● Monitor oxygenation status. ● Educate the patient about the importance of taking these medications at regularly scheduled times. ● Teach the patient and his family how to monitor pulse rate and blood pressure.

Antihypertensives

Angiotensin-converting enzyme inhibitors: captopril (Capoten), enalapril (Vasotec) *Beta-adrenergic blockers:* atenolol (Tenormin), metoprolol (Lopressor), nadolol (Corgard), propranolol (Inderal) *Calcium channel blockers:* diltiazem (Cardizem), nicardipine (Cardene), nifedipine (Procardia), verapamil (Isoptin) *Central-acting adrenergic inhibitors:* clonidine (Catapres), methyldopa (Aldomet) *Diuretics:* (see page 365) *Peripheral-acting adrenergic inhibitors:* guanethidine sulfate (Ismelin), reserpine (Serpasil)	● Hypertension	● Heart failure ● Bradycardia ● Hypotension	*Life-threatening* ● Hemolytic anemia ● Hepatic necrosis ● Leukopenia *Commonly seen* ● Dry mouth ● Drowsiness ● Dizziness ● Impotence ● Nasal congestion ● Nausea ● Orthostatic hypotension ● Skin rash	● Assess blood pressure before administering the drug. ● Monitor pulse rate and blood pressure. ● Assess the patient for orthostatic hypotension; supervise ambulation if orthostatic hypotension occurs. ● Monitor daily weight and intake and output.

Common drugs	Indications	Contraindications	Adverse reactions	Nursing implications

Drugs that affect the cardiovascular system *(continued)*

Antihypertensives *(continued)*

Common drugs	Indications	Contraindications	Adverse reactions	Nursing implications
Peripheral vasodilators: diazoxide (Hyperstat), hydralazine (Apresoline), nitroprusside sodium (Nipride), prazosin (Minipress), terazosin (Hytrin)				

Antilipemics

Common drugs	Indications	Contraindications	Adverse reactions	Nursing implications
atorvastatin (Lipitor), cholestyramine (Questran), colestipol (Colestid), ezemtimibe (Zetia), fluvastatin (Lescol), lovastatin (Mevacor), niacin (Nicobid), pravastatin (Pravachol), rosuvastatin (Crestor), simvastatin (Zocor)	● Reduce serum lipid levels when dietary measures haven't been successful ● Primary prevention of cardiac events (atorvastatin, fluvastatin, lovastatin, pravastatin, rosuvastatin, simvastatin)	● Fat-soluble vitamin deficiency ● Severe constipation or bowel obstruction ● History of GI disorders and impaired liver function (use with caution)	● Abdominal discomfort ● Diarrhea ● Nausea and vomiting (cholestyramine, colestipol) ● Muscle pain ● Increased liver enzyme levels (atorvastatin, ezemtimibe, fluvastatin, lovastatin, pravastatin, rosuvastatin, simvastatin) ● Constipation (cholestyramine)	● Assess the patient's dietary habits. ● Monitor bowel elimination patterns, and document changes. ● Report changes in GI status. ● Teach the patient and his family how to reduce other risks of cardiac disease.

Cardiac glycoside

Common drugs	Indications	Contraindications	Adverse reactions	Nursing implications
digoxin (Lanoxin)	● Heart failure ● Atrial tachyarrhythmias (to control ventricular rate)	● Uncontrolled ventricular arrhythmias ● Complete heart block ● MI, cardiac myopathy, and renal impairment (use with caution)	● Nausea and vomiting ● Bradycardia ● Hypotension ● Weakness and fatigue	● Monitor the apical pulse before administering the drug. ● Check for signs and symptoms of toxic reaction (anorexia, nausea, vomiting, fatigue, weakness, and bradycardia). ● Monitor electrolyte levels (imbalances increase the potential for toxic reaction, especially hypokalemia).

Diuretics

Common drugs	Indications	Contraindications	Adverse reactions	Nursing implications
Carbonic anhydrase inhibitors: acetazolamide (Diamox) *Loop diuretics:* bumetanide (Bumex), ethacrynic acid (Edecrin), furosemide (Lasix) *Osmotic diuretics:* mannitol (Osmitrol), urea (Ureaphil) *Potassium-sparing diuretics:* spironolactone (Aldactone), triamterene (Dyrenium)	● Heart failure, edema, and hypertension ● Cerebral edema (mannitol) ● Glaucoma (acetazolamide, mannitol)	● Hypotension ● Kidney failure (anuria) ● Hypovolemia ● Hypokalemia (for non-potassium-sparing diuretics)	● Dehydration ● Hypotension and orthostatic hypotension ● Electrolyte imbalances ● Hypokalemia ● Arrhythmias ● Muscle cramps ● Photosensitivity	● Monitor weight, fluid balance, blood pressure, and electrolyte levels. ● Assess the patient for signs of fluid overload. ● Administer diuretics at times that don't disturb the patient's sleep. ● Review drug interactions, especially those involving digoxin and lithium.

Common drugs	Indications	Contraindications	Adverse reactions	Nursing implications

Drugs that affect the cardiovascular system *(continued)*

Diuretics (continued)

Common drugs	Indications	Contraindications	Adverse reactions	Nursing implications
Thiazide diuretics: chlorothiazide (Diuril), chlorthalidone (Hygroton), hydrochlorothiazide (HydroDIURIL, Oretic), indapamide (Lozol)				• Be aware that hypokalemia can lead to arrhythmias, muscle cramps, and digoxin toxicity. • Keep in mind that lithium excretion is decreased with concomitant use of loop, potassium-sparing, or thiazide diuretics; this can cause lithium toxicity. • Teach the patient about diet restrictions.

Anticoagulants and thrombolytics

Common drugs	Indications	Contraindications	Adverse reactions	Nursing implications
Anticoagulants: dalteparin (Fragmin), enoxaparin (Lovenox), heparin, warfarin (Coumadin) *Thrombolytics:* alteplase (Activase), anistreplase (Eminase), streptokinase (Streptase)	• Treat and prevent clotting disorders, such as deep vein thrombosis, phlebitis, pulmonary embolus, peripheral vascular disease, and disorders arising from prolonged bed rest (anticoagulants) • Used in emergent situations, such as dissolving clots in coronary arteries, pulmonary arteries, and deep veins and preventing the extension of MI (thrombolytics)	• Bleeding or coagulation disorders • Active bleeding and blood dyscrasias • Active ulcer disease • Cancer	• Bleeding and thrombocytopenia • Potentially severe allergic responses (thrombolytics)	• Monitor partial thromboplastin time (heparin) and prothrombin time (warfarin). • Monitor the patient for signs and symptoms of bleeding (such as bleeding gums or presence of blood in stool). • Reduce the number of punctures; apply pressure to puncture sites. Make sure thrombolytics are administered only in settings in which the patient can be closely monitored. • If the patient is taking dalteparin and enoxaparin, educate him about subcutaneous drug administration. • Educate the patient and his family about necessary precautions when taking anticoagulants, such as using a soft toothbrush and an electric razor, returning for routine laboratory tests, avoiding aspirin and ibuprofen, and informing other physicians and dentists about anticoagulant therapy.

Common drugs	Indications	Contraindications	Adverse reactions	Nursing implications

Drugs that affect the cardiovascular system *(continued)*

Antianemics

Iron products: ferrous gluconate (Fergon), ferrous sulfate (Feosol), iron dextran (DexFerrum, InFeD) *Vitamins:* cyanocobalamin (vitamin B12), folic acid (Folvite) *Other:* darbepoetin alfa (Aranesp), epoetin alfa (Epogen, Procrit)	● Iron deficiency anemia (iron products) ● Pernicious anemia and vitamin B12 deficiency (cyanocobalamin) ● Folic acid deficiency (folic acid) ● Anemia of chronic disease (epoetin alfa, darbepoetin alfa)	● Don't administer until type of anemia has been diagnosed ● GI disturbances	● Constipation, diarrhea, dark stools, GI upset, and staining at the injection site of I.M. preparations (iron products) ● Allergic reactions and peripheral vascular thrombosis with cyanocobalamin ● Hyperkalemia, hypertension, arthralgia, edema (epoetin alfa, darbepoetin alfa)	● Assess the patient's nutritional status. ● Assess hemoglobin level and hematocrit and total body stores of iron. ● Teach the patient and his family the importance of a balanced diet. ● Tell the patient and his family that oral preparations are best absorbed on an empty stomach. ● Tell the patient and his family that iron products turn the stools black or dark green. ● Teach the patient and his family how to administer subcutaneous injections (epoetin alfa, darbepoetin alfa)

Drugs that affect the respiratory system

Bronchodilators

albuterol (Ventolin, Proventil), aminophylline (Phyllocontin), epinephrine (Adrenalin, Sus-Phrine), isoetharine (Bronkosol), isoproterenol (Isuprel), metaproterenol (Metaprel, Alupent), salmeterol (Serevent), terbutaline (Brethine), theophylline (Theo-Dur)	● Bronchospasm associated with asthma, bronchitis, and other chronic obstructive pulmonary diseases ● Acute bronchospasm	● Untreated cardiac arrhythmias ● Coronary artery disease	● Tachycardia and arrhythmias ● Nervousness ● Headache	● Assess breath sounds, respiratory status, sputum production, and vital signs. ● Teach the patient and his family how to administer inhaled medications. ● Monitor serum levels (theophylline).

Antitussives, expectorants, and mucolytics

Antitussives: codeine, dextromethorphan (Pertussin), diphenhydramine (Benadryl) *Expectorants:* guaifenesin (Robitussin), *Mucolytics:* acetylcysteine (Mucomyst), potassium iodide saturated solution (Pima, SSK1, Thyro-Block)	● Unproductive or excessive cough ● Promote rest	● Hypersensitivity ● Chronic obstructive pulmonary disease	● Nausea ● Drowsiness	● Assess respiratory status, cough, and sputum production. ● Encourage increased fluid intake to reduce mucous viscosity.

Common drugs	Indications	Contraindications	Adverse reactions	Nursing implications

Drugs that affect the GI system

Antacids

aluminum hydroxide (Amphojel); aluminum hydroxide and magnesium hydroxide (Maalox); aluminum hydroxide, magnesium hydroxide, and simethicone (Gelusil, Mylanta); calcium carbonate (Rolaids, Tums); magaldrate and simethicone (Riopan)	• Hyperacidity • Gastroesophageal reflux • Peptic ulcer disease	• Undiagnosed abdominal pain • Renal failure (antacids with magnesium, which can't be excreted and may produce hypermagnesemia and toxic drug levels) • Impaired GI motility	• Stomach cramps • Diarrhea (magnesium) • Constipation (aluminum)	• Assess bowel elimination patterns. • If the patient is on a sodium-restricted diet, instruct him and his family to check the sodium content of antacids.

Antidiarrheals

attapulgite (Kaopectate), bismuth subsalicylate (Pepto-Bismol), diphenoxylate with atropine (Lomotil), loperamide (Imodium)	• Acute diarrhea • Chronic diarrhea	• Undiagnosed abdominal pain • Hypersensitivity reactions • Infectious diarrhea	• Constipation • Drowsiness (Lomotil, Imodium)	• Assess bowel elimination patterns. • Assess fluid and electrolyte balance.

Antiemetics

dimenhydrinate (Dramamine), granisetron (Kytril), meclizine (Antivert), metoclopramide (Reglan), ondansetron (Zofran), prochlorperazine (Compazine), promethazine (Phenergan), scopolamine (Transderm-Scōp), trimethobenzamide (Tigan)	• Depress the vomiting center in the medulla by acting on the chemoreceptor trigger zone (metoclopramide, prochlorperazine, promethazine, trimethobenzamide, ganistron, ondansetron) • Decrease the effects of motion on the vomiting center (dimenhydrinate, meclizine, scopolamine)	• Intestinal obstruction • Sedative use (use with caution)	• Drowsiness • Hypotension • Extrapyramidal reactions (metoclopramide, prochlorperazine, promethazine)	• Assess the patient for symptoms of nausea and vomiting. • Assess GI status, including bowel sounds and presence of abdominal pain. • Monitor intake and output. • Ensure adequate hydration.

Antiulceratives

Histamine-2 (H$_2$) antagonists: cimetidine (Tagamet), famotidine (Pepcid), nizatidine (Axid), ranitidine (Zantac) *Prostaglandin-like:* misoprostol (Cytotec)	• *H$_2$- antagonists:* treat and prevent gastric and duodenal ulcers, treat gastric hypersecretion • *Prostaglandin-like:* inhibit gastric acid secretion in patients taking high doses of NSAIDs by synthetically mimicking prostaglandin	• *H$_2$- antagonists:* impaired liver or kidney function (use with caution), hypersensitivity reactions • *Prostaglandin-like:* pregnancy (has an oxytocic action)	• *H$_2$- antagonists:* confusion, dizziness, headache • *Prostaglandin-like:* diarrhea and abdominal pain	• Assess the patient for changes in mental status (H$_2$- antagonists). • Don't administer antiulceratives with antacids; antacids can interfere with the absorption of H$_2$- antagonists. • Instruct the patient to take misoprostol with meals and at bedtime to help decrease diarrhea.

Common drugs	Indications	Contraindications	Adverse reactions	Nursing implications

Drugs that affect the GI system *(continued)*

Proton pump inhibitor

omeprazole (Prilosec), lansoprazole (Prevacid) pantoprazole (Protonix)	● Peptic ulcer disease ● Gastroesophageal reflux disease ● Erosive esophagitis	● Lactation	● Nausea ● Diarrhea ● Headache	● Treatment course is about 8 weeks. The long-term effects of this amount of acid suppression are unknown at this time.

Pepsin inhibitor

sucralfate (Carafate)	● Peptic ulcer disease (forms a protective coating over the ulcer)	● Safe use in pregnancy or lactation not established	● Constipation ● Impaired absorption of other drugs	● Give on an empty stomach about 1 hour before meals and at bedtime.

Laxatives

Bulk-forming agents: methylcellulose (Citrucel), psyllium (Metamucil) *Lubricants:* hyperosmolar agents, lactulose (Cephulac), magnesium citrate, magnesium hydroxide, magnesium sulfate (Epsom salts), mineral oil, phosphates and biphosphates (Fleet Phospho-Soda) *Stimulants:* bisacodyl (Dulcolax), castor oil, cascara sagrada, senna (Senokot) *Stool softeners:* docusate calcium (Surfak), docusate sodium (Colace, Dialose)	● Constipation associated with many conditions and medications ● Straining during defecation (stool softeners)	● GI conditions, such as abdominal pain, nausea, and vomiting ● Diarrhea	● Cramping ● Nausea and vomiting ● Damage to the bowel or rectum with chronic use ● Electrolyte imbalance and dehydration	● Assess bowel elimination patterns. ● Assess the patient for previous use of laxatives. ● Monitor stools. ● Teach the patient and his family that a high fiber diet, fluids, and exercise promote regular patterns of elimination.

Common drugs	Indications	Contraindications	Adverse reactions	Nursing implications

Drugs that affect the endocrine system

Antidiabetics

Insulins: rapid-acting (Humalog, Humulin R), intermediate-acting (NPH insulin, Humulin N), mixed (Humulin 70/30), basal or long-acting (insulin detemir [Levemir], insulin glargine [Lantus]) *Oral antidiabetics:* acetohexamide (Dymelor), chlorpropamide (Diabinese), glimepiride (Amaryl), glipizide (Glucotrol), glyburide (Micronase), tolazamide (Tolinase), tolbutamide (Orinase) *Biguanide:* metformin (Glucophage) *Alpha glucosidase inhibitors:* acarbose (Precose), miglitol (Glyset) *Meglitinide:* repaglinide (Prandin) *Thiazolidinedione:* rosiglitazone (Avandia)	• *Insulin:* type 1 and type 2 diabetes mellitus when oral antidiabetics, diet, and weight control are ineffective • *Oral antidiabetic:* type 2 diabetes mellitus • *Biguanide:* type 2 diabetes (used to decrease hepatic production of glucose) • *Alpha glucosidase inhibitor:* type 2 diabetes (blocks absorption of carbohydrate) • *Meglitinide:* type 2 diabetes (stimulates release of insulin from pancreas) • *Thiazolidinedione:* type 2 diabetes (reduces cellular insulin resistance)	• Hypersensitivity to a specific insulin • Hypoglycemia • Renal impairment, hepatic dysfunction, alcohol abuse (metformin) • Concomitant administration of other drugs with renal tubular excretion such as cimetidine (metformin) • Impaired liver function (acarbose) • Type 1 diabetes (repaglinide) • New York Heart Association (NYHA) class III or IV cardiac status (rosiglitazone)	• Hypoglycemia • Lipodystrophy (insulin) • Weight gain, GI upset, anorexia, nausea, and diarrhea (metformin) • Vitamin B12 malabsorption (metformin) • Risk of lactic acidosis with kidney disease (metformin) • Flatulence, abdominal distention, and diarrhea (acarbose) • May increase liver function test results (acarbose)	• Monitor blood glucose levels. • Assess the patient for signs and symptoms of hypoglycemia and hyperglycemia. • Assess dietary habits and the patient's knowledge of diet restrictions. • Monitor actual dietary intake. • Make sure the patient and his family are taught about diabetes and its treatment, including medications, diet, insulin monitoring, hypoglycemia and hyperglycemia, and the effects of illness and stress.

Antithyroids

methimazole (Tapazole), potassium iodide, propylthiouracil, sodium iodide	• Hyperthyroidism • Graves' disease	• Pregnancy and lactation • Hypersensitivity to iodine or iodide preparations	• Rash • Nausea and vomiting • Anorexia • Hypothyroidism	• Assess the patient's nutritional status. • Monitor T3 and T4 levels. • Monitor weight weekly. • Tell the patient to take the medication at the same time every day.

Thyroid hormones

levothyroxine (Synthroid), thyroid (Thyrar)	• Supplement or replace natural thyroid hormone • Hypothyroidism, myxedema, goiter, postthyroidectomy	• Hyperthyroidism • Thyrotoxicosis • Untreated adrenal insufficiency • Acute MI	• Tachycardia • Nervousness • Insomnia • Increased appetite • Weight loss	• Assess the patient's nutritional status. • Monitor T3 and T4 levels. • Administer the drug in the morning on an empty stomach to prevent insomnia and increase absorption. • Assess the patient for symptoms of cardiovascular disease

Common drugs	Indications	Contraindications	Adverse reactions	Nursing implications

Drugs used to treat inflammation, allergy, and organ rejection

Adrenocorticosteroids

Common drugs	Indications	Contraindications	Adverse reactions	Nursing implications
cortisone acetate (Cortone), dexamethasone (Decadron), hydrocortisone sodium succinate (Solu-Cortef), methylprednisolone (Medrol), methylprednisolone sodium succinate (Solu-Medrol), prednisolone (Prelone), prednisone (Deltasone), triamcinolone (Aristocort)	● Replacement therapy in patients with adrenal insufficiency ● Shock (to increase cardiac output and blood pressure) ● Inflammatory disorders, such as joint diseases, GI disorders, and skin allergies ● Cerebral edema	● Peptic ulcer disease ● Tuberculosis ● Severe infections ● Autoimmune disorders, heart failure, diabetes, and glaucoma (use with caution)	● Water and sodium retention ● Mood swings ● Hyperglycemia ● Acne and facial hair growth ● GI distress ● Masked signs of infection ● Hypokalemia	● Monitor weight, blood pressure, and blood counts. ● Administer oral doses with milk or food to decrease the risk of GI distress. ● Assess the patient for signs and symptoms of fluid retention, hypokalemia, hyperglycemia, and mental changes. ● Wean the patient from steroid therapy. ● Tell the patient to avoid infected people, immunizations, vaccinations, and skin testing.

Antihistamines

Common drugs	Indications	Contraindications	Adverse reactions	Nursing implications
brompheniramine (Dimetane), cetirizine (Zyrtec), chlorpheniramine (Chlor-Trimeton), desloratadine (Clarinex), diphenhydramine (Benadryl), fexofenadine (Allegra), loratadine (Claritin), promethazine (Phenergan)	● Allergic symptoms from common allergies, drug allergies, and severe allergic reactions ● Nausea and vomiting ● Motion sickness ● Increase effect of analgesics and promote sedation	● Drug hypersensitivity ● Glaucoma ● Emphysema ● CNS depression and seizure disorders (use with caution)	● Sedation and drowsiness ● Dry mouth ● Hypotension ● GI upset	● Assess the patient for known allergies. ● Protect a sedated patient from injury. ● Provide adequate hydration. ● Tell the patient to avoid activities that require mental alertness, to avoid alcohol, to take the drug with food to prevent GI distress, and to maintain adequate fluid intake.

Immunosupressants

Common drugs	Indications	Contraindications	Adverse reactions	Nursing implications
azathioprine (Imuran), cyclosporine (Neoral, Sandimmune)	● Prevent rejection of organ transplants ● Severe rheumatoid arthritis	● Bone marrow suppression ● Severe infections ● Kidney and liver disease (use with caution)	● Anorexia ● Nausea and vomiting ● Chills and fever ● Anaphylactic reactions ● Oral inflammation	● Assess the patient for signs and symptoms of infection. ● Protect the patient from exposure to infectious agents. ● Educate the patient and family about the signs and symptoms of infection. ● Warn the patient not to use cyclosporine products interchangeably without physician supervision. ● Tell the patient to avoid people with infections and to practice strict oral hygiene.

Common drugs	Indications	Contraindications	Adverse reactions	Nursing implications

Drugs used to treat infection

Antibacterials

Common drugs	Indications	Contraindications	Adverse reactions	Nursing implications
Aminoglycosides: amikacin (Amikin), gentamicin (Garamycin), kanamycin (Kantrex), neomycin (Mycifradin), netilmicin (Netromycin), streptomycin, tobramycin (Nebcin) *Cephalosporins:* cefaclor (Ceclor), cefazolin (Ancef), cefixime (Suprax), cefoxitin (Mefoxin), ceftazidime (Fortaz), ceftriaxone (Rocephin), cefuroxime sodium (Zinacef), cephalexin (Keflex) *Penicillins* *Macrolides:* azithromycin (Zithromax), clarithromycin (Biaxin), erythromycin (Erythrocin) *Sulfonamides:* co-trimoxazole (Bactrim), sulfamethoxazole (Gantanol), sulfisoxazole (Gantrisin) *Tetracyclines:* demeclocycline (Declomycin), doxycycline (Vibramycin), oxytetracycline (Terramycin), tetracycline (Achromycin) *Other:* chloramphenicol (Chloromycetin), clindamycin (Cleocin), methenamine mandelate (Mandelamine), nitrofurantoin (Macrodantin), vancomycin (Vancocin)	• Bacterial infections • Infections caused by spirochetes, rickettsiae, and other organisms • Urinary tract infections (sulfonamides, cephalosporins, methenamine mandelate, nitrofurantoin)	• Hypersensitivity • Liver or renal failure	• Superinfections, especially with broad-spectrum agents • Allergic reactions • GI distress	• Assess the patient for signs and symptoms of infection. • Check for a history of allergy. • Withhold the medication if an allergic response occurs.

Antifungals

Common drugs	Indications	Contraindications	Adverse reactions	Nursing implications
amphotericin B (Fungizone), amphotericin B lipid products (ABELCET, AmBisome, Amphotec), clotrimazole (Lotrimin), fluconazole (Diflucan), miconazole (Monistat), nystatin (Mycostatin)	• Systemic and local fungal infections • Candida infections • Ringworm infections	• Hypersensitivity • Renal failure	• Nausea and vomiting • Blood dyscrasias • Headache, fever, and chills • Skin irritation • Hypersensitivity reactions	• Assess the patient for signs and symptoms of infection. • Assess the infected areas. • Wear gloves when applying topical preparations. • Be aware of proper dosing. Doses of amphotericin B lipid products aren't interchangeable with conventional amphotericin B.

Common drugs	Indications	Contraindications	Adverse reactions	Nursing implications

Drugs used to treat infection *(continued)*

Anthelmintics

Common drugs	Indications	Contraindications	Adverse reactions	Nursing implications
iodoquinol (Diquinol), lindane (Kwell), mebendazole (Vermox), metronidazole (Flagyl), quinine sulfate	• Malaria • Roundworm, pinworm, whipworm, hookworm, tapeworm, lice, and other parasitic infections	• Myasthenia gravis (quinine) • Pregnancy and lactation	• GI disturbances • Dizziness • Eczema (lindane)	• Teach the patient how to take the medication properly. • Emphasize basic hygiene, such as regular hand washing and no sharing of personal items with others. • If the patient is receiving metronidazole, assess him for signs of candidal overgrowth. • Advise the patient that all sexual partners should be treated with metronidazole. • Administer quinine with food to prevent GI irritation.

Antituberculotics

Common drugs	Indications	Contraindications	Adverse reactions	Nursing implications
ethambutol (Myambutol), isoniazid (Laniazid, Nydrazid), rifampin (Rifadin), rifapentine (Priftin), streptomycin	• Tuberculosis (TB) prevention in those who are exposed to it • Active TB	• Hypersensitivity • Liver disease	• Nausea and vomiting • Risk of damage to the liver, kidneys, and optic nerve	• Assess the patient's pulmonary status. • Keep in mind that antacids can delay the absorption of isoniazid and that isoniazid inhibits phenytoin metabolism. • Tell the patient that rifampin may cause the saliva, sputum, sweat, urine, and stools to appear reddish brown or reddish orange. • Educate the patient and his family about the importance of continuing long-term multi-dose therapy even after symptoms have subsided.

Antivirals

Common drugs	Indications	Contraindications	Adverse reactions	Nursing implications
acyclovir (Zovirax), amantadine (Symmetrel), didanosine (Videx), famciclovir (Famvir), foscarnet (Foscavir), ganciclovir (Cytovene), indinavir (Crixivan), oseltamivir (Tamiflu), valacyclovir (Valtrex), zalcitabine (HIVID), zidovudine (Retrovir)	• Viral infections • Genital, encephalic, and ophthalmic herpes simplex • Influenza A and influenza B virus prevention • Human immunodeficiency virus	• Hypersensitivity • Pregnancy	• Dizziness • Headache • Nausea and vomiting • Diarrhea • Hypotension • Renal failure • Peripheral neuropathy • Pancreatitis	• Assess the patient for signs and symptoms of infection. • Maintain adequate fluid intake. • Wear gloves when applying topical preparations.

Common drugs	Indications	Contraindications	Adverse reactions	Nursing implications
Drugs used to treat infection *(continued)*				
Antihyperuricemics				
Anti-inflammatory: colchicine *Uric acid synthesis inhibitor:* allopurinol (Zyloprim) *Uricosurics:* probenecid (Benemid)	● Uric acid buildup prevention (probenecid, allopurinol) ● Decrease acute joint inflammation from increased uric acid (colchicine)	● History of renal calculi (probenecid) ● Hypersensitivity ● Impaired liver or kidney function ● Peptic ulcer disease	● GI irritation ● Skin reactions ● Bone marrow depression	● Encourage the patient to drink at least 2 qt (2 L) of fluid per day. ● Administer after meals to decrease GI distress. ● Tell the patient that he should discontinue allopurinol and call the physician if a rash develops.

Posttest

This posttest has been designed to evaluate your readiness to take the certification examination for medical-surgical nursing. Similar in form and content to the actual examination, the posttest consists of 50 questions based on brief clinical situations. The questions will help sharpen your test-taking skills, while assessing your knowledge of medical-surgical nursing theory and practice.

You'll have 50 minutes to complete the posttest. To improve your chances for performing well, consider these suggestions:

● Read each clinical situation and question closely. Weigh the four options carefully, then select the option that best answers the question. (*Note:* In this posttest, options are lettered A, B, C, and D to aid in later identification of correct answers and rationales. These letters won't appear on the certification examination.)

● Completely darken the circle in front of the answer that you select using a #2 pencil. (You must use a #2 pencil when taking the certification examination.) Don't use check marks, Xs, or lines.

● If you decide to change your answer, erase the old answer completely. (The certification examination is scored electronically; an incomplete erasure may cause both answers to be scored, in which case you won't receive credit for answering the question.)

● If you have difficulty understanding a question or are unsure of the answer, place a small mark next to the question number and, if time permits, return to it later. If you have no idea of the correct answer, make an educated guess. (Only correct answers are counted in scoring the certification examination, so guessing is preferable to leaving a question unanswered.)

After you complete the posttest, or after the 50-minute time limit expires, check your responses against the correct answers and rationales provided on pages 387 to 395.

Now, select a quiet room where you'll be undisturbed, set a timer for 50 minutes, and begin.

Questions

1. Prevention and early treatment of Lyme disease are crucial because late complications of this disease include:

○ **A.** sterility.

○ **B.** renal failure.

○ **C.** lung abscess.

○ **D.** arthritis.

2. A patient, age 28, is admitted with a suspected malignant melanoma on his left shoulder. When performing the physical assessment, the nurse would expect to find which of the following?

○ **A.** A brown birthmark that has lightened in color

○ **B.** An area of petechiae

○ **C.** A brown or black mole with red, white, or blue areas

○ **D.** A red birthmark that has recently become darker

3. A patient, age 32, is admitted with a tentative diagnosis of acquired immunodeficiency syndrome (AIDS). The practitioner orders a biopsy of his facial lesions; the preliminary biopsy report indicates Kaposi's sarcoma. Which of the following would be the nurse's *best* approach?

○ **A.** Tell the patient that Kaposi's sarcoma is common in people with AIDS.

○ **B.** Pretend not to notice the lesions on the patient's face.

○ **C.** Inform the patient of the biopsy results, and support him emotionally.

○ **D.** Explore the patient's feelings about his facial disfigurement.

4. A patient, who is human immunodeficiency virus (HIV)-positive, begins zidovudine therapy. Which statement *best* describes the action of this drug?

○ **A.** It eliminates the virus that causes AIDS.

○ **B.** It interferes with viral replication.

○ **C.** It stimulates the immune system.

○ **D.** It clears up skin lesions.

5. During routine hygiene care for a patient with AIDS, a nurse following standard precautions would take which action?

○ **A.** Use reverse isolation.

○ **B.** Place the patient in a private room.

○ **C.** Put on a mask, gloves, and a gown.

○ **D.** Wear gloves when giving mouth care.

6. When assessing the skin of a patient with deep partial-thickness burns, what would the nurse expect to find?

○ **A.** Dry, pale areas with no blister formation

○ **B.** Blisters of varying sizes, with areas of charred tissue

○ **C.** Cherry-red areas with weeping blisters

○ **D.** Pearly-white areas with charred tissue

7. A patient, age 23, underwent a rhinoplasty 6 hours ago. After administering his pain medication, the nurse notes that he's swallowing frequently. What's the most likely cause of the swallowing?

○ **A.** Oral dryness caused by nasal packing

○ **B.** Bleeding posterior to the nasal packing

○ **C.** An adverse reaction to the analgesic

○ **D.** A normal response to the analgesic

8. A patient, age 72, has otosclerosis and is scheduled for a stapedectomy. During preoperative teaching, the nurse should give him which instruction?

○ **A.** "Cough and sneeze with your mouth closed."

○ **B.** "Try to get up and walk around as soon as you return from the operating room."

○ **C.** "Lie on the bed with your operative ear facing up."

○ **D.** "Turn your head rapidly to prevent dizziness."

9. During an eye assessment, a patient complains that "a curtain seems to be coming down in front of my eye." This complaint suggests which condition?

○ **A.** Glaucoma

○ **B.** Retinal detachment

○ **C.** Cataract

○ **D.** Blepharitis

10. A patient, age 64, is receiving treatment for heart failure. The nurse should plan to teach about which drugs?

○ **A.** Vasodilating agents, digoxin, and anti-inflammatory agents

○ **B.** Digoxin, vasodilating agents, and diuretics

○ **C.** Vasoconstricting agents, beta-adrenergic blockers, and digoxin

○ **D.** Antibiotics, vasopressors, and steroids

11. When assessing the patient with an acute dissecting thoracic aortic aneurysm, the nurse would expect which finding?

○ **A.** Hypertension

○ **B.** Decreased hemoglobin level and hematocrit

○ **C.** Severe chest pain

○ **D.** Slow respiratory rate

12. A patient, age 72, has vascular disease. Which nursing intervention would be appropriate?

○ **A.** Encourage him to avoid caffeine and nicotine.

○ **B.** Advise him to wear knee-length stockings.

○ **C.** Instruct him to soak both feet in cool water.

○ **D.** Caution him not to exercise daily.

13. A patient, age 38, has acute bronchitis. The nurse formulates a nursing diagnosis of *Ineffective airway clearance*. After implementing the care plan, the nurse would expect which outcome?

○ **A.** The patient maintains a respiratory rate of 24 breaths/minute.

○ **B.** The patient maintains an arterial oxygen saturation of 90%.

○ **C.** The patient maintains clear breath sounds.

○ **D.** The patient exhibits increased anxiety.

14. A patient, age 27, is admitted with complaints of severe fatigue, muscle weakness, and anorexia. He states he's recovering from the flu and has had severe nausea, frequent vomiting, and diarrhea. Blood is drawn for serum electrolyte measurements. Based on the patient's symptoms, which finding should the nurse expect the laboratory report to show?

○ **A.** Below normal calcium level

○ **B.** Below normal sodium level

○ **C.** Below normal potassium level

○ **D.** Above normal calcium level

15. The nurse who elicits a positive Chvostek's sign would suspect that the patient has which condition?

○ **A.** Hyperkalemia

○ **B.** Hypocalcemia

○ **C.** Hypercalcemia

○ **D.** Hypernatremia

16. A patient, age 18, develops diabetes insipidus after a severe closed head injury. Which assessment findings would indicate that he also has hypernatremia?

○ **A.** Anorexia, muscle cramps, and a serum sodium level greater than 135 mEq/L

○ **B.** Numbness, muscle cramps, and a positive Trousseau's sign

○ **C.** Cardiac arrhythmias, muscle weakness, nausea, and vomiting

○ **D.** Thirst, dry and swollen tongue, and disorientation

17. A patient, age 63, is resuscitated successfully after cardiac arrest. Blood studies show he's acidotic—a common finding in patients who have suffered cardiac arrest. What's the most likely explanation for the acidic serum pH?

○ **A.** Decreased tissue perfusion causes lactic acid production.

○ **B.** The patient typically has an irregular heartbeat.

○ **C.** The patient was treated inappropriately with sodium bicarbonate.

○ **D.** Fat-forming ketoacids are broken down.

18. A patient, age 52, is admitted with a diagnosis of Cushing's syndrome. When analyzing the patient's laboratory data, what would the nurse expect to find?

○ **A.** Hyperglycemia, an increased white blood cell (WBC) count, and elevated cortisol and 17-ketosteroid levels

○ **B.** A decreased WBC count, hyponatremia, metabolic acidosis, and hyperglycemia

○ **C.** Glycosuria, hyperkalemia, a decreased cortisol level, and metabolic alkalosis

○ **D.** Decreased 17-ketosteroid levels, an elevated serum glucose level, hypocalcemia, and hyponatremia

19. A patient, age 68, has benign prostatic hyperplasia. He's admitted for cystoscopy and transurethral resection of the prostate (TURP). During preoperative teaching, the nurse notes that the patient seems very anxious. Exploring the patient's anxiety, the nurse learns he's sexually active and is worried about becoming impotent. How should the nurse deal with his concerns?

○ **A.** Advise him to speak with the surgeon.

○ **B.** Tell him not to worry because he won't become impotent after surgery.

○ **C.** Advise him that TURP seldom causes impotence.

○ **D.** Refer him to the psychiatric clinical nurse specialist.

20. Six hours after undergoing TURP, a patient complains of severe bladder spasms. The nurse notes that his urinary drainage is burgundy-colored and contains large clots, his skin feels cool to the touch, and a rounded swelling is palpable above his symphysis pubis. Which action should the nurse implement *first*?

○ **A.** Assess the patency of the continuous irrigation system.

○ **B.** Assess the patient for indications of shock.

○ **C.** Administer ordered antispasmodic agents.

○ **D.** Notify the attending practitioner.

21. A patient, age 34, is scheduled for discharge after undergoing a modified retroperitoneal lymph node dissection for testicular cancer. He seems quiet and depressed, and the nurse asks if he has anything on his mind. "Now that I'm ready to go home," he says, "I keep thinking about the practitioner telling me I'll be sterile. I'm worried about how my wife will react, even though we didn't plan to have children." What would be the nurse's *best* response?

○ **A.** "Don't worry about being sterile if you didn't plan on having children anyway."

○ **B.** "Sterility is an expected result of the treatment. You can feel comforted by the fact that this disease has a high cure rate."

○ **C.** "What does being sterile mean to you? Tell me more about how you feel."

○ **D.** "I think you should ask the surgeon to talk with you and your wife about your concerns."

22. A patient, age 32, is admitted with a diagnosis of endometriosis. Which of the following is the nurse *most* likely to find during an assessment of a patient with endometriosis?

○ **A.** Chronic, severe pain related to menstruation

○ **B.** Loss and grieving associated with infertility problems

○ **C.** Changes in body image, self-concept, and sexuality

○ **D.** High anxiety with a need for perfection and control

23. A patient, age 49, returns from the postanesthesia care unit after a total abdominal hysterectomy and bilateral salpingo-oophorectomy to treat cervical cancer. Which nursing intervention has the highest priority at this time?

○ **A.** Monitor the patient for indications of hemorrhage.

○ **B.** Assess the patient's pain level and response to analgesics.

○ **C.** Encourage the patient to do deep breathing and leg exercises.

○ **D.** Provide emotional support to the patient.

24. A patient, age 64, is found on the floor of his bathroom in his apartment after apparently falling and hitting his head on the bathtub. On admission to the neurologic unit, he has a decreased level of consciousness (LOC). The practitioner's orders are to elevate the head of the bed; keep the patient's head in neutral alignment, with neck flexion on head rotation; avoid sharp hip flexion; give an acetaminophen suppository, 300 mg, every 6 hours if the patient's temperature exceeds 99.8° F (37.7° C); and give dextrose 5% in water (D_5W) at 20 ml/hr. Which statement *best* describes the rationale for the positioning order?

    ○ **A.** It decreases cerebral arterial pressure.

    ○ **B.** It doesn't impede venous outflow.

    ○ **C.** It prevents flexion contractures.

    ○ **D.** It prevents aspiration of stomach contents.

25. A patient with a head injury and reduced LOC is placed on a hypothermia blanket and given antipyretic medication. Which statement *best* describes the therapeutic value of these interventions?

    ○ **A.** They prevent hypoxia associated with diaphoresis.

    ○ **B.** They promote the integrity of intracerebral neurons.

    ○ **C.** They promote equalization of osmotic pressures.

    ○ **D.** They reduce brain metabolism and limit hypoxia.

26. A patient, age 76, is transferred to the medical-surgical unit from the emergency department (ED) with a diagnosis of left-sided stroke in evolution. On admission to the unit, he has a blood pressure of 150/90 mm Hg, an apical pulse of 78 beats/minute and regular, a respiratory rate of 20 breaths/minute, and a rectal temperature of 100° F (37.8° C). The practitioner orders oxygen by nasal cannula at 2 L/minute; vital sign assessment every hour for the first 4 hours, every 2 hours for the next 4 hours, and then every 4 hours; I.V. D_5W in half-normal saline solution at a rate of 100 ml/hour, and no oral intake. When helping to transfer the patient to his bed, the nurse notices a snoring quality to his respirations. Which nursing action is the highest priority at this time?

    ○ **A.** Place the patient in Fowler's position.

    ○ **B.** Assess the patient's ability to communicate his needs.

    ○ **C.** Position the patient on his side, with the head of the bed elevated slightly.

    ○ **D.** Place items the patient may need to the left side of the bed.

27. Two hours after a patient with left-sided stroke in evolution was admitted to the unit, the nurse measures his blood pressure at 170/80 mm Hg, apical pulse at 58 beats/minute and regular, respiratory rate at 14 breaths/minute, and axillary temperature at 101° F (38.3° C). What's the *first* action the nurse should take at this time?

○ **A.** Report the patient's vital signs to the practitioner.

○ **B.** Assess the patient's vital signs more frequently.

○ **C.** Assess the patient for a distended bladder.

○ **D.** Assess the patient for signs of overhydration.

28. A patient, age 68, has a primary brain tumor. During the past 18 months, he has been admitted to the neurologic unit several times for surgery, radiation therapy, and chemotherapy. Today, he's admitted to investigate a recent onset of seizures. The nurse notes that the patient has become listless and sleepy. Which action should the nurse take *first*?

○ **A.** Assess the patient's verbal and motor responses and ability to open his eyes.

○ **B.** Ask the patient how he's feeling.

○ **C.** Call the practitioner and report the findings.

○ **D.** Continue observing the patient's behavior, which may be an adverse effect of phenytoin.

29. A patient, age 16, has type 1 diabetes mellitus and is in the hospital for regulation of his disease. He tells the nurse he feels hungry, thirsty, tired, and weak, and he frequently asks to use the bathroom. What should the nurse do *first*?

○ **A.** Administer the patient's prescribed insulin.

○ **B.** Notify the practitioner immediately.

○ **C.** Determine the patient's blood glucose level.

○ **D.** Give an additional snack with the patient's next meal.

30. A patient, age 39, has type 1 diabetes mellitus. When he arrives at the ED complaining of dizziness, the nurse notes that he seems weak, confused, and disoriented. His wife states that he took his usual morning dose of 6 units of regular insulin and 15 units of NPH insulin, but ate little of his breakfast. What's the most likely cause of the patient's signs and symptoms?

○ **A.** Ketoacidosis

○ **B.** Hyperglycemia

○ **C.** Hyperlipidemia

○ **D.** Hypoglycemia

31. A patient, age 19, is HIV-positive. When would a diagnosis of AIDS be confirmed?

○ **A.** When the enzyme-linked immunosorbent assay (ELISA) test is positive

○ **B.** When the Western blot test is positive

○ **C.** When he's diagnosed with malignant (non-Hodgkin's) lymphoma

○ **D.** When seroconversion takes place

32. A patient, age 60, is admitted to the hospital with a diagnosis of pneumonia in the left lower lobe. His arterial blood gas (ABG) findings include pH, 7.35; Pa_{O_2}, 60 mm Hg; Pa_{CO_2}, 40 mm Hg; and HCO_3^-, 34 mEq/L. Based on these results, which nursing diagnosis has the highest priority?

○ **A.** Ineffective breathing pattern

○ **B.** Impaired gas exchange

○ **C.** Ineffective airway clearance

○ **D.** Risk for infection

33. A patient, age 54, seeks medical attention for low-grade afternoon fevers, night sweats, loss of appetite, and a productive cough. The practitioner suspects pulmonary tuberculosis (TB), especially after the patient remarks that his wife recently was diagnosed with TB. A positive acid-fast bacillus sputum culture confirms that the patient has TB. Which nursing diagnosis has the highest priority?

○ **A.** Deficient knowledge related to spread of infection

○ **B.** Imbalanced nutrition: Less than body requirements related to not eating

○ **C.** Anxiety related to hearing the diagnosis

○ **D.** Risk for injury related to infection

34. A patient is taking isoniazid to treat TB. Which instruction should the nurse give him about this drug?

○ **A.** Drinking alcohol daily can cause drug-induced hepatitis.

○ **B.** Taking isoniazid with aluminum hydroxide minimizes GI upset.

○ **C.** Isoniazid is best absorbed when taken on an empty stomach.

○ **D.** Prolonged use of isoniazid causes dark, concentrated urine.

35. A patient, age 41, undergoes a right upper lobectomy. Postoperatively, he has a chest tube connected to an underwater seal with suction. One day after surgery, the nurse detects no bubbling in the suction compartment. What would be the *best* nursing action at this time?

○ **A.** Milk the chest tube, using slow, even strokes.

○ **B.** Add more sterile water to the suction compartment.

○ **C.** Check the practitioner's order for amount of suction, and increase pressure until gentle bubbling occurs.

○ **D.** Check the practitioner's order for amount of suction, and increase the water seal by 3.9"(10 cm).

36. A patient, age 63, is admitted with acute bronchopneumonia. The nurse notes that he's in moderate respiratory distress. The patient has a history of emphysema-type chronic obstructive pulmonary disease (COPD). The practitioner orders strict bed rest. Which position would help the patient feel most comfortable?

○ **A.** Semi-Fowler's position with legs elevated

○ **B.** High Fowler's position, using the bedside table as an arm rest

○ **C.** Sims' position with the head elevated 90 degrees

○ **D.** Side-lying position with the head elevated 45 degrees

37. A patient, age 58, is brought to the ED complaining of chest pain and light-headedness. He has a history of stable angina pectoris. Blood is drawn for analysis and an electrocardiogram (ECG) is done. A change in which component of the ECG tracing would alert the nurse that the patient is having a myocardial infarction (MI)?

○ **A.** P wave

○ **B.** R wave

○ **C.** QRS complex

○ **D.** ST segment

38. The practitioner orders I.V. streptokinase for a patient with an evolving MI. During streptokinase therapy, which nursing assessment is *most* important?

○ **A.** Assess the patient for cardiac arrhythmias.

○ **B.** Assess the patient for signs of bleeding.

○ **C.** Assess the patient for increased chest pain.

○ **D.** Assess the patient for signs of pulmonary edema.

39. A patient develops left ventricular dysfunction secondary to an MI. During the physical assessment, the nurse would expect to find:

○ **A.** bilateral basilar crackles.

○ **B.** elevated central venous pressure.

○ **C.** pitting sacral edema.

○ **D.** hepatojugular reflux.

40. While monitoring a patient's cardiac rhythm, the nurse observes seven multifocal premature ventricular contractions (PVCs) on a 1-minute rhythm strip. What should the nurse do *first*?

○ **A.** Change the ECG leads.

○ **B.** Administer lidocaine as prescribed.

○ **C.** Continue to monitor the patient.

○ **D.** Have the patient change position.

41. A patient, age 48, is recovering from an MI. When preparing him for discharge, the nurse should include all of the following instructions *except:*

○ **A.** "Avoid extremes of heat and cold."

○ **B.** "Monitor your pulse during physical activity."

○ **C.** "Eat several small meals each day."

○ **D.** "Lift weights daily to strengthen your arms."

42. A patient is admitted with a diagnosis of hepatitis B. To prevent the spread of this infection, which measure is appropriate?

○ **A.** Respiratory precautions

○ **B.** Enteric precautions

○ **C.** Blood and body fluid precautions

○ **D.** Contact precautions

43. For a patient with hepatitis B, which nursing intervention *isn't* appropriate?

○ **A.** Provide rest periods after meals.

○ **B.** Provide a low-protein diet.

○ **C.** Give frequent, small meals.

○ **D.** Assess the skin for excoriation.

44. A patient, age 53, comes to the ED short of breath. His respiratory rate is 45 breaths/minute; he can't speak because of severe dyspnea. The patient's history reveals an MI and several episodes of heart failure. When auscultating his chest, what would the nurse expect to hear?

○ **A.** A friction rub and clear breath sounds

○ **B.** A murmur and crackles

○ **C.** A friction rub and crackles

○ **D.** An S_3 gallop and crackles

45. A patient, age 55, is admitted with cor pulmonale secondary to advanced COPD. He has been a coal miner for 35 years. When performing the physical assessment, what would the nurse expect to find?

○ **A.** Dyspnea, cyanosis, and increased respiratory excursion

○ **B.** Distended neck veins, cyanosis, and reduced expiratory phase

○ **C.** Dyspnea, cyanosis, and reduced respiratory rate

○ **D.** Distended neck veins, right upper quadrant tenderness, and dependent edema

46. Which nursing intervention would be *most* effective in improving the breathing of a patient with COPD?

○ **A.** Administering oxygen as prescribed

○ **B.** Alternating rest and activity

○ **C.** Teaching pursed-lip breathing

○ **D.** Implementing postural drainage and percussion

47. A patient, age 64, is ready for discharge after hospitalization for an exacerbation of COPD. Which statement by the patient would indicate that he understands his discharge instructions?

○ **A.** "I should take my medicine at bedtime to prevent insomnia."

○ **B.** "I should do my most difficult activities when I first get up in the morning."

○ **C.** "I'll eat several small meals during the day."

○ **D.** "I should plan to do my exercises after I eat."

48. A patient, age 65, is admitted with thyrotoxicosis. His history reveals hyperthyroidism. Laboratory results show that he has elevated T_3 and T_4 levels. The nurse would expect to administer which drugs?

○ **A.** Dexamethasone, cortisol, and levothyroxine

○ **B.** Iodine, propylthiouracil, and propranolol

○ **C.** Epinephrine, dopamine, and norepinephrine

○ **D.** Aminophylline, ephedrine, and theophylline

49. This patient undergoes a subtotal thyroidectomy. Which interventions should the nurse implement for him immediately after surgery?

○ **A.** Assess vital signs every 4 hours; maintain the patient in a supine position; withhold all oral intake; maintain strict intake and output; keep a tracheostomy set at the bedside.

○ **B.** Assess vital signs every hour until stable; provide a liquid diet; maintain the patient in Trendelenburg's position; use mist inhalation.

○ **C.** Assess vital signs every 15 minutes until stable; maintain the patient in semi-Fowler's position; give fluids as tolerated; keep a tracheostomy set at the bedside.

○ **D.** Assess vital signs every 2 hours; keep the patient in a lateral recumbent position; provide the house diet; maintain strict intake and output.

50. A patient, age 58, is admitted with complaints of anorexia, weight loss, and general body wasting. After a diagnostic workup, he's diagnosed with Addison's disease. Which statement *best* describes the pathophysiology of Addison's disease?

○ **A.** Release of adrenocortical hormones is increased.

○ **B.** Release of adrenocortical hormones is decreased.

○ **C.** Release of adrenal medullary hormones is decreased.

○ **D.** A tumor develops in the adrenal gland.

Answers and rationales

1. Correct answer: D If Lyme disease goes untreated, arthritis, neurologic problems, and cardiac abnormalities may arise as late complications. The first sign of Lyme disease is typically a skin lesion that enlarges and has a characteristic red border. However, not all patients develop this lesion. Options A, B, and C are incorrect because they aren't complications of Lyme disease.

2. Correct answer: C Melanomas have an irregular shape and lack uniformity in color. They may appear brown or black with red, white, or blue areas. Options A, B, and C contain inaccurate information.

3. Correct answer: D Facial lesions can contribute to decreased self-esteem and an altered body image. Kaposi's sarcoma is among the many psychosocial and physical traumas that may confront the patient with AIDS; anxiety, anger, grief, and depression are common emotional responses. The nurse who works with patients who have AIDS must develop excellent listening skills. The patient may be especially concerned that others will realize he has Kaposi's sarcoma. Option A doesn't provide emotional support to the patient. Option B ignores the patient's concerns. Option C is incorrect because the practitioner should inform the patient of the biopsy results, not the nurse.

4. Correct answer: B Zidovudine inhibits deoxyribonucleic acid synthesis within the virus that causes AIDS, interfering with viral replication. Options A, C, and D inaccurately describe the drug's action.

5. Correct answer: D Standard precautions stipulate that a health care worker who anticipates coming into contact with a patient's blood or body fluids must wear gloves; this protects the health care worker. Option A is incorrect because reverse isolation is used to protect the patient from the health care worker. Option B is incorrect because a private room doesn't provide a method of barrier protection, which is needed for standard precautions. Option C is incorrect because a mask and gloves are needed only for anticipated contact with airborne droplets of blood or body fluids; a gown is needed only for anticipated contact with splashes of blood or body fluids.

6. Correct answer: C In partial-thickness burns, skin color varies from pink to cherry-red. Deep second-degree burns appear cherry-red and may have blisters that ooze fluid. Options A and D are incorrect because they describe full-thickness burns. Option B is incorrect because it describes superficial partial-thickness burns.

7. Correct answer: B In a patient who has nasal packing in place, frequent swallowing may indicate bleeding in the posterior pharynx. Option A is incorrect because mouth dryness causes thirst, not frequent swallowing. Options C and D are incorrect because frequent swallowing isn't a response to analgesics.

8. Correct answer: C To prevent pressure on the graft site, which may cause graft displacement, the nurse should instruct the patient to lie on the nonoperative side. Option A is incorrect because the patient should cough or sneeze with his mouth open, not closed, to prevent increased pressure through the eustachian tube into the middle ear (which could displace the graft). Option B is incorrect because the patient should remain in bed for 24 hours after surgery to prevent graft displacement. Option D is incorrect because rapid head movement could cause vertigo.

9. Correct answer: B With extensive, rapidly developing retinal detachment, a patient may report the sensation of a curtain dropping down in front of his eye. Options A, C, and D are incorrect because glaucoma, cataracts, and blepharitis don't cause this sensation.

10. Correct answer: B The practitioner may prescribe digoxin for the patient with heart failure to increase contractility and slow the heart rate (and thus improve cardiac function); a vasodilating agent to decrease afterload; and a diuretic to reduce peripheral resistance (and thus improve cardiac output). Option A inaccurately suggests that anti-inflammatory agents are used to treat heart failure; option C inaccurately suggests that vasoconstricting agents are used. None of the drugs listed in option D are prescribed for the patient with heart failure.

11. Correct answer: C When the dissecting aneurysm begins, severe chest pain (described as a tearing in the chest) develops; typically, the patient also has signs and symptoms of respiratory distress and ischemia of the central nervous system, limbs, kidneys, and mesentery. Option A describes a possible cause—not a symptom—of the dissecting aneurysm. Options B and D aren't associated with this disorder.

12. Correct answer: A The nurse should encourage the patient to avoid caffeine and nicotine because they constrict vessels and would further impair his circulation; this includes encouraging the patient to quit smoking or chewing tobacco, avoid drinking caffeine-containing beverages, and avoid ingesting such drugs as amphetamines. Option B is incorrect because it would impair circulation. Option C is incorrect because the patient with peripheral vascular disease should keep the extremities warm and dry. This patient also should exercise daily, unless pain is experienced, not avoid daily exercise, as option D suggests.

13. Correct answer: C Maintaining clear breath sounds would indicate that the patient has effective airway clearance. The respiratory rate in Option A is too high for an adult. The pulse oximetry reading in Option B is too low. Option D is incorrect because increased airway clearance would help decrease—not increase—the patient's anxiety.

14. Correct answer: C Lack of potassium intake (related to anorexia and nausea) plus potassium loss by way of gastric secretions (from vomiting) and intestinal fluids (from diarrhea) puts this patient at high risk for a below-normal serum potassium level. Options A and D are incorrect because vomiting and diarrhea don't alter the body's calcium level; calcium is stored in bone and isn't affected by GI changes. Option B is incorrect because vomiting may increase the serum sodium level.

15. Correct answer: B A positive Chvostek's sign (contraction of facial muscles when the facial nerve is tapped) indicates neuromuscular irritability, a sign of hypocalcemia. Options A, C, and D are incorrect because a positive Chvostek's sign doesn't appear with those conditions.

16. Correct answer: D Diabetes insipidus results from lack of antidiuretic hormone, which causes significant urine losses. Such losses, in turn, lead to hypernatremia (an elevated serum sodium level), which causes dry and sticky mucous membranes, thirst, swollen tongue, and disorientation. Option A is incorrect because a serum sodium level of 135 mEq/L falls within the normal range and muscle cramps are a sign of hyponatremia. Option B is incorrect because numbness and a positive Trousseau's sign indicate hypocalcemia. Option C is incorrect because muscle irritability—not weakness—is characteristic of hypernatremia.

17. Correct answer: A Cardiac arrest leads to ischemia (resulting from decreased tissue perfusion) and to subsequent cardiac insufficiency; cardiac insufficiency causes anaerobic metabolism (metabolism occurring without oxygen), leading to lactic acid production. Ischemia of any organ or body part can cause an increase in the lactic acid level. Option B is incorrect because an irregular heartbeat doesn't necessarily cause acidosis. Option C is incorrect because sodium bicarbonate treatment causes alkalosis. Option D is incorrect because this type of acidosis occurs in diabetes mellitus.

18. Correct answer: A In patients with Cushing's syndrome (hyperadrenalism), laboratory findings typically include sustained hyperglycemia, elevated cortisol and 17-ketosteroid levels, elevated WBC count, hypernatremia, hypokalemia, and metabolic alkalosis. Option B is incorrect because a decreased WBC count, hyponatremia, and metabolic acidosis aren't seen in Cushing's syndrome. Cushing's syndrome doesn't cause decreased cortisol level and hyperkalemia (option C) or hyponatremia and hypocalcemia (option D).

19. Correct answer: C The nurse should tell the patient that only 5% of patients experience impotence after TURP. If the patient continues to seem worried, however, the nurse should advise him to speak with his surgeon. Options A and B wouldn't give the patient a chance to express his concerns. Option D is incorrect because the nurse should help the patient express his concerns initially as well as give him appropriate information; this doesn't require a referral to a psychiatric clinical nurse specialist.

20. Correct answer: B The nurse first should check for indications of shock by taking the patient's vital signs. Clots in the urinary drainage indicate bleeding, which is common after TURP (especially during the first 2 postoperative hours). *After* making sure the patient isn't in shock, the nurse should check the irrigation system (option A) notify the practitioner (option D), and administer ordered antispasmodic agents (option C), because spasms can precipitate bleeding.

21. Correct answer: C The nurse should elicit the patient's concerns and listen actively as he expresses these concerns. Option A is incorrect because although the patient didn't plan to have children, he may view his sterility as yet another threat to his masculinity. The testicular cancer probably already has threatened his self-concept. Option B is incorrect because it invalidates the patient's feelings. Option D isn't the *best* response because the nurse can and should help the patient explore his feelings. At a later time, the nurse may suggest that the patient talk with his practitioner.

22. Correct answer: A Pain is the most common symptom of endometriosis. Option B is incorrect because infertility is a possible consequence of endometriosis. Options C and D don't refer to the most likely assessment finding for a patient with endometriosis.

23. Correct answer: A   Although all of the options are important nursing interventions, monitoring for hemorrhage is the highest priority. Hemorrhage can lead to a life-threatening situation for the patient. The nurse should assess for signs and symptoms of hemorrhage every 15 minutes for the first 2 hours, then at least hourly for the next 8 hours.

24. Correct answer: B   Any activity or position that impedes venous outflow from the patient's head may increase blood volume inside the skull, possibly raising intracranial pressure (ICP). Increased ICP can cause brain damage and impair vital physiologic functions. Option A is incorrect because cerebral arterial pressure is affected by the balance between the arterial oxygen level and the arterial carbon dioxide level—not by the position ordered. Option C is incorrect because preventing flexion contractures isn't a priority at this time. Option D is incorrect because the ordered position doesn't prevent aspiration of stomach contents.

25. Correct answer: D   The hypothermia blanket and antipyretic medication can induce hypothermia, which in turn decreases brain metabolism and makes the brain less vulnerable to hypoxia by decreasing the need for oxygen. Option A is incorrect because diaphoresis doesn't cause hypoxia; antipyretic medication may cause diaphoresis as vasodilation occurs. The integrity of intracerebral neurons (option B) and osmotic pressure equalization (option C) depend on an adequate supply of oxygen, carbon dioxide, and glucose, and may occur as a result of decreased cerebral metabolism and hypoxia.

26. Correct answer: C   Stroke in evolution refers to continuing neurologic changes over 24 to 48 hours. The patient should be placed on his side because leaving a patient on his back may cause the tongue to fall backward and the aspiration of secretions, resulting in airway obstruction that in turn may induce atelectasis and pneumonia. Option A is inappropriate for this patient because weakness on the right side (resulting from his left-sided lesion) would make him unable to maintain this position. Options B and D aren't priorities.

27. Correct answer: A   A brain injury, such as the one this patient has suffered, can cause increased ICP. Slow respirations, a slow pulse, and elevated pulse pressure are associated with compromised cerebral circulation. These changes signal increasing ICP—a condition that calls for practitioner notification so that prompt medical intervention can help prevent additional damage. Although options B, C, and D also are important, the nurse should take these actions only *after* notifying the practitioner.

28. Correct answer: A   Listlessness and sleepiness suggest the patient has a decreased LOC—the earliest sign that his condition is deteriorating. Option A describes the components of the Glasgow Coma Scale, which the nurse should use to obtain an objective determination of the patient's LOC. Options B, C, and D are appropriate but don't take precedence over objective determination of the patient's LOC.

29. Correct answer: C Polyphagia (increased appetite), polydipsia (increased thirst), lethargy, and polyuria (increased urination) signal hyperglycemia and indicate a need to determine the patient's glucose level. Option A is incorrect because giving insulin won't affect the blood glucose level immediately. Option B is incorrect because the practitioner need not be notified of these common symptoms. Option D would worsen the patient's hyperglycemia.

30. Correct answer: D Dizziness, weakness, confusion, and disorientation signal an insulin reaction and severe hypoglycemi—a common finding in diabetic patients who take insulin but miss a meal. Ketoacidosis (option A) and hyperglycemia (option B) are rare in a patient with diabetes who takes insulin and decreases his nutritional intake. Option C is incorrect because hyperlipidemia (an excessive blood fat level) doesn't cause ketoacidosis.

31. Correct answer: C AIDS isn't diagnosed until an AIDS-indicator condition occurs. Options A and B are incorrect because the ELISA test and the Western blot test identify HIV antibodies in the blood; a patient who is HIV-positive has already tested positive for HIV antibodies. Being HIV-positive *isn't* synonymous with a diagnosis of AIDS. Option D is incorrect because seroconversion is the basis for establishing that a patient is HIV-positive, not for diagnosing AIDS.

32. Correct answer: B Because the patient's ABG measurements reveal hypoxemia, impaired gas exchange has the highest priority. Option A isn't relevant because the patient has a normal $Paco_2$ level, which means that breathing isn't a problem. Option C is incorrect because the data don't indicate a problem with the patient's airway. Option D is incorrect because the patient with pneumonia already has an infection.

33. Correct answer: A Because the patient isn't in acute distress, the highest-priority nursing diagnosis is *Deficient knowledge related to spread of the infection.* Options B, C, and D must be addressed but aren't priorities at this time; as the nurse gives the patient information about TB, these other nursing diagnoses may diminish in importance.

34. Correct answer: A Drinking alcohol daily during isoniazid therapy can induce drug-related hepatitis. Option B is incorrect because the patient should avoid concomitant use of aluminum-containing antacids with isoniazid because they impair isoniazid absorption. Option C is incorrect because the patient should take isoniazid with meals for maximal absorption and to decrease GI upset. Option D gives false information.

35. Correct answer: C When a chest tube is attached to suction, gentle bubbling should appear in the suction compartment continuously. Increasing the pressure should cause bubbling. None of the other options would correct the suction problem.

36. Correct answer: B   High Fowler's position elevates the clavicles and helps the lungs to expand, thereby easing respirations. The other options wouldn't promote more comfortable breathing.

37. Correct answer: D   An active ischemic injury in the myocardium causes displacement of the ST segment. Options A, B, and C aren't associated with an MI.

38. Correct answer: B   Bleeding is a major complication associated with streptokinase therapy. Streptokinase promotes systemic thrombolysis by activating plasminogen, which degrades fibrin clots; this can cause bleeding. Another complication to streptokinase is an allergic response. Although streptokinase may cause reperfusion arrhythmias, option A is incorrect because these arrhythmias usually require no treatment. Streptokinase isn't associated with chest pain (option C) or pulmonary edema (option D).

39. Correct answer: A   Signs and symptoms of acute left ventricular dysfunction are associated primarily with pulmonary congestion, which is characterized by bilateral, bibasilar crackles. Options B, C, and D are signs of right-sided heart failure.

40. Correct answer: B   Various protocols are available for managing ventricular arrhythmias. Typically, the patient with more than five or six PVCs per minute is treated, especially if the PVCs are multifocal; lidocaine is the most commonly used agent. Options A, C, and D don't address the patient's immediate needs.

41. Correct answer: D   Exercising the upper extremities—especially with heavy lifting—can strain the myocardium. Options A, B, and C are appropriate discharge instructions for a patient recovering from an MI.

42. Correct answer: C   Blood and body fluid precautions are needed because hepatitis B is transmitted through the serum and body fluids. Options A, B, and D are inappropriate for a patient with this disease.

43. Correct answer: B   The patient with hepatitis B needs a high-protein—not low-protein—diet to enhance the recovery of injured liver cells. Options A, C, and D are inappropriate for a patient with hepatitis B.

44. Correct answer: D   An S_3 gallop is characteristic of heart failure; crackles indicate the presence of intra-alveolar fluid, which may result from left-sided heart failure. Option A is incorrect because this patient wouldn't have clear breath sounds. Option B is incorrect because heart failure doesn't cause a murmur. Option C is incorrect because pleurisy, not heart failure, causes a friction rub.

45. Correct answer: D Cor pulmonale is a form of right-sided heart failure caused by pulmonary disease; only option D lists signs of right-sided heart failure. Option A is incorrect because respiratory excursion is reduced with COPD. Option B is incorrect because the patient with diagnosed COPD will have a prolonged expiratory phase. Option C is incorrect because the patient with COPD and cor pulmonale will have an increased respiratory rate.

46. Correct answer: C Pursed-lip and diaphragmatic breathing, which increase carbon dioxide elimination, are the most effective ways to improve this patient's breathing. Option A must be done cautiously in patients with COPD because their breathing stimulus depends on a low arterial oxygen content. Option B would improve the patient's activity tolerance but not his ventilation. In conjunction with breathing exercises, option D is used to remove retained secretions and thus improve gas exchange.

47. Correct answer: C Because this patient may feel full after even a small meal, he should eat smaller, more-frequent, high-calorie meals to obtain the energy he needs for breathing. Option A is incorrect because taking a bronchodilator at bedtime may contribute to insomnia. Option B is incorrect because most patients with COPD tolerate activity better if it's spaced throughout the day with frequent rest periods. Option D is incorrect because the patient should exercise before eating to obtain the energy for digestion.

48. Correct answer: B Iodine reduces thyroid vascularity and prevents release of thyroid hormone into the circulation. Propylthiouracil, which blocks thyroid hormone synthesis, is the drug most commonly used to treat hyperthyroidism; methimazole has similar effects and can be used in patients allergic to propylthiouracil. Propranolol, a beta-adrenergic blocker, is used to decrease patient anxiety and the cardiac effects of hyperthyroidism. Option A is incorrect because levothyroxine is used to treat hypothyroidism, not hyperthyroidism. The adrenergic agents listed in option C are inappropriate for the hyperthyroid patient because they would further stimulate the cardiovascular system, which is already under stress from hypermetabolism. The drugs listed in option D are used primarily to treat asthma and may lead to increased excitability and tachycardia in a patient with hyperthyroidism.

49. Correct answer: C Because hemorrhage and respiratory obstruction can develop after a subtotal thyroidectomy, the nurse must monitor vital signs every 15 minutes until the patient is stable, then every 30 minutes to 1 hour for the next several hours. Semi-Fowler's position promotes comfort and breathing and allows immobilization, which is needed to prevent strain on the suture line. Fluids should be given unless the patient experiences nausea and vomiting or has difficulty swallowing. A tracheostomy set is needed because airway obstruction may result from edema. Options A and D are incorrect because vital signs should be monitored more frequently, and the patient should be in semi-Fowler's position. Option B is incorrect because Trendelenburg's position would cause a decreased number of respirations and edema at the surgical site.

50. Correct answer: B   In Addison's disease (adrenocortical insufficiency), the release of adrenocortical hormones diminishes. Option A is incorrect because adrenocortical hormone release decreases rather than increases. Option C is incorrect because Addison's disease doesn't affect hormones produced by the adrenal medulla. Option D is incorrect because Addison's disease is thought to have an autoimmune etiology.

Analyzing the posttest

Total the number of *incorrect* responses to the posttest. A score of 1 to 9 indicates that you have an excellent knowledge base and that you're well prepared for the certification examination; a score of 10 to 14 indicates adequate preparation, although more study or improvement in test-taking skills is recommended; a score of 15 or more indicates the need for intensive study before taking the certification examination.

For a more detailed analysis of your performance, complete the self-diagnostic profile worksheet.

Self-diagnostic profile for posttest

In the top row of boxes, record the number of each question you answered incorrectly. Then beneath each question number, check the box that corresponds to the reason you answered the question incorrectly. Finally, tabulate the number of check marks on each line in the right-hand column marked "Totals." You now have an individualized profile of weak areas that require further study or improvement in test-taking ability before you take the Medical-Surgical Nursing Certification Examination.

Question number																					Totals
Test-taking skills																					
1. Misread question																					
2. Missed important point																					
3. Forgot fact or concept																					
4. Applied wrong fact or concept																					
5. Drew wrong conclusion																					
6. Incorrectly evaluated distractors																					
7. Mistakenly filled in wrong circle																					
8. Read into question																					
9. Guessed wrong																					
10. Misunderstood question																					

Selected references

2005 American Heart Association Guidelines for Cardiopulmonary Resuscitation and Emergency Cardiovascular Care, *Circulation* 112:24(Suppl IV):IV-1–IV-203, December 2005.

Black, J.M., and Hawks, J.H. *Medical-Surgical Nursing: Clinical Management for Positive Outcomes,* 7th ed. Philadelphia: W.B. Saunders Co., 2004.

Burrows-Hudson, S., "Chronic Kidney Disease: An Overview," *AJN* 25(2):40-49, February 2005.

Gambrell, M., and Flynn, N. "Seizures 101," *Men in Nursing* 1(1):18-24, February, 2006.

Hess, C.T. *Clinical Guide: Wound Care,* 5th ed. Philadelphia: Lippincott Williams & Wilkins, 2005.

Ignatavicius, D.D., and Workman, M.L. *Medical-Surgical Nursing: Critical Thinking for Collaborative Care,* 5th ed. Philadelphia: W.B. Saunders Co., 2005.

McCance, K.L., and Heuther, S.E. *Pathophysiology: The Biologic Basis for Disease in Adults and Children,* 5th ed. St. Louis: C.V. Mosby, 2005.

Nursing2007 Drug Handbook, 27th ed. Philadelphia: Lippincott Williams & Wilkins, 2007.

Porth, C. *Essentials of Pathophysiology: Concepts of Altered Health States,* 7th ed. Philadelphia: Lippincott Williams & Wilkins, 2005.

Pravikoff, D.S., et al. "Evidence-Based Practice," *AJN* 105(9):40-51, September 2005.

Professional Guide to Pathophysiology, 2nd ed. Philadelphia: Lippincott Williams & Wilkins, 2007.

Seaback, W.W. *Nursing Process: Concepts and Application,* 2nd ed. Albany, N.Y.: Thomson Delmar Learning, 2006.

Skidmore-Roth, L. *Mosby's 2007 Nursing Drug Reference,* 20th ed. St. Louis: C.V. Mosby, 2007.

Smeltzer, S.C., and Bare, B.G. *Brunner & Suddarth's Textbook of Medical-Surgical Nursing,* 10th ed. Philadelphia: Lippincott Williams & Wilkins, 2004.

Tortora, G.J., and Derrickson, B.H. *Principles of Anatomy and Physiology,* 11th ed. Hoboken, N.J.: John Wiley & Sons, 2005.

Yarbro, C.H., et al., eds. *Cancer Nursing: Principles and Practice.* Sudbury, Mass.: Jones and Bartlett Publishers, 2005.

Index